PRACTICAL ASPECTS OF URINARY INCONTINENCE

DEVELOPMENTS IN SURGERY

J.M. Greep, H.A.J. Lemmens, D.B. Roos, H.C. Urschel, eds., Pain in Shoulder and Arm: An Integrated View
ISBN 90 247 2146 6

B. Niederle, Surgery of the Biliary Tract
ISBN 90 247 2402 3

J.A. Nakhosteen & W. Maassen, eds., Bronchology: Research, Diagnostic and Therapeutic Aspects
ISBN 90 247 2449 X

R. van Schilfgaarde, J.C. Stanley, P. van Brummelen & E.H. Overbosch, eds., Clinical Aspects of Renovascular Hypertension
ISBN 0 89838 574 1

G.M. Abouna, ed. & A.G. White, ass. ed., Current Status of Clinical Organ Transplantation. With some Recent Developments in Renal Surgery
ISBN 0 89838 635 7

A. Cuschieri & G. Berci, Common Bile Duct Exploration
ISBN 0 89838 639 X

F.M.J. Debruyne & Ph.E.V.A. van Kerrebroeck, Practical Aspects of Urinary Incontinence
ISBN 0 89838 752 3

PRACTICAL ASPECTS OF URINARY INCONTINENCE

edited by

F.M.J. DEBRUYNE and Ph.E.V.A. VAN KERREBROECK

Department of Urology, University Hospital St. Radboud, Nijmegen, The Netherlands

1986 **MARTINUS NIJHOFF PUBLISHERS**
a member of the KLUWER ACADEMIC PUBLISHERS GROUP
DORDRECHT / BOSTON / LANCASTER
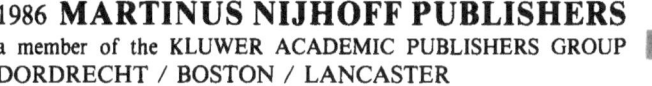

Distributors

for the United States and Canada: Kluwer Academic Publishers, 190 Old Derby Street, Hingham, MA 02043, USA
for the UK and Ireland: Kluwer Academic Publishers, MTP Press Limited, Falcon House, Queen Square, Lancaster LA1 1RN, UK
for all other countries: Kluwer Academic Publishers Group, Distribution Center, P.O. Box 322, 3300 AH Dordrecht, The Netherlands

Library of Congress Cataloging in Publication Data

ISBN-13: 978-94-010-8381-2   e-ISBN-13: 978-94-009-4237-0
DOI: 10.1007/978-94-009-4237-0

Contents

CHAPTER ONE: INVESTIGATIONS FOR URINARY INCONTINENCE

CHAPTER TWO: GENUINE URINARY STRESS INCONTINENCE

CHAPTER THREE: RECURRENT URINARY STRESS
INCONTINENCE

CHAPTER FOUR: INCONTINENCE AND RESOLUTIONS
OF VAGINAL PROLAPSE

CHAPTER FIVE: VESICO-VAGINAL FISTULAE

CHAPTER SIX: MALE INCONTINENCE

CHAPTER SEVEN: ARTIFICIAL SPHINCTERS IN THE MANAGEMENT OF URINARY INCONTINENCE

CHAPTER EIGHT: PAST AND FUTURE OF URINARY INCONTINENCE

Preface

Urinary incontinence is becoming an increasingly dominant condition in daily urological and gynaecological practice, although the total number of patients suffering from the different forms of incontinence remains unclear. An estimated figure for The Netherlands, with a population of 14 500 000, has been given as between 500 000 and 600 000 patients, showing that approximately 4% of the total population suffer from this condition, the majority being female. The impact of this number is tremendous, not only regarding health care costs, but even more with regard to the psycho-social consequences. It is obvious that continuing efforts must be made to understand more fully the different forms of urinary incontinence.

An exact diagnosis is the first step necessary for adequate therapy. We all know how disastrous it can be to institute inappropriate treatment as a consequence of misunderstanding the proper aetiology in each individual case.

What has happened in the past 15 years? During that time we have developed sophisticated machinery to diagnose in more detail the exact origin of each type of urinary incontinence, and on entering a urodynamic laboratory, one is struck by the complexity of measuring equipment. But how reliable are all these measurements and how can they be translated into an effective therapy? This still remains one of the major problems, although continuing progress has been made and will be made by the research work of many experts in the field of urinary incontinence.

In June 1984 a symposium was held at the Department of Urology, University of Nijmegen Medical School. The symposium was dedicated to Dr. W.A. Moonen, the first professor and chairman of our department, on the occasion of his 65th birthday and many of these experts were present.

The aims of the symposium were twofold. First, to give a detailed insight into the surgical aspects in the management of different forms of urinary incontinence and second, to discuss in detail the rationale or irrationality of the diagnostic work-up and therapeutic approach. The present book compiles the most important contributions to this symposium.

In the process of preparing a new book, the question arises as to whether

another publication in the field of urinary incontinence is necessary or mandatory. The overwhelming amount of literature in this field rather predicates the contrary. However, reviewing the surgical demonstrations together with the papers presented at the symposium, we feel justified in publishing the views of such experts as a monograph, focusing on the practical aspects of urinary incontinence. Practical aspects are dealt with in two forms:
a. practical views in diagnostic work-up;
b. practical surgical approach to curable forms of urinary incontinence.

Therefore this volume contains a considerable amount of information and practical tips for use in every-day urologic and gynaecological practice. Where necessary, the practical points are elicited and supported by fundamental and theoretical arguments which play a role in the total approach to the problem.

Using this concept we hope to have contributed in a valuable way to a better understanding of the management of urinary incontinence and to have given to the interested reader a practical overview that he can consult and use when in doubt about how to manage an individual patient. And one knows how often we still are in doubt!

Acknowledgements

We would like to thank the many authors and contributors. Through their efforts, based on vast experience in the field of urinary incontinence, we were able to realize the idea of publishing a book on the 'Practical Aspects of Urinary Incontinence'.

We would also like to express our gratitude to Mrs. A.M.A. Zick-van Ruiten, who did all the difficult and time consuming secretarial work necessary to put this book together.

We would also like to thank Mr. B.F. Commandeur of Martinus Nijhoff Publishers, whose excellent advice stimulated us to finish our work.

Frans M.J. Debruyne,

March 1985　　　　　　　　　　　　　　　Philip E.V.A. van Kerrebroeck

List of contributors

Baert, L., Urologic Centre of Kortrijk, Hospital 'O.L. Vrouw', Budastraat 37, B-8500 Kortrijk, Belgium
* Beck, L., Department of Obstetrics and Gynaecology, University of Düsseldorf, Moorenstrasse 5, D-4000 Düsseldorf, F.R.G.
Blok, C., Department of Urology, University Hospital, P.O. Box 16250, 3500 CG Utrecht, The Netherlands
* Bressel, M., Department of Urology, General Hospital 'Harburg', Eissendorfer Pferdeweg 52, D-2100 Hamburg 90, F.R.G.
* Brillenburg Wurth, G.H., Department of Urology, Hospital 'Diaconessenhuis', Ds. Theodor Fliednerstraat 1, 5631 BM Eindhoven, The Netherlands
* Camp, K. van, Department of Urology, University of Antwerp, B-2610 Wilrijk/Antwerp, Belgium
Colstrup, H., Department of Urology, Gentofte and Herlev Hospitals, University of Copenhagen, Niels Andersens Vej 65, DK-2900 Hellerup, Denmark
* Coolsaet, B.L.R.A., Department of Urology, University Hospital, P.O. Box 16250, 3500 CG Utrecht, The Netherlands
* Debruyne, F.M.J., Department of Urology, University Hospital 'St. Radboud', P.O. Box 9101, 6500 HB Nijmegen, The Netherlands
* Denis, L., Department of Urology, General Hospital 'Middelheim', Lindendreef 1, B-2020 Antwerp, Belgium
* Dony, J.M.J., Department of Obstetrics and Gynaecology, University Hospital 'St. Radboud', P.O. Box 9101, 6500 HB Nijmegen, The Netherlands
* Frimodt-Møller, C., Department of Urology, Gentofte and Herlev Hospitals, University of Copenhagen, Niels Andersens Vej 65, DK-2900 Hellerup, Denmark
* Geelen, J.M. van, Department of Obstetrics and Gynaecology, Hospital 'St. Anna', Joannes Zwijsenlaan 1, 5342 BR Oss, The Netherlands
Gijsegem, M. van, Department of Obstetrics and Gynaecology, General Hospital 'H. Familie', B-9000 Gent, Belgium

Hadley, H.R., Division of Urology, Department of Surgery, University of California School of Medicine, 10833 Le Conte Avenue, Los Angeles, CA 90024, USA

* Hald, T., Department of Urology, Herlev Hospital, University of Copenhagen, Herlev Ringvej, DK-2730 Herlev, Denmark

* Haspels, A.A., Department of Obstetrics and Gynaecology, University Hospital, P.O. Box 16250, 3500 CG Utrecht, The Netherlands

* Hauri, D., Urologic Clinic, University Hospital, CH-8091 Zürich, Switzerland

Hohenfellner, R., University Clinic for Urology, Langenbeckstrasse 1, D-6500 Mainz, F.R.G.

* Janssens, J., Department of Obstetrics and Gynaecology, University Hospital, Oostersingel 59, 9713 EZ Groningen, The Netherlands

* Jonas, U., Department of Urology, University Hospital, Rijnsburgerweg 10, 2333 AA Leiden, The Netherlands

Jonge, M.C. de, Department of Medical Physics, University Hospital, Oostersingel 59, 9713 EZ Groningen, The Netherlands

Kauer, F.M., Department of Obstetrics and Gynaecology, University Hospital, Oostersingel 59, 9713 EZ Groningen, The Netherlands

Kerrebroeck, Ph.E.V.A. van, Department of Urology, University Hospital 'St. Radboud', P.O. Box 9101, 6500 HB Nijmegen, The Netherlands

* Kramer, A.E.J.L., Department of Urology, University Hospital, Rijnsburgerweg 10, 2333 AA Leiden, The Netherlands

* Kroovand, R.L., Section of Pediatric and Reconstructive Urology, Bowman Gray School of Medicine of Wake Forest University, Winston-Salem, NC 27103, USA

* Madersbacher, H., Department of Urology, Innsbruck University Hospital, Anichstrasse 35, A-6020 Innsbruck, Austria

* Mattelaer, J.J., Urologic Centre of Kortrijk, Hospital 'O.L. Vrouw', Budastraat 37, B-8500 Kortrijk, Belgium

Meyhoff, H.-H., Department of Urology, Gentofte and Herlev Hospitals, University of Copenhagen, Niels Andersens Vej 65, DK-2900 Hellerup, Denmark

Minnaert, H., Department of Urology, University Hospital, De Pintelaan 135, B-9000 Gent, Belgium

* Montauban van Swijndregt, L., Department of Obstetrics and Gynaecology, General Hospital 'H. Familie', B-9000 Gent, Belgium

* Moonen, W.A., Department of Urology, University Hospital 'St. Radboud', P.O. Box 9101, 6500 HB Nijmegen, The Netherlands

Nollin, P. de, Urologic Centre of Kortrijk, Hospital 'O.L. Vrouw', Budastraat 37, B-8500 Kortrijk, Belgium

Oosterlinck, W., Department of Urology, University Hospital, De Pintelaan 135, B-9000 Gent, Belgium

* Petri, E., University Clinic for Obstetrics and Gynaecology, Langenbeck-strasse 1, D-6500 Mainz, F.R.G.

* Raz, S., Division of Urology, Department of Surgery, University of California School of Medicine, 10833 Le Conte Avenue, Los Angeles, CA 90024, USA

Sansen, W., Department of ESAT, Catholic University of Leuven, Brusselsestraat 69, B-3000 Leuven, Belgium

* Schreiter, F., Urological Clinic, Hospital of Schwelm, University Witten-Herdecke, Dr. Möllerstrasse 15, D-5830 Schwelm, F.R.G.

* Shortliffe, L.M. Dairiki, Division of Urology S-287, Stanford University School of Medicine, Stanford, CA 94305, USA

Stamey, Th.A., Division of Urology, Stanford University School of Medicine, Stanford, CA 94305, USA

* Stanton, S.L., Urodynamic Unit, Department of Obstetrics and Gynaecology, St. George's Hospital Medical School, Lanesborough Wing, Cranmer Terrace, London SW17 ORE, United Kingdom

* Sy, W. de, Department of Urology, University Hospital, De Pintelaan 135, B-9000 Gent, Belgium

* Tanagho, E.A., Department of Urology, U-518, University of California School of Medicine, San Francisco, CA 94143, USA

* Turner Warwick, R.T., The London University Institute of Urology, 61 Harley House, Marylebone Road, London NW 1, United Kingdom

Venrooy, G.E.P.M. van, Department of Urology, University Hospital, P.O. Box 16250, 3500 CG Utrecht, The Netherlands

* Vereecken, R.L., Department of Urology, Catholic University of Leuven, Brusselsestraat 69, B-3000 Leuven, Belgium

Vervecken, W., Department of Urology, General Hospital Stuivenberg, Antwerp, Belgium

Zimmern, Ph.E., Division of Urology, Department of Surgery, University of California School of Medicine, 10833 Le Conte Avenue, Los Angeles, CA 90024, USA

* These contributors were active participants in the symposium held in Nijmegen, The Netherlands, on 21-23 June 1984.

Introduction

Problems in the management of urinary incontinence

E.A. TANAGHO

It is a special privilege to present the introduction of this book. I will review the basic elements of female urinary incontinence, its aetiology, means of presentation, and guidelines for management. In so doing, we can pinpoint the problems and discuss their avoidance.

Diagnosis

To limit the causes of urinary incontinence to one particular entity would be simplistic; we must first differentiate each and address it accordingly. Urinary incontinence has many variations: anatomic stress incontinence; neuropathic incontinence (directly related to neurologic lesions); congenital incontinence; false incontinence (which can be misleading); and iatrogenic or traumatic incontinence (surgical or otherwise). I will stress a few aspects about each.

Anatomic stress incontinence is probably the most common; fortunately, it is easy to recognize and cure. What should be emphasized is that, in this instance, the sphincteric mechanism itself is intact; there is nothing intrinsically wrong. Primarily, this is a pelvic floor problem: a weakness in the pelvic floor support leads to incontinence. Here, if one restores anatomy, one will restore function. This is probably one of the easiest things for a surgeon to handle; we know how to restore anatomy and restoration of function will follow.

Some basic urodynamic features of anatomic stress incontinence are quite well known and are essential for diagnosis. Uniformly, you will find low closure pressure, a short functional length of the urethra on the expanse of the proximal segment, and, most importantly, abnormal responses to stress. Even if the first two are not immediately apparent, evidence of abnormality in response to stress will be seen, and this will be your guide for diagnosis.

If you proceed further, you will find that there is almost always a drop in the closure pressure with changes in position on bladder filling, as during evaluation of the hold maneuver or of the activity of the external sphincter. These features, associated with evidence of anatomic abnormality, make the diagnosis quite clear.

True urge incontinence is primarily detrusor hyperreflexia and is not associated with any anatomic abnormality. Sphincteric function is normal. Most importantly, there is no neuropathy. Urodynamically, one can easily differentiate this entity from anatomic stress incontinence. However, a combination of the two is quite common, and this is where we get into trouble, ignoring one and putting all the emphasis on the other. With detailed urodynamic study, one can quantify the contribution of each and determine which is primary and which secondary.

In *neuropathic incontinence,* a neurologic deficit is often evident. This form of incontinence varies in its manifestation, but correct diagnosis is essential because what might be an appropriate treatment for anatomic stress incontinence or for combined stress and urge incontinence will never succeed with the neurogenic bladder. There are two basic defects: either a flaccid sphincteric mechanism or a hyperreflexive bladder consequent to the neuropathic lesions. However, a combination of the two is not uncommon.

Congenital incontinence is quite varied. Some anomalies are easy to identify and treat, while others are quite challenging. Although the ectopic ureter is probably the easiest, it must be anticipated. All of us have had cases that have been misdiagnosed: the ectopic ureter is missed until the child is in her early teens; she may be receiving extensive psychiatric therapy for her wetness, while the problem is congenital – the ureter opening just a bit below the sphincteric mechanism. Ectopy in duplicated urinary systems, with a non-functioning upper unit, is probably the most common entity but is easily missed because the lower unit will function normally and one will not suspect an ectopic ureter draining an upper unit. Ectopy of a single system is rather rare but must be looked for; if it is bilateral, the bladder might never develop fully and the patient will be wet all the time. Female epispadias, an almost ignored entity, is not uncommon. A careful examination of the external genitalia will reveal the characteristic bifid clitoris, as well as the lack of formation of the anterior commissure; on endoscopic examination, this entity becomes quite clear. Cloacal malformation in all its varieties can also be a problem and a challenging one to treat.

False or overflow incontinence, although rare in females, is an easy entity once you think about it; if you do not, then you might be misled. Congenital obstruction is not that common. Iatrogenic obstruction may be much more common than other causes. Not infrequently, this is a purely myogenic problem. Detrusor activity is defective, leading to increased residual urine and the resultant overflow.

Iatrogenic incontinence, whether of our own doing or from some other cause, presents a problem. It can arise after pelvic surgery, ureteral, vesical, or urethral surgery, but one must identify the correct site to treat it appropriately. The problem arises with a combined injury: e.g. in the patient with a vesical fistula as well as a ureteral fistula, the former is the one attacked surgically, while the latter is completely ignored, only to present itself after the failure of the first procedure.

The level of the urethral fistula or diverticulum will determine the extent of the muscular involvement. In repair, one must keep in mind that the more proximal the fistula or diverticulum, the more likely the risk of damage to the sphincteric mechanism.

Traumatic incontinence is a major entity, and we are largely responsible. Fracture of the pelvis and rupture of the urethra are not of our own doing, but these are not that common. What is more common is our surgical damage to the sphincteric mechanism. Formerly, some surgeons undertook transurethral resection of the bladder neck (which should probably never have been done in some female patients) or extensive internal urethrotomy with deep cuts throughout the entire length of the sphincter, damaging its musculature. What is more common now is damage from urethral surgery. Not infrequently, we will casually undertake fistula repair or excision of a urethral diverticulum, damaging what remains of the sphincteric mechanism in the process. We have to be very careful about the dissection and treatment of the fistulae or diverticula in the urethral sphincteric segment. The structure of the sphincter is so delicate, so close and compact, that any rough handling of the tissue or loss of anatomical planes will easily damage and destroy it. Should one not sufficiently respect the delicate urethral musculature, coming too close and handling it indiscriminately, a scarred, fibrosed, sphincteric segment will result that is beyond hope of repair. Such injury represents the most challenging manifestation of urinary incontinence because the basic sphincteric mechanism has already been lost or damaged.

It cannot be emphasized too strongly that, because iatrogenic and traumatic incontinence are of our own doing, every attempt should be made at avoidance. When we damage and scar the sphincteric mechanism, recurrent urinary incontinence will always ensue. With careful regard for the sphincteric mechanism and awareness of its basic elements and physiologic function, this should never happen.

Treatment

What are the available therapeutic techniques to manage urinary incontinence? I will list them and discuss each separately: anatomic repair (probably the easiest and most successful); pharmacologic manipulation (limited in its use); reconstructive surgery (for serious congenital anomalies or after severe traumatic or iatrogenic injury); and neurostimulation (now assuming a major role in managing sphincteric weakness and detrusor hyperreflexia). Another modality, the artificial sphincter, will be discussed fully during the program.

Anatomic repair, with proper patient selection and adherence to basic principles, should be uniformly successful. There is no real excuse for failure. If we know what's wrong anatomically, we can correct it surgically. The result should also be permanent; there should be no reason for the repair to fail two or five years down the line. If it does, there is something wrong with the basic surgical technique.

Pharmacologic manipulation can be directed toward the bladder wall itself and achieve a certain degree of success in reducing detrusor hyperreflexia. Improving sphincteric function by building up tonus of the sphincteric element is relatively disappointing and of very limited benefit, but it is always worth trying.

Reconstructive surgery is a last resort and should never be undertaken unless there is no intrinsic sphincteric element left. This can be encountered in congenital anomalies, in severe trauma and complete disruption of the sphincteric mechanism, or after extensive scarring and fibrosis induced by ill-advised or ill-performed surgical techniques. There are several choices for reconstructive surgery, using either the anterior bladder wall or the trigonal or bladder base technique and modifications of these.

The success rate for reconstructive surgery is quite satisfactory. Although it is never as good as anatomic repair, it can give a favorable result in 70% to 80% of patients.

Neurostimulation, which is promising to be quite useful and successful, can handle most neuropathic or functional incontinence, and can also deal with the bladder as well as the sphincter.

For detrusor hyperreflexia, it can alleviate both sensory and motor urge incontinence. It can modulate the activity of the entire pelvic floor and has broad potential. At the University of California, San Francisco, we have been interested in this field for many years and are just now appreciating the potential of electrical stimulation to modulate function of the entire lower urinary tract, be it sphincteric weakness or detrusor hyperreflexia.

With stimulation, one can activate the external sphincter, actually changing the histologic nature of its musculature by converting pure striated muscle to something between striated and smooth muscle. Repeated bursts of pulses to the external sphincter from stimulation of the pudendal nerve or any sacral root will activate this muscle, which will be fatigue-resistant and maintain tonus for a long period of time, thus achieving continence. One can build up this mechanism to provide permanent sphincteric control.

Neurostimulation has great potential, and we should be looking forward to it.

The artificial sphincter is available if reconstructive surgery is not feasible or if scarring and trauma have already destroyed everything and one has no alternative but a mechanical device to try to maintain continence. Careful patient selection will play a major role in its success or failure. One also has to realize that it does have definite limitations, especially in the female.

Urinary diversion is a treatment that we hope never to see again. It may have been acceptable a decade or two ago, but not with today's understanding and abilities. As for neurectomy, I mention it only to comment that we should no longer interfere with the normal neural pathways now that they can easily be manipulated by other techniques, especially stimulation. These two treatment choices should be condemned.

Problems in management

What are the major problems in management? If I had to single one out, it would be inappropriate patient selection. If you misdiagnose, confusing the causes of incontinence, you are bound to have a very high rate of failure and recurrent incontinence. With proper patient selection, identification of the site, and an appropriate choice for repair, your success rate will be quite high and the problems much, much less. Beware the ill-advised surgical approach and rationale! Don't undertake one approach simply because it has been reported to be effective. Rationalize it. Make some sense of it in relation to the basic cause of the incontinence after you have identified it.

The last problem, which I have stressed all along, is iatrogenic damage. When operating for urinary incontinence, do not interfere with the basic sphincteric element. If you start to damage it, if you work on it directly to try to improve it, the end result will be iatrogenic scarring and fibrosis and eventual loss. Most of these major problems are really our own doing. We can avoid them if we are careful.

These are my guidelines:
1. Conduct a proper evaluation. Don't rush into surgery before evaluating your patient properly.
2. Adhere to rational principles. Be extremely critical of any surgical technique that doesn't make sense to you.
3. Avoid any iatrogenic damage whenever possible. (This is definitely in our power; we are the ones responsible.)
4. Respect neuroanatomy and neurophysiology. If you find it intact, leave it.
5. Avoid irreversible steps, particularly neurectomy.

CHAPTER ONE

Investigations for urinary incontinence

I.1. Practical equipment for office urodynamics

A.E.J.L. KRAMER

Introduction

Urodynamic investigations have found their place among the diagnostic armamentarium in urology and uro-gynaecology. Proper urodynamic test procedures can answer specific clinical questions, guide towards effective treatment by clear definition of the underlying pathology and objectify the results of treatment. In this way urodynamics has a greater meaning than just an objective or quantitative recording of the patient's symptoms.

While highly sophisticated machinery may be necessary to perform urodynamic studies in selected patients in whom the lower urinary tract symptoms cannot be objectified without multi-channel telemetry or video-urodynamics, simpler studies like uroflowmetry or cystometry alone or in combination will elucidate the cause of urinary incontinence in a vast majority of patients. The first group of patients should be referred to specialized centres both for economical use of the equipment and for expertise in the interpretation of the results. Other authors in this chapter deal with these specialized techniques.

In the clinical office these patients can be selected for referral if their history is complicated, if the simpler urodynamic tests fail or if therapy is compromised. Office urodynamics should include at least a recording of the urinary flow rate and favourably also of the detrusor pressure during filling. A combined filling and voiding study with bladder and abdominal pressure and flow rate recorded synchronously greatly enhances the quality of the study. In some patients urethral recordings can be performed in the office as well, although it must be appreciated that the technique of urethral measurements is more vulnerable to errors. Electromyography is a too complicated technique for use in the office but surface EMG to monitor overall pelvic floor activity may be of limited value in the hands of an experienced clinician.

The principles of the various measurement and recording techniques will be discussed together with the practical implications for the planning of an office urodynamics system. The clinical indications for and implications of urodynamic investigations in incontinent patients are described by other authors in this chapter. The International Continence Society's Standardization Committee has published various reports, compiled in a monograph in 1984, on The Standardization of Terminology of Lower Urinary Tract Function in which urodynamic terms and interpretation of measurements are defined. For technical specifications the reader is referred to the report: 'Urodynamic Equipment – technical aspects' that is produced by a Working Party of this Standardization Committee for publication in 1985.

Flow rate and bladder and abdominal pressure measurement will be discussed first, followed by a section on recorders as they are common to both types of measurement. In a last section urethral measurements and EMG will be mentioned briefly as their use in office urodynamics has a limited significance only.

Urinary flow rate measurement

Uroflowmetry or measurement of the rate of expelled urine is the simplest urodynamic investigation. Because of its non-invasivity and of the possibility of measuring in the relative privacy of an ordinary toilet it can be used easily as a first screening. For the same reasons a lot of research is directed towards an extensive clinical interpretation of flow patterns.

Flow meters measure and indicate the quantity of urine passed per time unit. A trend curve can be plotted and various parameter values can be extracted or calculated from the recording. Although the flow rate is indicated always as a volume rate (ml/s) not all available flow meters take the measurement directly in this way. Depending on the transducer technique two physical properties may be measured: volume or mass, and each of them in two ways: as a rate proper or as an accumulated amount (Table 1).

Mass metering is converted to a volume reading by division of the output value by the fluid density. All mass type meters provide the user with a density dial that corrects the electronic circuitry amplification to the recorder. Although in principle the setting cannot be effectuated without a separate measurement of the urine density a value near 1.02 will be accurate within a few percent in most cases. If the urine density deviates significantly from this value a correction to the recorded values must be made afterwards.

Continuous measurement of the accumulated amount of fluid present in the collecting vessel allows a curve of increasing output volume to be recorded. The steepness of this curve represents the flow rate. Most flow meters of this type use an electronic differentiating technique to present the flow rate directly during the voiding. Without proper precautions, that can be of electronic nature also, small random variations that may occur in the volume readings will be over-emphasized in the differentiated flow rate signal. The total voided volume is directly available from this type of measurement but is given in most rate-type flow meters also by electronic integration of the flow rate curve.

Table 1 presents a grouping of commonly used uroflowmeters according to the measured property and the principle of measurement.

The various types of modern flow meters are all of sufficient accuracy to enable their use in urodynamic investigations (about 5%). The working principles of the various transducers are discussed underneath.

Rotating disc uroflowmeter. The voiding takes place into a funnel which directs the urine onto a horizontal disc that is rotating at constant speed. The disc is rimmed so that a small amount of urine will be kept and rotates with the disc until the urine is projected off the disc again into a collecting chamber and vessel. A feed-back mechanism keeps the disc rotation speed at a constant value despite the increased inertia presented by the urine. The energy necessary to maintain a constant disc rotation is uniquely related to the mass of urine entering the disc. Thus this energy is a measure of the mass flow rate of urine. Integration of this figure represents the total mass voided.

Gravimetric flowmeters. These types of flowmeters measure the accumulated mass of urine in the collecting vessel either directly as total weight via a load cell or by sensing the pressure in a vessel of known geometry. The flow is directed into the vessel by means of a funnel mostly and the latter also acts often as a mechanical filter to avoid a direct stream into the vessel. This prevents the stream force to be added to the weight measurement in the first type or unwanted oscillations of the fluid surface and thus of the pressure sensed in the second type of measurement. Because of the necessary differentiation these artefacts would be amplified in the flow rate readings.

Table 1. Transducer types and properties of different flowmeters*.

		Technique of measurement	
		Flow rate	Accumulated amount
Metered physical property	Mass	Rotating disc	Gravimetric (weight, pressure)
	Volume	Air displacement electromagnetic	Capacitance dip stick collecting vessel height

* Mass meter outputs are divided by fluid density to give volume readings. Accumulated amounts are differentiated to give flow rates. Flow rates can be integrated to give total voided amount.

Air displacement flow meters. The urine is directed into a closed vessel and expels the air from this vessel through an anemometer tube. The air flow is passing a hot wire and the energy needed to keep this wire at a fixed temperature is a measure for the volume flow rate. The funnel ends below the fluid level in the vessel to ensure an airtight lock and the flushing outlet of the vessel also needs to be airtight.

Electromagnetic flowmeters. The principle of electricity generation by moving a conductor in a magnetic field, rendering a voltage proportional to both the field strength and the velocity is used in this type of flowmeters. An annular cuff containing an electromagnetic field generator and sensing electrodes is placed around the end of the funnel. The urine passing through this funnel acts as the conductor. Depending on the geometry of the magnetic field and of the funnel ending the voltage developed over the electrodes is a measure of the urine velocity across the cross-section and thus of the volume flow rate.

Dip stick flowmeters. This type of measuring is comparable to the pressure gravimetric one in that an open long-line capacitor is placed vertically in a vessel of known geometry. The capacitance changes because of the filling of the vessel and this change is a measure of the filling height and thus in this case of the volume collected.

Collecting vessel height flowmeter. Other types of measurement of the height of urine in a defined vessel have been described among which ultrasonic detection of the fluid-air boundary or detection of a floating device. These techniques also give a measure of the volume collected.

One general problem with all kinds of flowmeters is the collection of the urine expelled. Mostly a funnel and often some kind of tubing is used to direct the urine to the transducer or the collecting vessel and this leads to a delay time between the physical onset of voiding and the first detection of flow by the flowmeter. This delay is mostly not constant but depends on the actual flow rate also, leading to an unwanted filtering of possible physiological variations in the flow rate before they can be detected. This drawback that might be accepted as it is for single flow rate studies should be appreciated however if the flow rate measurement is to be correlated with any synchronously measured other event as e.g. in combined pressure-flow studies.

Pressure measurements in the bladder (and the abdomen)

All practical types of pressure measurement that enable direct recording of the pressures are based on the same principle. The pressure is sensed by the mechanical deformation of a sensor membrane that is exposed to the pressure on one side and to a known reference pressure on the other side. The size of the deformation is related to the pressure difference and is transduced to an electrical signal that can be processed and recorded. The reference pressure is often the atmospheric pressure in which case the reference side of the membrane is communicating with the open air. The membrane may be mounted on a closed vacuum chamber so that the reference pressure is the vacuum. This type of measurement is called absolute pressure measurement.

The pressure detector can be positioned outside the patient and connected to the bladder or (mostly the saline-filled rectal ampulla for) the abdominal cavity by appropriate tubing. Alternatively, if the transducer is small enough, the transducer itself can be mounted on the catheter and measure from inside the organ.

For the sake of simplicity in the following discussion the measurement of abdominal pressure will not be mentioned as a separate item because no essential difference exists between this and the intravesical pressure measurement.

Four types of transducer are available of which only two are fit to be so far miniaturized that they will allow catheter mounting also. These last are
— the resistive or strain gauge type, that has gained most popularity;
— the opto-electronic type, that is marketed recently in catheter form.
The other two types are less popular in the urodynamics field although available as external transducers,
— the inductive type;
— the capacitive type.

Resistive type transducers. A strain gauge is mounted onto the membrane and due to the deformation its resistance is changing. This change is a measure of the applied pressure. As only the sensor itself and the wires need to be mounted one catheter allows for multiple transducers (4 to 5 in a 10 French catheter). Because the resistance change is sensed by applying a voltage across the transducer electrical safeguarding is essential in this type of measurement.

Opto-electronic type transducers. The membrane mirrors a light source onto a light-sensitive device. Deformation of the membrane will change the lighting of the sensor and thus measure the pressure. Using a fibre-optics catheter with a bifurcated fibre bundle the light of an external source is projected onto a membrane that is mounted in the catheter and the mirrored light sensed also externally by transmission through the other part of the fibres. Multiple sensors are not available yet in one catheter.

Inductive type transducers. The membrane's deformation is mechanically transformed into the movement of the shaft in a displacement transformer coil.

Capacitive type transducers. The membrane acts as the moving plate of a variable capacitor.

External transducers are connected to the bladder by means of various types of catheters and extension tubing. The bladder pressure is transmitted to the membrane via this connection that is accomplished as either:
— an open-end system. The bladder contents and the membrane chamber are in physical contact to one another;
— a sealed system. The contents of the catheter and the tubing are sealed to the bladder mostly by means of a latex balloon. These systems are not practical in the case of gas (carbondioxide) cystometry.

Special precautions have to be taken for these connections if the bladder and/or the catheter system is fluid-filled. The inertia of the mass of fluid in the connections together with the elasticity of the tubing will filter the pressure variations before they can be transduced. Especially if the channels are too narrow or if air bubbles are not completely flushed out this will adversely affect the quality of the measurement.

All pressure measurements described here measure the total pressure in the bladder. This pressure contains two components: one is generated by the passive and contractile properties of the detrusor itself, the other is the static head of the filling medium. If the detrusor is filled with gas the last component is negligible. In fluid cystometry this component must be accounted for as e.g. position changes of the patient or increasing filling of the bladder are reflected in the pressure measured.

In external cystometry the external transducers therefore are always positioned at the upper edge of the symphysis pubis, as for most patients in each position this is the best estimation of the anatomical upper level of the bladder. The recorded pressure thus is the difference with the static pressure at this level. Any change of position within the bladder of the pressure lumen of an open-end system or the balloon of a sealed system filled with a fluid of equal density as the bladder's contents will not be reflected in the pressure sensed because the horizontal plane of equal pressure in the fluid projected from the transducer will always be at the reference level (Fig. 1). When a sealed system is filled with a liquid of unequal density (oil, air) a pressure difference will be noted equal to the difference of the pressures of the two liquid columns of the same height.

Intravesical measurement of the pressure is in principle independent of the patient's position as the transducer has a defined anatomical position already. However in this case the changes in static head caused by inadvertent movement of the catheter within the bladder are not correctable if no monitoring of this position is performed (Fig. 1). Experience with normal catheter-tip transducers indicated no serious errors in this aspect but superflexible types might be more susceptible.

While fluid cystometry is generally accepted to give more reliable clinical results than gas (carbondioxide) cystometry, the latter procedure has the advantage for office urodynamics that it is a fast and technically easier pro-

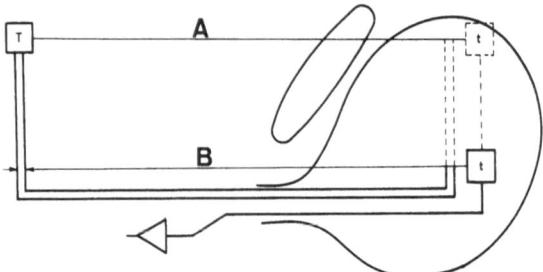

Fig. 1. If a fluid connection of equal density exists between the bladder and the external transducer a lowering of the balloon or the opening of the catheter does not affect the pressure
reading: the plane of equal pressure stays at the same place. Different densities give rise to a
change. Taking the fluid density as 1 and the shift as 10 cm the plane B has a 10 cmH20 higher
pressure than plane A. This is corrected to the transducer again as the tubing column from B to
A represents 10 cmH20 as well. If a sealed catheter is oil-filled (density .8) this correction does
not take place fully and the transducer will read a 2 cmH20 higher pressure.

The intravesical transducer will always read a 10 cmH20 higher pressure when changing from
position A to B. T: external transducer; t: intravesical transducer.

cedure. It however cannot be combined with a flow study, it necessitates fast
filling always and thus will give inadequate quantitation of bladder capacity
and eventual instabilities, and it is difficult to combine with synchronous
abdominal pressure measurement.

This last combination is essential to be able to distinguish between detrusor contractions and abdominal straining. Care should be taken before automatic electronic substraction of intravesical and abdominal pressure is prac-
tized, because autonomic contractions and relaxations of the rectum or the
dampening effect of rectal contents cannot be appreciated then. When electronic subtraction is performed at least one of the original signals should be
recorded too.

The combined pressure-flow studies enable the differentiation between
detrusor failure or other causes for an impaired urinary flow. As mentioned
before the flow meter delay should be accounted for here, either by shifting
the flow rate measurement accordingly or by interpreting only a steady flow
episode.

Comparing the technology of pressure sensors and the activities to be
measured it can be stated that no difficulties are to be expected in this
respect. Some transducers even are so fast that their responses are damped
for urodynamic applications to prevail high-frequency artefacts.

Recorders

The recorders that will be dealt with in this section are used for producing a permanent copy of the investigation and its results, mostly on a paper chart. They might be coupled directly to the registration equipment, but electronic storage e.g. on magnetic tape recorders or in computer memory can be an intermediate step. This will allow then later copying of the same investigation, perhaps on a different time scale, or in the case of computer storage even full editing of the curves and automatic calculation of important parameters.

Because the signals that have to be reproduced from uroflowmetry and pressure measurements will not show very fast changes even the simplest types of commercially available paper recorders will function adequately for direct registration. Recorders that will be coupled to tape recorders or computers may need some special specifications that however are beyond the scope of this section. Most recorders will present curves that follow the trend of the variable in the time but it is possible also to make recordings of two variables plotted perpendicularly to each other. Time chart recorders offer the possibility of changing the speed of forwarding of the paper along the time (X) axis.

The recorders writing technique can be either by moving pens writing directly on the paper (inked or by heat or electric charge), by moving an ink jet, a UV-beam or charged particles over the paper or by heating or charging the appropriate spot underneath the paper. The pen recorders often write curvilinear as the pen driving mechanism is at some distance from the writing point in the plane of the paper. This is somewhat embarrassing in the interpretation of the recordings.

Single-channel recorders are in use for flowmetry only and gas cystometry. Most of these are the simplest type of pen recorders. Using multichannel recorders of the pen type problems will occur if every channel must have access to the full paper width. This problem is resolved either by limiting each pen's excursion to a proportional part of the paper width, in which case the different channels are written synchronized according to the time axis, or by using pens of different lengths that overlap each other on the paper and can write over the full width. In the last case of course the timing of the curves is shifted on the paper and this will impair the readability of the curves. As however the multi-channel recorders of the non-pen type are far more expensive than the pen types any one of the mentioned drawbacks is often acceptable for use in the office.

Other office urodynamics

Some other types of urodynamic investigations might be performed in the office also but mostly need more expertise from the side of the investigator to be performed in a correct fashion.

Pelvic floor electromyography

It is generally accepted that clinical meaningful electromyography in urodynamics should be acquired from intramuscular recordings in the urethral sphincter. However, in the office some information might be gained from pelvic floor or anal sphincter surface EMG, especially to confirm the suspicion that a patient is not able to relax the pelvic floor adequately. For general office urodynamics yet this will not be a routine examination as the extra technical equipment necessary and the vulnerability of EMG-measurements to artefacts are relatively prohibitive to its use.

Urethral pressure measurement

Urethral pressures can be measured either with a catheter- or sealed external type of pressure transducer as described in the section on bladder pressure or by a perfusion technique. In the last method a slow perfusion is maintained through a catheter with side holes ending in the urethra and the pressure to maintain a constant flow rate is measured. This pressure reflects the closure pressure of the urethra at the site of the holes. As the recent opinion is that the static measurement of the urethral pressure profile by withdrawal of the catheter bears little clinical significance and probably the closure pressure measurements, found by subtracting the concurrently measured intravesical pressure, are more valuable the balloon and perfusion techniques are slowly abandoned. Unless a suprapubic measurement of the bladder pressure is performed only the resistive type of microtransducers can be used for this measurement. This technique is however open to criticism as mechanical contact between the walls of the urethra and the sensor element may give rise to serious artefacts.

Fluid bridge test

Although originally more a clinical test than a recording technique a description of this method seems on its place here. The test is used to find out whether the proximal urethra is opening in a patient when coughing. A pressure measuring catheter is placed in the partially filled bladder. A second hole in the catheter is positioned at a known distance from the meatus and the patient asked to cough. When urine is lost from the catheter obviously the position of the second hole had an open connection with the bladder at that moment.

Two variations have been described for the recording of this test. Brown and Sutherst [1] originated the test and used a second pressure transducer connected to the proximal urethral lumen. Plevnik et al. [2] replaced the proximal urethral opening by a measurement of the electrical impedance of the proximal urethral area.

When a double fluid pressure measuring system is available already in the office the first technique can be applied easily without much extra burden to the patient.

Abstract

Uroflowmetry and cystometry are routine investigations in the detection of lower urinary tract disorders. Urethral pressure profilometry and fluid bridge tests might be a valuable addition to office urodynamics. Extensive procedures including multichannel measurements, combined cine-fluoro-scopic investigations (video-urodynamics), sphincter electromyography and neurological tests should be confined to specialized centres.

The physical variable to be measured is sensed by a transducer and the electrical output signal processed and recorded. Technical aspects and the practical set-up of various measuring and recording devices that find their place in contemporary office urodynamics will be discussed.

References

1. Brown M. and Sutherst J.R. A test for bladder neck competence: the fluid-bridge test. Urol. Int. 34 (1979): 403–409.
2. Plevnik S., Vrtacnik P. and Janez J. Detection of fluid entry into the urethra by electric impedance measurement: electric fluid bridge test. Clin. Phys. Physiol. Meas. 4 (1983): 309–313.

I.2. The role of radiology in urodynamics

H.R. HADLEY, P.E. ZIMMERN & S. RAZ

Introduction

This chapter will discuss the indications for and the interpretation of various radiological procedures available to most urologists and gynecologists for the assistance in the management of the incontinent patient. Because it provides the physician with objective anatomical information that can be corroborated with the patient's historical and physical findings, we feel that radiography of the lower urinary tract is an important adjunct to the evaluation of the incontinent patient. We will discuss the role of conventional radiology in the female and male in separate sections of this chapter. We will then devote the last section to the use of videourodynamics, which combines and simultaneously records the urodynamics and radiography of the lower urinary tract.

The role of radiology in the incontinent female

Initially, we will discuss the technique we prefer for the radiological evaluation of the lower urinary tract. Later, we will outline the important aspects in the interpretation of these films.

Technique

After the patient has done her best to empty her bladder, a preliminary (scout) upright film that includes the kidneys, bladder, and 4–5 cm below the ischial tuberosities is obtained. A urethral catheter is then inserted and the volume of residual urine is measured and recorded. Under low gravity pressure (less than 30 cm of water) the bladder is filled. Films are obtained when the patient notes the first sensation of fullness and at the volume which the patient is unable to tolerate further filling. These two films are referred to as the filling phase of the cystogram. The patient is then asked to stand up. With the catheter still in place, relaxing and straining films are obtained in the anteroposterior, oblique and lateral views. The catheter is then removed. With the patient in the oblique position; resting, coughing and straining films are taken. In the oblique position, films are obtained while the patient is voiding and immediately after the patient is asked to interrupt her urinary stream (stop-flow film). Finally, a post-void film is taken. All of the above films are exposed with the patient in the standing position.

Important aspects of the various films obtained

Preliminary (scout) film. The bony structure abnormalities that will interest the urodynamicist include spinal dysraphisms (spina bifida, myelomeningocele, etc.), intravertebral narrowing due to degenerative disease, evidence of a prior operative procedure (spinal fusion, laminectomy, etc.), and osteoblastic or osteolytic changes suggestive of primary or metastatic disease to the spinal column. All these aforementioned findings may affect the neurologic status of the bladder and urethra and therefore, assist in the evaluation of the incontinent patient. In the region of the kidneys and ureters the scout film will give evidence of radioopaque urinary stones, which may be due to or the cause of recurrent or persistent urinary tract infections. Renal or pelvic calculi may occur because of ureteral obstruction or vesicoureteral reflux associated with a neurogenic or obstructed bladder. In the true pelvis the scout film may demonstrate bladder or urethral calculi. The former is not uncommonly seen in patients with either anatomical or functional (detrusor-sphincter dyssynergia) bladder outlet obstruction. The use of a long term indwelling catheter in an immobilized patient commonly results in the formation of bladder calculi. Urethral calculi are usually associated with urethral diverticuli, which are commonly manifest by urgency, dysuria, dyspareunia and urethral dribbling.

Other abnormalities noted on the scout film may be a soft tissue pelvic mass indicating a large uterus, ovarian cyst, or a full bladder in a patient with urinary retention. A colon filled with stool may be an indication of a neurologic abnormality to the pelvic floor.

The filling phase. This section will outline the important findings that may be noted during the filling phase.

Bladder diverticuli are not an uncommon finding and may be the cause of frequency, postvoid fullness, and recurrent urinary tract infections. Acquired bladder diverticuli may be due to high detrusor voiding pressures that are secondary to anatomical outlet obstruction or detrusor-sphincter dyssynergia. In the female, however, bladder diverticuli or trabeculation have been observed in an unstable bladder without obstruction.

The presence of vesicoureteral reflux seen on the static cystogram may be congenital or due to a bladder with high filling pressures. Vesicoureteral reflux may explain recurrent urinary tract infection in the patient with incontinence. Although mild reflux is not an absolute contraindication to an operation for incontinence, severe reflux is best managed with further evaluation and a possible ureteral reconstructive operative procedure.

Filling defects in the contrast can be due to a ureterocele, tumor, bladder stone, or foreign body. A uterocele may be associated with urinary incontinence that is due to an ectopic ureter emanating into the vagina or overflow incontinence due to bladder outlet obstruction. Bladder neoplasia (especially in the region of the bladder neck), bladder stone, and foreign body can cause urinary urgency and frequency.

Bladder capacity can be estimated during the filling phase of the cystogram. Because it is less physiologic, filling of the bladder should not be done with pressures greater than 30 cm. A limited capacity may be the result of poor bladder compliance, motor instability, or sensory instability. *Poor bladder* compliance is a result of intrinsic disease of the bladder wall and may be caused by chronic infection, radiotherapy, chemotherapy (cyclophosphamide), interstitial cystitis, chronic obstruction, and others. *Motor instability* is stated to occur when a bladder contraction of greater than 15 cm water occurs during a filling cystometrogram. It has a myriad of aetiologies which can be found in other chapters of this text. If associated with a neurologic disorder, motor instability is referred to as bladder hyperreflexia. *Sensory instability* occurs when the patient's functional bladder capacity is diminished because of urgency and pain that occurs early during the bladder filling [1].

Trabeculation may be seen on the filling phase of the cystogram (Fig. 1). A normal bladder should have a smooth wall without trabeculation. Patients with uninhibited bladder contractions, urgency, and urgency incontinence but normal activity of the pelvic floor may develop trabeculation because the patient contracts the pelvic floor simultaneous to the uninhibited bladder contraction. This temporary functional obstruction may result in trabeculation. Trabeculation may also be seen in bladders that have poor compliance without motor instability. In the poorly compliant bladder there is an abnormally rapid rise in the true detrusor pressure with relatively small bladder volumes. This is not an uninhibited contraction but rather a lack of bladder distensibility. Trabeculation, therefore, in the female is not always a sign of obstruction, but may be seen because of an overactive or poorly compliant bladder.

Films with *the urethral catheter.* In the standing position, anteroposterior, oblique and lateral films of the bladder are taken when the patient is at rest and during straining. The following abnormalities may be identified.

If the bladder base falls below the level of the inferior ramus of the sym-

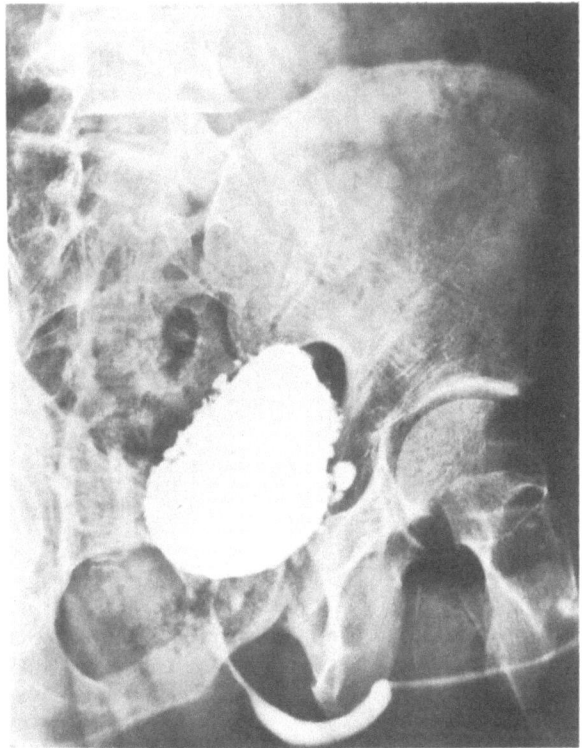

Fig. 1. Oblique view of a trabeculated bladder.

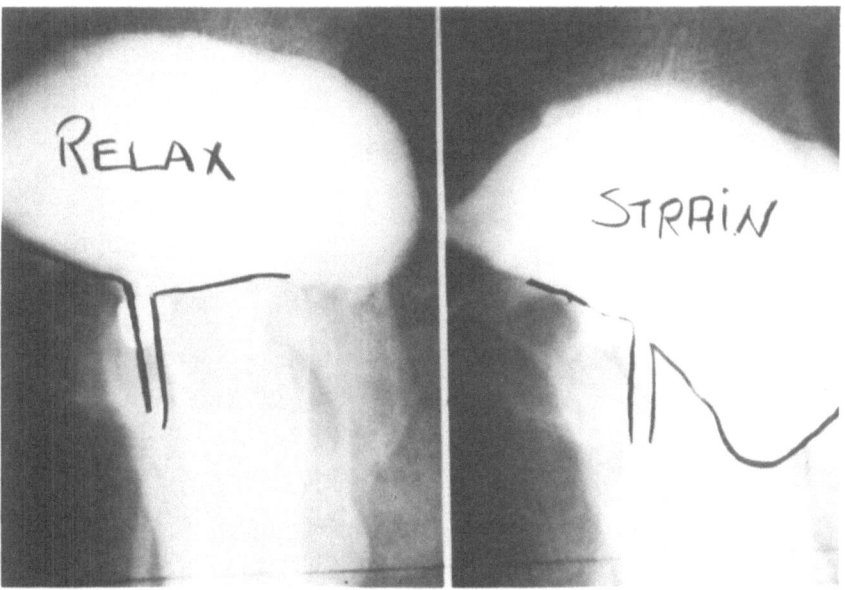

Fig. 2. Lateral view of a cystocele. Note that the bladder has dropped below the level of the inferior edge of the symphysis pubis. The urethra is not hypermobile.

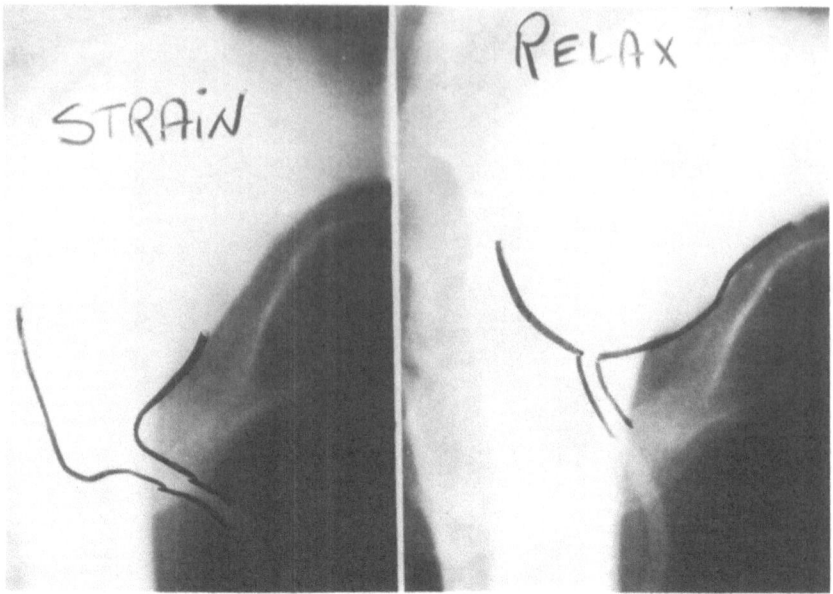

Fig. 3. Lateral view of a cystourethrocele. Note that both the bladder and the urethra drop below the symphysis pubis during straining. There is funneling of the bladder neck.

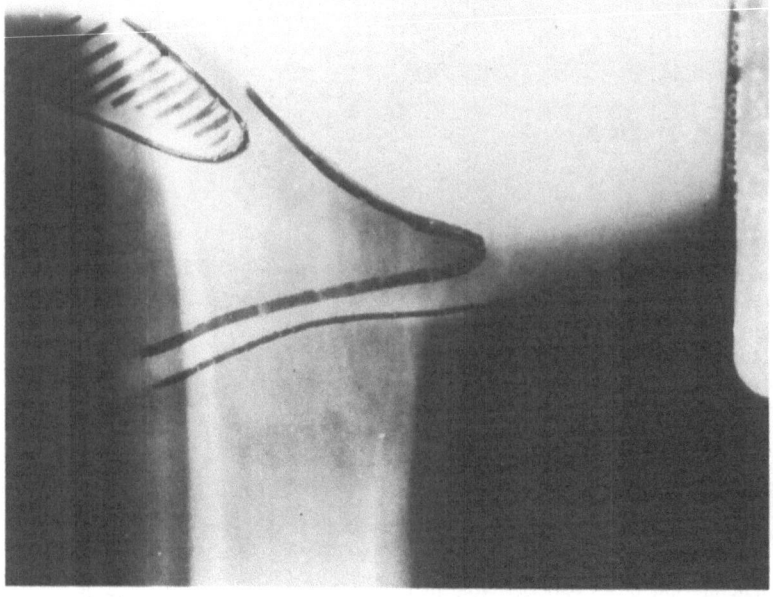

Fig. 4. Urethrocele.

physis pubis, a cystocele is said to be present (Fig. 2). If a cystocele is present, the bladder neck and urethra are obscured on the AP film, and their true position can be appreciated only on the lateral or oblique film. Many times, what appears to be descent of the bladder neck and urethra on the AP film is found to be only a cystocele on the lateral view. If the bladder neck drops below the level of the inferior ramus of the symphysis pubis, it is likely to see funneling of the bladder neck (Fig. 3). If the urethra has descended below the symphysis, it is referred to as a urethrocele (Fig. 4).

Although there has been considerable interest in the urethral axis and the urethrotrigonal angles, we have not placed a significant importance on these values for the evaluation of the incontinent patient. The urethral axis is normally perpendicular (plus or minus 5–10 degrees) to the horizontal axis of the patient (Fig. 5). With multiple deliveries and age, there may be displacement and posterior rotation of the axis of the uretha. Unfortunately, this observed rotation is only an indication of the support of the urethra and bladder and not necessarily a cause of urinary incontinence. If the resting

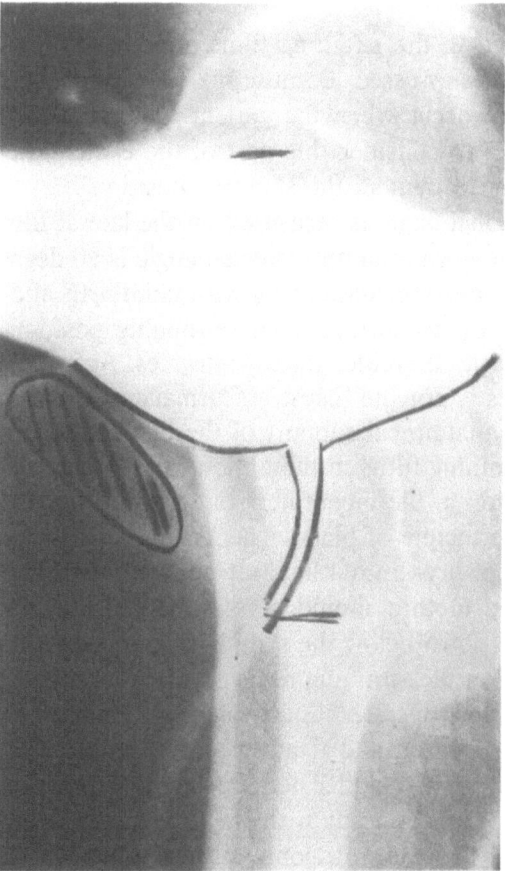

Fig. 5. Normal vertical axis of the urethra as seen on the lateral view.

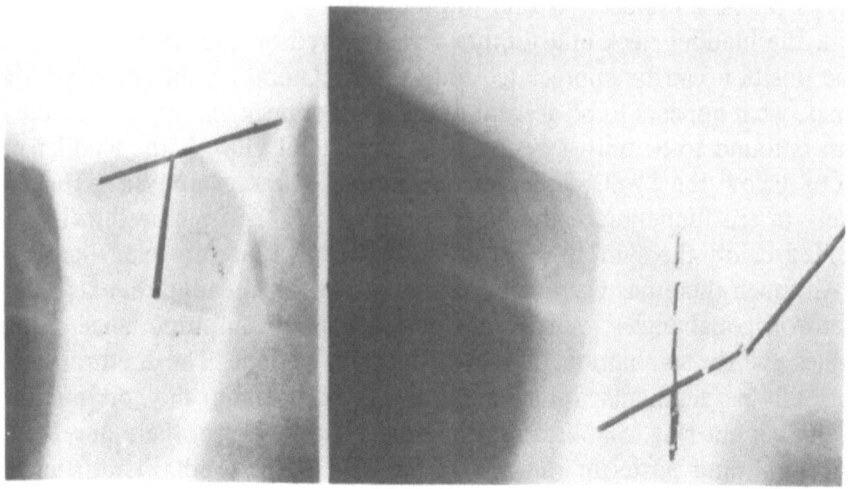

Fig. 6. The normal urethrotrigonal angle is approximately 90 degrees as demonstrated on the left radiograph. The right radiograph demonstrates a urethrotrigonal angle greater than 180 degrees.

films are compared to the straining films, mobility of the urethra and the bladder neck may be assessed. Because the changes of the bladder and urethral anatomy that occur when the patient is upright are best assessed by these radiographs, we consider this part of the evaluation as the 'physical examination of the patient in the standing position'.

The urethrotrigonal angle is measured on the lateral film with a catheter in the urethra. The normal urethrotrigonal angle is 90 degrees (Fig. 6). With the pelvic floor relaxation that occurs with childbirth and age, the urethra may descend out of its normal fixed retropubic position and 'open' the urethrotrigonal angle to greater than 90 degrees. Again, the change in urethrotrigonal angles is not the 'cause' of urinary incontinence but rather an indication of the anatomical support of the bladder and urethra.

Resting and straining films in the oblique and lateral views may be helpful in the evaluation of the incontinent patient who has failed bladder neck suspension. The principle of bladder neck surgery is to replace and fix the urethra and bladder neck into a high retropubic position. Radiographically, the well supported urethra should be seen behind the symphysis pubis. If the urethra is still down below the symphysis pubis or if there is significant urethral mobility on the straining films of a patient who has failed bladder neck suspension, post-operative incontinence is most likely due to the failure of adequate elevation and fixation to the urethra.

When funneling of the bladder neck occurs, it is best seen on the oblique and lateral views. Concomitant with the development of urethral descent and a widening of the urethrotrigonal angle the bladder neck will begin to funnel. It is important to be reminded that funneling of the bladder neck may also be seen in patients who are incontinent because of an overactive or poorly compliant bladder. In the overactive or poorly compliant bladder there is an increase in the tensile forces on the trigone during filling, which effectively opens and funnels the bladder neck. Funneling of the bladder neck may also be observed in the patient with detrusor-sphincter dyssynergia. Funneling of the bladder neck in these patients is most likely due to the high distal urethral sphincteric pressures, which cause proximal urethral dilatation. If proper cystometric examination demonstrates a stable compliant bladder in a patient who is suffering from stress urinary incontinence, funneling of the bladder neck is suggestive of urethral sphincter incompetence. The urodynamic evaluation that will best differentiate genuine stress urinary incontinence from incontinence due to an overactive bladder is videourodynamics (see below).

It is important to remember that the loss of the urethrotrigonal angle and the development of funneling of the bladder neck can be seen in patients who are *continent*. It is rare, however, to see a cystogram without funneling of the bladder neck and with normal urethrotrigonal angle in a patient who has genuine stress urinary incontinence. The vast majority of patients with true stress urinary incontinence due to sphincter insufficiency will demonstrate certain degrees of anatomic abnormality of the bladder neck and urethra. Careful urodynamic evaluation, therefore, is indicated in patients complaining of 'stress incontinence' but who do not have a funneled bladder neck noted on the cystogram.

A vesicovaginal fistula can also be seen on the lateral view of the cystogram. It is important that the urodynamicist suspects this diagnosis, when the patient complains of continuous urinary leakage not related to stress or urgency.

Films without *the urethral catheter.* After the catheter is removed, films are obtained in the oblique position while the patient is at rest, straining, and coughing.

Funneling of the bladder neck is again assessed. It is not uncommon that a patient who appeared to have a normal bladder neck on the films with the catheter in place may demonstrate funneling of the bladder neck on the films without the catheter. An erroneously apparent competent bladder neck may be due to the spastic influence the catheter has on the bladder neck muscle fibers. It is important to remember that an open or funneled bladder neck may be demonstrated in women without urinary complaints, with genuine stress urinary incontinence, and/or an overactive bladder. Remember to evaluate with caution the patient does not have an open or funneled bladder neck yet complains of 'stress incontinence'.

During straining or coughing, objective radiographic evidence of stress urinary incontinence may be seen. Again, this finding is suggestive of genuine stress incontinence but does not rule out the possibility of an over-active or poorly compliant bladder. It is rare for patients with clinically significant genuine stress incontinence not to be incontinent under the sti-mulus of cough. When the clinical history is ambiguous, coughing films will many times provide objective evidence of stress urinary incontinence and help to differentiate urge incontinence from stress incontinence. Occasional-ly, we will see a patient with true sphincter insufficiency and urethral incompetence fail to demonstrate leakage during coughing. This is because of reflex contraction of the pelvic floor that results from pain and discom-fort from the insertion of the urethral catheter. In such cases incontinence should be demonstrated during the physical examination before catheteriza-tion.

It is important to relate the incontinence to the time of stress. If there is a delay between the cough and incontinence, or if there is continuous incon-tinence after stress, we must suspect an overactive bladder. Stress hyperre-flexia or unstable stress incontinence is manifested by a cough causing an uninhibited bladder contraction and sudden relaxation of the pelvic floor with a subsequent loss of urine. This is *not* sphincter insufficiency, and bladder neck suspension will not correct this condition. One can make the diagnosis with close observation, even without urodynamic equipment. Patients with stress incontinence due to sphincter insufficiency leak urine only at the time of cough and not beyond the time of stress. Once the leakage occurs, the patient is asked to stop flow. Many patients with 'stress hyperreflexia' will lose practically all the urine at the time of cough, a find-ing that can also be used to differentiate these patients from those with true sphincter insufficiency. Patients with sphincter insufficiency are usually able to interrupt the leaking flow.

The stop-flow film. Additional information concerning the competency of the bladder neck is obtained by taking a film just after the patient is asked to interrupt her stream. Under fluoroscopy, voluntary closure of the normal urethra usually results in a retrograde 'milking' effect of the contrast mate-rial into the bladder. Patients with severe urethral dysfunction or an over-active bladder may be incapable of developing urethral or bladder neck competence in spite of voluntary elevation of the pelvic floor.

Voiding film. A film is obtained in the oblique position while the patient is voiding. During this phase of the study we may observe outlet obstruction, urethral diverticuli, distal sphincter dysfunction (detrusor-sphincter dyssy-nergia) (Fig. 7) or unmask vesicoureteral reflux.

Postvoid film. Large postvoid residuals may be seen in patients with func-tional or anatomical outlet obstruction. Functional obstruction is seen in

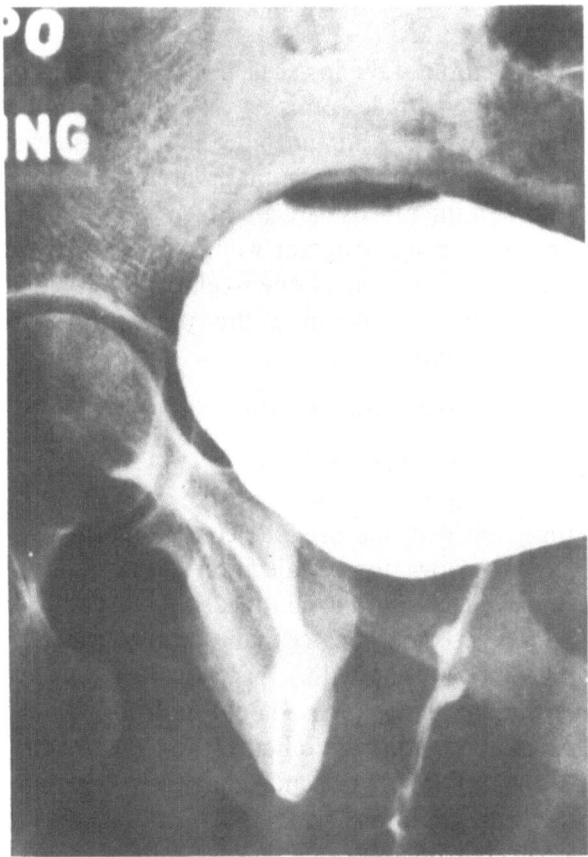

Fig. 7. Urethral diverticulum.

patients with detrusor-sphincter dyssynergia. Anatomical obstruction may be observed in patients with severe urethral descent because of urethral kinking. With abdominal straining or attempted voiding the kinking worsens and may obstruct the bladder outlet. Another type of outlet obstruction in the female is urethral strictures, which although rare, may occur after repeated dilation or internal urethrotomy. Other causes of urethral obstruction are an atrophic urethra and urethral valves (rare).

Large residuals of urine may be due to an acontractile bladder secondary to diabetes or a previous pelvic operation that effectively denervates the bladder. These patients may have overflow incontinence due to a urinary retention and relative urethral insufficiency.

The postvoid film may demonstrate vaginal 'trapping' of urine. This occurs when part of the voided urine is sequestered in the vaginal vault. Urinary leakage is noted by the patient soon after she arises from the toilet.

Radiological evaluation of male incontinence

A full radiological evaluation of the lower urinary tract should be performed routinely in the incontinent male, utilizing an injecting urethrogram and voiding cystourethrogram [2, 3]. An injecting urethrogram should not be performed subsequent to minimally traumatic urethral endoscopy or manipulation. Small tears in the mucosa are a frequent event after urethral manipulation, and an injecting urethrogram will easily show extravasation of contrast in these patients. A period of one week or more will elapse before healing is complete. Whenever possible, this procedure should be done before endoscopic manipulation.

Injecting (retrograde) urethrogram

An injecting urethrogram with the Brodney clamp or with a Foley catheter at the tip of the urethra allows for visualization of the anterior urethra and membranous urethra. Injection of the contrast should be done only with the use of pressure by gravity of not greater than 40 cm of water. The injecting urethrogram should not be done with a piston syringe. During retrograde flow of the contrast material the penis should be held with slight outward traction at 30 degrees above the horizontal. If the patient is at high risk for extravasation, fluoroscopy is recommended for early detection of contrast extravasation. The anterior urethra and the membranous urethra in the injecting films should be checked for integrity. False passages from catheters, sinus, and diverticula may be seen as a contributory factor in the incontinent patient. To prevent superposition of the bulbar urethra over the membranous urethra, films are obtained in the 30 degree oblique position.

If the urethra is found to be radiographically normal, the catheter is passed into the bladder.

Cystogram

The bladder is filled with contrast material at a pressure not greater than 30 cm water. Bladder capacity should be checked during the cystogram. Patients with urinary incontinence caused by sphincteric insufficiency should, in most cases, have adequate bladder capacity. In contrast, those with an overactive bladder usually have small functional capacities. Some patients with sphincteric insufficiency and severe incontinence will experience an early desire to void, owing to the leakage of urine through the distal urethral sphincter (DUS). The early sensation of urinary incontinence gives a false indication of small bladder capacity. By pulling the balloon of the Foley catheter into the posterior urethra (allowing only the bladder to be distended while preventing contrast to enter the distal urethra), the urodynamicist is more likely to obtain a true cystometric capacity.

When a patient's bladder has been filled, he should be checked for vesicoureteric reflux, bladder diverticulum, or bladder fistula. In the standing relaxed position, the patient's level of continence is determined. If the patient is incontinent after a prostatectomy and the cystogram shows the level of continence to be in the bladder neck area, bladder neck obstruction with overflow incontinence should be suspected. It is important to remember, however, that the radiographic assessment of the distal urethral sphincter can not be accurate in the presence of a concurrent bladder neck obstruction.

Attention should also be paid to the prostatic fossa. Any filling defects, especially in the apical area, may represent residual adenoma and can be an important factor in the persistence of incontinence. When the patient is standing and the level of continence has been determined, leakage of urine under stress should be checked by asking the patient to cough and strain. Films obtained during these maneuvers may provide objective evidence of urinary stress incontinence. Some patients who experience urinary incontinence while they are relaxed may note that when coughing they are continent. This may occur because reflex contraction of the somatic skeletal portion of the distal urethral sphincter that effectively shuts off the membranous urethra during coughing. Although some patients with minimal urinary stress incontinence demonstrate these findings, most will leak urine only when coughing and straining, and the urine stops flowing immediately with and simultaneously to the cessation of the stress. Patients with an overactive bladder, however, are not only unable to halt the urinary stream, but usually completely empty their bladder after the coughing or straining event has induced an involuntary bladder contraction.

Voiding films

Because the ability of the distal urethra to open properly is crucial, voiding films are valuable. Patients with sphincteric insufficiency have a wide-open distal urethral sphincter mechanism. Filling defects in the area may represent raised flaps from the previous resection or residual tissue that does not allow perfect coaptation of the DUS mechanism. Further resection will substantially improve the symptomatology of these patients.

Films should be taken when voiding has been stopped voluntarily. Although the sphincter voluntarily contracts, this does not indicate that the patient is free of sphincteric insufficiency. On the contrary, most patients with sphincter insufficiency have excellent voluntary sphincter activity, suggesting that the chief damage has been to the inner layer, smooth muscles and/or 'slow-twitch' skeletal muscles of the DUS and not to the somatic 'fast-twitch' skeletal muscles. In normal patients following prostatectomy, voluntary contraction of the sphincter cuts off the urinary stream, dividing it into two parts: one part refluxes promptly to the prostatic urethra, and the other empties into the bulbar urethra. Patients suffering from post-prostatectomy incontinence partially or entirely lack this ability and there is a permanent filling of contrast in the DUS area after relaxation.

Postvoid films

Postvoiding films are subsequently obtained to rule out the presence of residual urine.

Summary

Because they are easily available, radiological studies are among the most practical tools in evaluation of the incontinent patient. If done at low pressure (no more than 40 cm water), these studies are parallel in value to the cystometrogram. It is possible to observe sensations, bladder capacity, and especially bladder compliance. (When a rapidly ascending cystometrogram is seen and high intravesical pressures develop, the flow of water stops, suggesting some dysfunction in the bladder stability).

Video urodynamics

Because the radiographic changes noted on cystourethrography are related not only to the changes in bladder volume but also to the changes in intraurethral and intravesical pressure, misinterpretation of the standard radiographs may occur. In order to obviate this pitfall, simultaneous urodynamic recordings and cystourethrographic exposures mixed on the same television monitor and recorded on a videotape may be done. Collectively, this is referred to as video urodynamics [4–8].

Video urodynamics requires a fluoroscopic image that is transmitted via a special effects generator to a television monitor. The generator splits the television monitor screen in two, allowing display of the fluoroscopic image and the urodynamic tracings to occur concomitantly. The urodynamic data reaches the monitor either directly or via a television camera, which is televising the tracing from the four channel recorder. A permanent record of the study is obtained by the use of a video cassette recorder.

Application of video urodynamics to urinary incontinence

Genuine stress urinary incontinence is defined as the unintentional loss of urine during abdominal straining without a simultaneous increase in the true detrusor pressure (true detrusor pressure equals intravesical pressure minus intraabdominal pressure). Genuine stress urinary incontinence, therefore, can only be definitively diagnosed only when incontinence occurs simultaneous to the measurement of true detrusor pressure. Videourodynamics offers objective radiographic evidence of incontinence with concurrent measurements of true detrusor pressures.

As mentioned in a previous section of this chapter bladder neck funneling is a common radiological finding in women with stress urinary incontinence. Bladder neck funneling, however, occurs normally during a detrusor contraction. Bladder neck funneling will also be demonstrated in the poorly compliant bladder where the high pressure associated with a relatively low volume tends to 'force' open the bladder neck, which will appear as bladder neck funneling on the standard radiograph. Simultaneous cystography and cystometry allows the differentiation of these various aetiologies of bladder neck funneling. Fluoroscopic evidence of an open bladder neck can, therefore, be correlated with the concurrent detrusor pressure. If the bladder neck funnels and the detrusor pressure is low, then primary urethral dysfunction is most likely. If the detrusor pressure rapidly rises and falls, the funneling of the bladder neck is most likely due to a detrusor contraction. If the open bladder neck is seen concomitant to a persistent unabating rise in detrusor pressure, poor bladder compliance should be suspected. To differentiate between a rise in detrusor pressure due to an uninhibited contraction and poor compliance, general anesthesia may be required in order to eliminate the neurological influence on bladder dynamics.

In the male, urinary incontinence is most commonly due to a prostatectomy. Video urodynamics will demonstrate objective evidence of urinary leakage through the posterior urethra with a simultaneous recording of detrusor pressure. If the incontinence is associated with an overactive bladder (a rise in detrusor pressure greater than 15 cm water) the patient may benefit from a trial of anticholinergic medications. If there is no rise in the detrusor pressure during the loss of urine, sphincter dysfunction due to operative damage is the most likely cause of the patient's incontinence.

References

1. Bates P. et al. First Report on the Standardisation of terminology of lower tract function. Br. J. of Urol. 48 (1976): 39.
2. Raz S. Diagnosis of urinary incontinence in the male. Urol. Clin. of N. Amer., 5 (1978): 305.

3. McCallum R.W. and Colapinto B. Urologic radiology of the adult male lower urinary tract. Springfield, Illinois, Charles C. Thomas, 1976.
4. Enhorning G., Miller E.R. and Hinman F. Jr. Urethral closure studied with cineroentgeno-graphy and simultaneous bladder-urethra pressure recording. Surg. Gynec. & Obstet., 118 (1964): 507.
5. Bates C.P. and Corney C.E. Synchronous cine-pressure-flow cystography: A method of routine urodynamic investigation. Br. J. Radiol., 44 (1971): 44.
6. McGuire E.J. Combined radiographic and manometric assessment of urethral sphincter function. J. Urol., 118 (1977): 632.
7. Whiteside G. and Bates P. Synchronous video pressure-flow cystourethrography. Urol. Cl. of N. Amer., 6 (1979): 93.
8. Webster, G.D. and Older R.A. Video urodynamics. Urology, XVI (1980): 106.

I.3. The value of the urethral pressure profile

J.M. van GEELEN

Introduction

The term 'urethral pressure profile' (UPP) denotes a recording of the intra-luminal pressure exerted by the urethral wall on a pressure measuring device as it is withdrawn from the bladder to the external meatus with the bladder at rest. Under normal conditions, during the filling phase of the bladder, the urethral lumen is closed and continence is maintained at the level of the bladder neck [1-5]. The intraluminal pressure within the urethra exceeds the bladder pressure over almost the entire urethral length [6].

Stimulated by the clinical problems encountered in the differential diag-nosis and treatment of urinary incontinence, the interest in studying urethral function by determining the urethral pressure profile has grown. Several techniques to record the urethral pressure profile have been developed du-ring the last two decades:

1. perfusion techniques utilizing constant water flow [7, 8];2.perfusion tech-niques utilizing gas or carbon dioxide [9, 10];3.fluid filled balloon cathet-ers with the pressure transducer located outside the urethra [11-15];4.pressure transducers placed intraluminally [16-18].

Until recently the open catheter perfusion system has been most commonly used for recording the urethral pressure profile [8]. The open catheter per-fusion system measures the resistance presented by the wall of the tubular structure to flow output from one or more openings in the catheter together with the pressure needed to maintain a constant flow within the system. An important disadvantage in routine measurements of the urethral pressure profile with a perfusion catheter is the slow response of the system to increasing pressures [19].

Recent technical advances have improved the recording equipment [20]. Microtransducers embedded in a thin semiflexible catheter are now avail-able which allow accurate and reliable measurements of the intravesical and intraurethral pressure under both static and dynamic conditions. With the aid of a mechanical withdrawal apparatus it is possible to record simulta-neously the intraurethral pressure in relation to the intravesical pressure at

34

every point throughout the urethra from the bladder neck to the external meatus. By subtraction the difference between maximum urethral pressure and total bladder pressure, i.e., urethral closure pressure, can be calculated. The microtransducer technique has proven to be an accurate and sensitive technique. The frequency response of the instrument is around 200 Hz [18]. The measurements are not influenced by inaccuracies inherent in a fluid filled or gas perfused system such as delayed response time, damping due to air bubbles and leakages. In addition, the small diameter of the catheter minimizes urethral distortion. Recording of the urethral pressure profile by the microtransducer technique gives greater consistency of results than by the techniques reported previously [21–24].

Definitions of urethral pressure profile variables

Simultaneous urethrocystometry, including measurement of the urethral pressure profile, provides recording of a number of variables of urethral function. Methods, definitions and units conform to the standards recommended by the International Continence Society (ICS) except where specifically noted [25].
* Functional urethral length (FUL): the length of the urethra along which the intraurethral pressure exceeds the total bladder pressure.
* Anatomic urethral length (AUL) or total profile length: the distance between the point in the urethra where intraurethral pressure exceeds the total bladder pressure and the point where the intraurethral pressure falls to atmospheric pressure.
* Bladder pressure or total bladder pressure (TBP): pressure within the bladder in relation to atmospheric pressure.
* Maximum urethral pressure (MUP): the maximum pressure of the urethral pressure profile recorded in relation to the atmospheric pressure.
* Urethral closure pressure (UCP): the difference between maximum urethral pressure and the simultaneously measured total bladder pressure.
In addition to the above measurements suggested by the ICS, two other features of the urethral pressure profile may be of clinical significance, i.e.:
* Point of maximum urethral pressure (PMP): distance from the internal meatus to the point of maximum urethral pressure.
* Integrated pressure (IP): surface of the area between the urethral pressure curve and the bladder pressure level (continence area).
These definitions are further illustrated in Fig. 1.

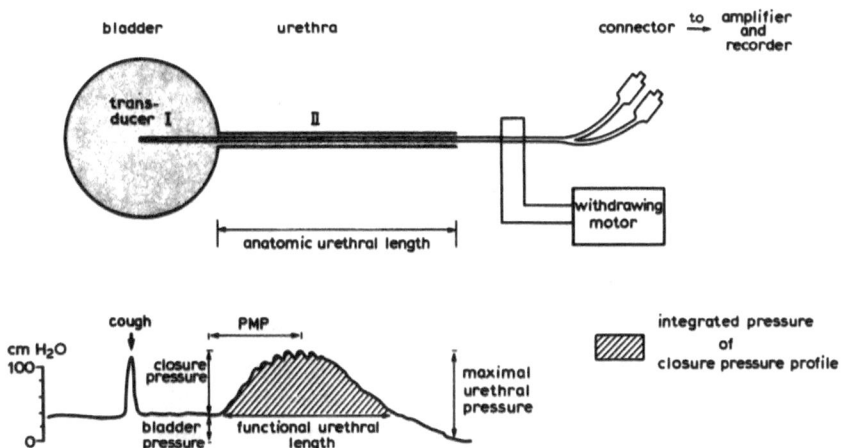

Fig. 1. Schematic representation of the urethral pressure profile showing definitions of the variables measured.

Factors determining the urethral pressure profile at rest

The urethral pressure profile represents a composite of the pressures produced by all of the components that are present in the urethral wall, i.e. the inner urethral wall composed of mucosa and submucosa, the smooth and striated urethral muscle, its binding fibro-elastic tissue and the periurethral striated muscle. The contribution of each component individually to the maintenance of the urethral closure pressure and their roles in the continence mechanism are not clear.

Inner urethral wall

The urethral mucosa and submucosa constitute a compressible and easily deformable layer. The spongy structure of this highly vascularized layer will under external compression ensure complete occlusion of the urethral lumen [26–28].

Mucosa. The epithelial lining in the distal third of the urethra consists of stratified squamous epithelium. More proximally the urethral epithelium gradually changes to pseudo-stratified cylindrical epithelium in the middle third and to transitional epithelium in the bladder neck and in the bladder [29]. Cytologic changes similar to those found in vaginal epithelial cells are observed in the urethral epithelium during the reproductive cycle. These changes result from differing levels of estrogen activity, both during the

menstrual cycle and from menarche to the reproductive years and postme-
nopause [30].

Submucosa. This layer consists of a loose areolar stroma in which a great
number of large thin-walled venous sinuses and arteriovenous anastomoses
can be observed. Berkow [31] and Huisman and Salomè [32] pointed out
that the blood supply and the number of venous sinuses in the urethral wall
is excessive in relation to the metabolic activity of this tissue. The vascular
bed is most prominent at midurethra and is most fully developed in the
reproductive period. Postmenopausally, the number of arteriovenous anastomoses declines whereas the diameter of the venous sinuses widens [29].
Clinical and experimental studies indicate that the urethral vascular bed
contributes considerably (up to 30%) to the total intra-urethral pressure [33–35]. Estrogens cause vasodilation and increased vascularisation in
the urethral vascular bed [37, 37].

The urethral smooth muscle

The anatomic structure of the bladder neck and proximal urethra is composed of several smooth muscle systems which together constitute the effective internal sphincter mechanism. The urethral smooth muscle consists of
an inner longitudinal and an outer circular smooth muscle layer which surround the urethra for almost its entire length. The urethral smooth musculature constitutes a tough and compact tubular structure consisting of relatively small muscle bundles embedded in dense fibro-elastic tissue [29, 38–
41].

The distal urethral sphincter is composed of the urethral smooth muscle
layers and the striated urethral and periurethral muscle. Pharmacological
experiments and clinical studies indicate that the innervation of the bladder
neck and urethral smooth muscle is mediated mainly by alpha adrenergic
receptors. The parasympathetic innervation seems of minor importance for
urethral closure function. The contribution of the smooth muscle component together with its binding fibroelastic elements to the resting urethral
closure pressure varies according to different investigators and ranges from
40 to 80% [14, 34, 42, 43].

The urethral striated muscle

The striated component of the urethra consists of the intrinsic urethral and
the extrinsic periurethral striated muscles. The intramural striated muscle
consists of circularly arranged muscle bundles which surround the urethra

like a horseshoe. These fibers cover the ventral and lateral aspects of the urethral wall and are most condensed in the midurethra. They are separated from the periurethral striated muscles of the pelvic floor by a continuous connective tissue septum [29, 40, 44]. Anatomic and neurohistochemical studies have demonstrated morphological differences and differences in innervation between the urethral striated muscles and the periurethral striated muscles. These observations suggest different functional activity of these separate components. The small diameter slow twitch fibres of the urethral striated muscle are functionally capable of maintaining tone over prolonged time periods without fatigue. The large diameter fast twitch and slow twitch fibres of the periurethral striated muscle of the pelvic floor allow for rapid, forceful muscle contraction and thus seem ideally suited to increase urethral resistance during those events which cause sudden increase in intraabdominal pressure (e.g. coughing, sneezing) and during voluntary interruption of micturition [45, 46].

Information as to the influence of the striated muscle component on intraurethral resistance is not consistent. From pharmacological and clinical studies, both in the experimental animal and in man, it may be derived that the striated component contributes up to 10 to 40 per cent of the urethral closure pressure at rest [7, 14, 34, 43, 47–50].

Factors determining the urethral pressure profile during stress

The proximal two-thirds of the urethra is located within the pelvic cavity above the urogenital diaphragm [29, 51]. Ventrally the urethra is attached to the symphysis pubis by the pubourethral ligaments. Dorsally, the urethra is supported along its course on the anterior vaginal wall by the levator ani muscles. Increased intraabdominal pressure is transmitted from the abdominal cavity to the bladder and urethra and through the urethral wall to the urethral lumen. From the topography of the pelvic organs one would expect the intraabdominal pressure rise to be transmitted equally to the bladder and to the intrapelvic segment of the urethra. However, even in asymptomatic women, transmission of pressure to the bladder and intrapelvic urethra is not equal and the pattern of transmission differs even between normal subjects. Several investigators observed in some women that transmission of intraabdominal pressure during stress resulted in an increase in urethral pressure which exceeded the increase in total bladder pressure, thus resulting in an increased urethral closure pressure. (Positive pressure transmission ratio or positive PTR) [13, 52–54]. In other normal subjects transmission of raised intraabdominal pressure gradually decreased from the bladder neck towards the external meatus thus resulting in a decrease in urethral closure pressure (negative PTR) [13, 52, 55, 56]. The decrease in urethral closure pressure during stress observed in continent women generally was not continuous along the entire urethral length and an increase in urethral closure pressure was often observed in the distal urethral segment [57, 58]. This distal response to stress preceded in time and exceeded in pressure the other pressure changes in the bladder and proximal urethra [13, 52, 53, 59]. Similar changes in urethral response to stress were observed in dogs [60].

These observations indicate that the urethral response to stress does not merely represent passive transmission of raised intraabdominal pressure but also involves, at least in the distal third of the functional urethra, an additional component, presumably active contraction of the urethral and periurethral striated muscles. This active mechanism magnifies the urethral pressure response and thus constitutes a secondary defence mechanism during stress.

Transmission of pressure to the bladder and intrapelvic urethra is governed by the anatomic position of these organs within the pelvic cavity and by the properties of the supporting tissue of the pelvic floor. Dislocation of the urethra, e.g., in prolapse of the anterior vaginal wall, dislocation of the bladder neck during stress and scarring of the urethral and periurethral tissue, may all impair proper transmission of pressure. The differing responses observed in healthy nulliparous women indicate that constitutional weakness of the supporting tissues in the anterior vaginal wall and in the pelvic floor may play a role as well.

Recording of the urethral pressure profile

Methodical and biological variables may affect the urethral pressure profile.

Methodical aspects

a) Degree of bladder filling: urethral length generally decreases and urethral closure pressure increases at increasing bladder volume [61–63]. The increase in urethral resistance during bladder filling is most probably mediated by both the sympathetically innervated urethral smooth muscle and by the striated urethral muscle [64].

b) Position of the patient: all urethral pressure profile variables increase when the subject changes from the supine to sitting or to standing position [65–67]. These postural changes must be explained by the increased pressure in the lower part of the abdomen exerted by the abdominal viscera and by the increased activity of the striated muscles of the pelvic floor which lengthen the urethra and compress the distal urethral segment. These changes are most obvious in the sitting position showing an increase in urethral closure pressure in the distal third of the functional urethra i.e. at the level where the striated muscles of the pelvic floor exert their effect.

c) Orientation of the recording catheter: the pattern of the urethral pressure profile is influenced by axial position of the recording catheter [67–72]. Urethral pressure profile recordings with the membrane of the transducer directed ventrally show shorter urethral length measurements and higher urethral pressures than recordings obtained with the transducer oriented laterally or dorsally. These effects of axial rotation are similar for the measurements in the supine and sitting positions and thus indicate an asymmetrical distribution of urethral closure forces in healthy women.

d) Catheter size: urethral pressure measurements increase with increasing catheter size. Generally, catheter sizes from 6 to 12 Charrière will not cause significant differences in urethral pressure profile measurements [21, 73].

e) Perfusion techniques: the rate of catheter withdrawal and the infusion flow rate influence the results of the urethral pressure profile recordings. Withdrawal rates of less than 20 cm/min and infusion flow rates above 1 ml/min in a fluid filled system, give rise to reproducible recordings [19, 21, 73].

Biological aspects

a) Age of the subject: the urethral pressure profile variables decrease with increasing age [13, 74]. As a rule of thumb, for continent women the value of the urethral closure pressure at rest can be calculated by the formula [73]:

amplitude in cm $H^2O = 100 - age$

b) Parity: vaginal delivery results in reduced urethral length and decreased urethral pressure variables. The postpartum changes are not substantially influenced by the duration of the second stage of labour nor by the presence or absence of an episiotomy nor are they correlated with the birthweight of the infant [75].

c) Hormonal status: Estrogens give rise to an increase in urethral length variables and to an increase in the amplitude of the vascular pulsations in the urethral wall. Urethral pressures at rest are not systematically correlated with changes in estrogen and progesterone levels within the range observed during the menstrual cycle [37]. Estrogens administered orally or intravaginally do not significantly change urethral pressure variables. The beneficial effect of estrogen therapy in cases of urinary stress incontinence can be explained by the stimulating effect of estrogens on the urethral mucosa and on the urethral vascular bed and by improved transmission of pressure over the urethra [76, 77]. Progestagens do not effect the urethral pressure profile [37, 77].

d) Uterovaginal prolapse: There is no evidence that prolapse of the anterior vaginal wall markedly influences the urethral pressure profile at rest. Severe uterovaginal prolapse may be associated with an increased urethral closure pressure [78]. Transmission of increased intra-abdominal pressure to bladder and proximal urethra most probably is determined by the mobility of the urethrovesical junction.

e) Degree of relaxation: the high degree of variability observed in successive urethral pressure profile measurements is probably due to activity of the striated musculature in the urethral wall and in the pelvic floor [79].

f) Use of drugs: the lower urinary tract is under control of both divisions of the autonomic nervous system. Drugs acting on the autonomic nervous system considerably influence the urethral pressure profile [14, 80].

It may be concluded that for proper comparison of the results of different urethral pressure profile studies complete and precise description of the recording equipment and methodology employed and of the study population is mandatory. Even when performed under strictly standardized conditions, normal values of urethral pressure profile variables vary over a wide range. The variability of the urethral pressure profile recordings as expressed by the coefficient of variation (CV) is in the same range for both the measurements within the same study session (short term reproducibility) and for those at one week intervals (long term reproducibility). Except for the PMP, the reproducibility is about the same for the recordings in the supine and sitting positions (Table 1) [67].

Table 1. Short term reproducibility and long term reproducibility of urethral pressure profile variables in healthy women. Mean standard deviations (SD) and coefficients of variation (CV) are given.

UPP-variable	SHORT TERM REPRODUCIBILITY					
	Supine			Sitting		
	Mean	SD	CV%	Mean	SD	CV%
FUL (mm)	33.5	1.9	5.7	40.3	2.1	5.1
AUL	41.2	1.5	3.6	4.7	2.1	4.4
PMP	16.7	1.6	9.6	21.2	3.3	15.4
UCP (cm H_2O)	82	6.5	7.9	104	8.4	8.2
MUP	96	6.7	6.9	135	8.3	6.2
IP/10 (continence area)	72	6.0	8.3	22	8.6	7.1

	LONG TERM REPRODUCIBILITY					
	Supine			Sitting		
UPP-variable	Mean	SD	CV%	Mean	SD	CV%
FUL (mm)	31.1	1.8	5.5	35.7	2.0	5.0
AUL	37.7	1.7	4.0	43.1	1.7	3.5
PMP	16.3	1.5	7.7	18.4	3.3	11.6
UCP (cm H_2O)	76	8.2	9.7	88	12.6	10.9
MUP	91	8.5	7.8	119	12.2	8.3
IP/10	68	10.2	13.5	89	14.6	14.7
(continence area)						

Clinical value of the urethral pressure profile

The urethral pressure profile in continent women

The clinical value of urethral pressure profile in diagnosing lower urinary tract disorders has been and still is the subject of many studies. Enhörning [13] first performed in a systematic way simultaneous measurements of intravesical and intraurethral pressures at rest and under dynamic conditions in normal women, in women suffering from stress incontinence and in puerperas. Since then, subsequent studies, utilizing different recording techniques, have assessed the diagnostic value of urethral pressure profile measurements for differentiation between different forms of urinary incontinence and to study the pathofysiology of lower urinary tract disorders [54–58, 69, 81–86]. All have confirmed or modified the results obtained by Enhörning [13]. In general, the results of these studies may be summarized as follows:

Under normal conditions the intraurethral pressure exceeds total bladder pressure from the bladder neck to almost as far as the external meatus. Maximum urethral pressures at rest are generally measured 1 to 1.5 cm from the urethrovesical junction, proximal to the site where the urethra perforates the urogenital diaphragm [51]. The closure function of the proximal urethra at rest is not governed by the intrapelvic position of the urethra at rest [4].

The urethral vascular bed probably plays an important auxiliary role in urethral closure mechanism. Vascular pulsations are generally observed in the urethral wall in nulliparous women. Usually the amplitude of these pulsations decreases after a vaginal delivery [75].

Passive continence is maintained at the level of the bladder neck. The bladder neck is competent, cough proof and strain proof and maintains continence without the assistance of the sphincter mechanism distal to it [5, 50]. The closure function of the bladder neck is determined by the tonus of the smooth muscle systems surrounding the bladder neck together with the inherent tension produced by the fibro-elastic tissue surrounding the smooth muscle bundles. The spongy structure of the inner urethral wall constitutes under external compression a watertight seal of the urethral lumen. During stress, the mode of transmission of increase intraabdominal pressure to bladder and urethra and the contractility of the striated urethral and periurethral muscles modify the pattern of the resting urethral pressure profile.

The clinical value of urethral pressure profile in urinary intontinence

There are 2 components in the mechanisms of continence and incontinence, i.e., the detrusor muscle and the urethra.

In clinical practice, the main point in the investigation of urinary incontinence is the differentiation of detrusor overactivity from incompetence of urethral closure mechanisms.

The results of the studies cited above almost all indicate that, when groups of women are compared, mean values of urethral pressure variables in stress incontinent women are significantly lower than those observed in continent women of the same age [13, 54–58, 63, 69, 73, 81–86]. Urethral length measurements, especially the functional urethral length (FUL) and the distance from the internal meatus to the point of maximum urethral pressure (PMP) are generally shorter in women suffering from stress incontinence than in continent women. A significant shortening of urethral length as the dominant sign in stress incontinence, cannot be ascertained by most clinical studies [81–89]. The decrease in urethral resistance generally correlates well with the degree of severity of incontinence [58, 90].

Because of the great variability of the values of the urethral pressure profile at rest, there is much overlap in the different measurements of the resting urethral pressure profile variables between continent and incontinent women. For this reason, the urethral pressure profile at rest alone can not serve to establish whether or not stress incontinence exists.

The most constant finding in women with stress incontinence, is a deficient transmission of increased intra-abdominal pressure to the urethra resulting in a sustained decrease in urethral closure pressure during stress. The mean decrease in urethral closure pressure along the urethra during stress is significantly greater in stress incontinent women than in continent women and the time necessary for recovery to normal resting values is also delayed [13, 57, 58, 69]. The decrease in urethral closure pressure during stress is most obvious when the patient is in upright position with full bladder.

In addition, the response in the distal third of the functional urethra, often observed in continent women during dynamic testing and positional changes, is usually absent in women with stress incontinence [57, 58, 66, 90].

Successful surgical correction of stress incontinence, irrespective of the surgical procedure applied, does not induce any significant changes in resting urethral pressure profile variables. Successful treatment of the condition is achieved by improvement of pressure transmission to the intrapelvic part of the urethra [91–95].

In conclusion, low urethral closure pressure and short functional urethral length in relation to the age of the subject certainly reflect decreased urethral resistance. Recording of the urethral pressure profile during stress will further reveal urethral incompetency as well as the degree of such incompetency. Defective transmission of raised intraabdominal pressure to the intrapelvic urethra is the primary factor in the pathogenesis of stress incontinence.

Recently the term 'urethral instability' has been introduced to describe the existence of prominent variations in urethral pressure of 20 cm H^2O or more in the absence of detrusor activity. The true nature of the unstable urethral pressure variations is unknown but the condition should be taken into consideration when evaluating patients with urinary incontinence without a specific diagnosis [96–98].

In detrusor overactivity, uninhibited detrusor contractions considerably influence the urethral pressure profile recordings and a reproducible pattern cannot be observed. In the absence of detrusor contractions, values of the resting urethral pressure profile variables as well as the response to stress are usually within normal limits. There is no correlation between values of urethral pressure profile variables at rest and the intensity of symptoms of frequency, urgency or urge incontinence. During a recording session uninhibited detrusor contractions may occur spontaneously or after provocation. The increase in intravesical pressure following uninhibited detrusor activity and the concomitant deterioration of the urethral pressure profile can be directly observed on the recording paper.

Conclusion

Recording of the urethral pressure profile under static and dynamic conditions has proven to be an invaluable tool for the assessment of urethral sphincter function and in the differentiation between different forms of urinary incontinence. The information it provides, however, is directly proportional to the care with which the test is performed [99].

44

References

1. Ardran G.M., Simmons C.A. and Stewart J.H. The closure of the female urethra. J. Obst. and Gynaec. Brit. Emp. 63 (1956): 26.
2. Caine M. and Edwards D. Peripheral control of micturition; a cineradiographic study. Brit. J. Urol., 30 (1958): 34.
3. Low, J.A. Role of the normal female urethra in the sphincter mechanism of the bladder. Am. J. Obstet. Gynecol. 82 (1961): 1.
4. Jeffcoate T.N.A. The principles governing the treatment of stress incontinence of urine in the female. Brit. J. Urol. 37 (1965): 633.
5. Turner-Warwick R. The treatment of female urinary incontinence. Proc. VI Annual Meeting I.C.S. Antwerp (1976).
6. Enhörning G., Miller E.R. and Hinman F. Urethral closure studied with cineroentgenography and simultaneous bladder-urethra pressure recording. Surg. Gynecol. & Obstet. 118 (1964): 507.
7. Lapides J., Ajemian E.P., Breakey B.A. and Lichtwardt J.R. Further observations on the kinetics of the urethrovesical sphincter. J. Urol. 84 (1960): 86.
8. Brown M. and Wickham J.E.A. The urethral pressure profile. Brit. J. Urol. 41 (1969): 211.
9. Robertson J.R. Gas cystometrogram with urethral pressure profile. Obst. Gynec. 44 (1974): 72.
10. Raz S. and Kaufman J.J. Carbondioxide urethral pressure profile. J. Urol. 115 (1976): 439.
11. Simons I. Studies in bladder function. The sphincterometer. J. Urol. 35 (1936): 96.
12. Hodgkinson C.P. Direct urethrocystometry. Am. J. Obstet. Gynecol. 79 (1960): 664.
13. Enhörning, G. Simultaneous recording of intravesical and intraurethral pressure. Acta Chir. Scand. Suppl. 276 (1961).
14. Donker P.J., Ivanovici F. and Noach E.L. Analysis of the urethral pressure profile by means of electromyography and the administration of drugs. Brit. J. Urol. 44 (1972): 180.
15. Tanagho E.A. and Jonas U. Membrane catheter: effective for recording pressures in the lower urinary tract. Urology 10 (1977): 173.
16. Karlsson S. Experimental studies of the functioning of the female urinary bladder and urethra. Acta Obstet. Gynec. Scand. 32 (1953): 285.
17. Shelley T. and Warrell D.W. Measurement of intravesical and intraurethral pressure in normal women suffering from incontinence of urine. J. Obstet. Gynecol. Br. Commonw. 72 (1965): 926.
18. Asmussen M. and Ulmsten U. Simultaneous urethrocystometry and urethra pressure profile measurements with a new technique. Acta Obstet. Gynec. Scand. 54 (1975): 1.
19. Abrams P.H., Martin S. and Griffith D.J. The measurement and interpretation of urethral pressures obtained by the method of Brown and Wickham. Brit. J. Urol. 50 (1978): 33.
20. Millar H.D. and Baker L.E. Stable ultraminiature catheter tip pressure transducer. Med. Biol. Eng. 11 (1973): 86.
21. Asmussen M. Urethrocystometry in women. Thesis, Lund, Studentlitteratuur (1975).
22. Furrer M. and Eberhard J. Vergleichende Untersuchungen zwischen der Zystourethromanometrie nach Heidenreich und der Mikrotransducer methode nach Ulmsten. Gynäk. Rdsch. 17 Suppl. 1 (1977): 105.
23. Erlandson B.E. and Fall M. Urethral pressure profile studied by two different microtip transducers and an open catheter system. Urol. Int. 33 (1978): 79.
24. Teague C.T. and Merrill D.C. Laboratory comparison of urethral Profilometry techniques. Urology 13 (1979): 221.
25. Bates P., Bradley W.E. and Hald, T. et al. First and second reports on the standardization of terminology of lower urinary tract function. Urology 9 (1977): 237.

26. Zinner N.R., Ritter R.C. and Sterling A.M. The mechanism of micturition. From: 'Scientific foundations of urology', Vol. II: 39. Eds.: D.I. Williams and G.D. Chisholm. William Heinemann. Medical books, Ltd. London (1976).

27. von Hayek H. Die Weibliche Harnröhre. Handbuch der Urologie II. Anatomie und Embryologie I, 315 (1969).

28. Zinner N.R., Sterling A.M. and Ritter R.C. Role of inner urethral softness in urinary continence. Urology 16 (1980): 115.

29. Huisman A.B. Morfologie van de vrouwelijke urethra. Thesis, Groningen, The Netherlands (1979).

30. Smith P.Ch.M. Age changes in the female urethra. Brit. J. Urol. 44 (1972): 667.

31. Berkow S.G. The corpus spongeosum of the urethra: its possible role in urinary control and stress incontinence in women. Am. J. Obstet. Gynecol. 65 (1953): 346.

32. Huisman A.B. and Salomé A.J. Morphology of the female urethra in relation to age. Proc. VII Annual Meeting I.C.S. Portoroz. P. 123 (1977).

33. Raz S., Caine M. and Zeigler M. The vascular component in the production of intraurethral pressure. J. Urol. 108 (1972): 93.

34. Rud T., Andersson K.E., Asmussen M., Hunting A. and Ulmsten U. Factors maintaining the intraurethral pressure in women. Invest. Urol. 17 (1980): 343.

35. Tulloch A.G.S. The vascular contribution to intra-urethral pressure. Brit. J. Urol. 46 (1974): 659.

36. Molnar G. and Nagy T. Die Bedeutung der Gefässverhältnisse der Weiblichen Harnröhre für die Funktion des Verschluss-systems der Harnblase. Z.f. Urol. 58 (1965): 825.

37. Van Geelen J.M., Doesburg W.H., Thomas C.M.G. and Martin Jr. C.B. Urodynamic studies in the normal menstrual cycle: The relationship between hormonal changes during the menstrual cycle and the urethral pressure profile. Am. J. Obstet. Gynecol., 141 (1981): 384.

38. Woodburne R.T. The sphincter mechanism of the urinary bladder and the urethra. Anat. Rec. 141 (1961): 11.

39. Bro-Rasmussen F., Halborg Sørensen H., Bredahl E. and Kelstrup A. The structure and function of the urinary bladder. Urol. Int. 19 (1965): 280.

40. Donker P.J., Dröes J.Th.P.M. and van Ulden B.M. Anatomy of the musculature and innervation of the bladder and the urethra. In: Williams D.I. and Chisholm G.D. (eds.) Scientific Foundations of Urology, Vol. II: 21. William Heinemann Medical Books, Ltd., London (1976).

41. Hutch J.A. Anatomy and physiology of the bladder, trigone and urethra. Butterworths Appleton Century Crofts, London (1972).

42. Tanagho E.A., Meyers F.H. adn Smith D.R. Urethral resistance: its components and implications. I. Smooth muscle components. Invest. Urol. 7 (1969): 136.

43. Awad S.A. and Downie J.W. Relative contributions of smooth and striated muscles to the canine urethral pressure profile. Brit. J. Urol. 48 (1976): 347.

44. Gosling J.A. and Dixon J.S. Light and electron microscopic observations on the human external urethral sphincter. J. Anat. 129 (1979): 216.

45. von Hayek H. Das Faser kaliber in den mm. transversus perinei und sphincter urethrae. Z. Anat. Entwickl. Gesch. 121 (1969): 455.

46. Gosling J.A., Dixon J.S., Critchley H.O.D. and Thompson S.A. A comparative study of the human external sphincter and periurethral levator ani muscles. Brit. J. Urol. 53 (1981): 35.

47. Cass A.S. and Hinman F.J. Constant urethral flow in the female dog. J. Urol. 90 (1968): 442.

48. Tanagho E.A., Meyers F.H. and Smith D.R. Urethral resistance: its components and implications. II. Striated muscle component. Invest. Urol. 7 (1969): 195.

49. Koff S.A. Striated muscle determinants of intra-urethral resistance. Invest. Urol. 15 (1977):

147.

50. McGuire E.J. and Wagner F.C. The effects of sacral denervation on bladder and urethral function. Surg., Gynec. Obst. 144 (1977): 343.

51. Westby M. and Asmussen M. The site of maximum urethral pressure and the location of the urogenital diaphragm in the female urethra as studied by simultaneous urethrocystometry and voiding urethrocystography. Proc. XI Annual Meeting I.C.S. Lund, p. 79 (1981).

52. Rud T. The striated pelvic floor muscles and their importance in maintaining urinary continence. Proc. 1st Joint. Meeting, X Annual Meeting I.C.S. – Urodynamics Society, Los Angeles, p. 79 (1980).

53. Constantinou C.E. and Govan D.E. Urodynamic analysis of urethral, vesical and perivesical pressure distribution in healthy female. Urol. Int. 35 (1980): 63.

54. Faysal M.H., Constantinou C.E., Rother L.F. and Govan D.E. The impact of bladder neck suspension on the resting and stress urethral pressure profile: a prospective study comparing controls with incontinent patients preoperatively and postoperatively. J. Urol. 125 (1981): 55.

55. Toews H.A. Intraurethral and intravesical pressures in normal and stressincontinent women. Obstet. Gynecol. 29 (1981): 613.

56. Bunne G. and Öbrink A. Urethral closure pressure with stress – A comparison between stress-incontinent and continent women. Urol. Research. 6 (1978): 127–134.

57. Heidler H., Wölk H. and Jonas U. Urethral closure mechanism under stress conditions. Eur. Urol. 5 (1979): 110.

58. Hilton P. and Stanton S.L. Urethral pressure measurement by microtransducer: the results in symptom-free women and in those with genuine stress incontinence. Brit. J. Obst. Gynec. 90 (1983): 919.

59. Van der Kooi J.B., van Wanroy P.J.S., de Jonge M.C., Kornelis J.A. and van den Berg J. Microtip-manometer measurement of the time separation of cough pulses from the bladder and urethra in women. Proc. XII Annual Meeting I.C.S. Leiden, P. 9 (1982).

60. Thüroff T.W., Bazeed M.A., Schmidt R.A. and Tanagho E.A. Mechanisms of urinary continence: an animal model to study urethral responses to stress conditions. J. Urol. 127 (1982): 1202.

61. Tanagho E.A., Miller E.R., Meyers F.H. and Corbett R.K. Observations on the dynamics of the bladder neck. Brit. J. Urol. 38 (1966): 72.

62. Griffith D.J. The mechanics of the urethra and of micturition. Brit. J. Urol. 45 (1973): 497.

63. Öbrink A., Bunne G. and Ulmsten U. Intraurethral and intravesical pressures in continent women. Acta Obstet. Gynec. Scand. 56 (1977): 525.

64. Kiruluta H.G., Downie J.W. and Awad S.A. The continence mechanisms: the effect of bladder filling on the urethra. J. Urol. 18 (1981): 460.

65. Henriksson L., Ulmsten U. and Andersson K.E. The effect of changes of posture on the urethral closure pressure in healthy women. Scand. J. Urol. Nephrol. 11 (1977): 201.

66. Witherow R.O. and Tiptaft R.C. The sitting and standing urethral pressure profile – a simple test for stress incontinence. Proc. VIII Annual Meeting I.C.S., Manchester (1978), p. 187.

67. Van Geelen J.M. The urethral pressure profile in continent women. Thesis Nijmegen. Publ.: Schriks Drukkerij B.V., Asten, The Netherlands (1983).

68. Ghoneim M.A., Rottembourg J.L., Fretin J. and Susset J.G. Urethral pressure profile. Standardization of Technique and Study of Reproducibility. Urology. V (1975): 632.

69. Bänninger U., Kunz J. and Reich P. Das Urethradruckprofil bei kontinenten und stressinkontinenten Frauen. Geburtsh. u. Frauenheilk. 40 (1980): 973.

70. Hilton P. and Stanton S.L. Urethral pressure measurements by microtransducer: II. An analysis of rotational variations. Proc. XI Annual Meeting I.C.S., Lund, p. 70 (1981).

71. Ward H.H. and Hosker G.L. Anisotropic urethral occlusive forces. Proc. XII Annual Meeting I.C.S. Leiden (1982), p. 163.

72. Martinez F.C. and Constantinou C.E. Axial asymmetry of the resting urethral pressure profile in the continent female. Proc. XII Annual Meeting I.C.S. Leiden (1982), p. 55.

73. Edwards L. and Malvern J. The urethral pressure profile: theoretical considerations and clinical application. Brit. J. Urol. 46 (1974): 325.

74. Rud T. Urethral pressure profile in continent women from childhood to old age. Acta Obstet. Gynecol. Scand. 59 (1980): 331.

75. Van Geelen J.M., Lemmens W.A.J.G., Eskes T.K.A.B. and Martin Jr. C.B. The urethral pressure profile in pregnancy and after delivery in healthy nulliparous women. Am. J. Obstet. Gynecol. 144 (1982): 636.

76. Hilton P. and Stanton S.L. The use of intravaginal oestrogen cream in genuine stress incontinence. Brit. J. Obst. Gynec. 90 (1983): 940.

77. Rud T. The effects of estrogens and gestagens on the urethral pressure profile in urinary continent and stress incontinent women. Acta Obstet. Gynecol. Scand. 59 (1980): 265.

78. Richardson D.A., Bent A.E. and Ostergard D.R. The effect of uterovaginal prolaps on urethrovesical pressure dynamics. Am. J. Obstet. Gynecol. 146 (1983): 901.

79. Plante P. and Susset J. Studies of female urethral pressure profile. Part I. The normal urethral pressure profile. J. Urol. 123 (1980): 64.

80. Mattiasson A. On the peripheral nervous control of the lower urinary tract. Thesis, Lund (1984).

81. Beck R.P. and Maughan G.B. Simultaneous intraurethral and intravesical pressure studies in normal women and those with stress incontinence. Am. J. Obst. Gynecol. 89 (1964): 746.

82. Low J.A. and Kao M.S. Patterns of urethral resistance in deficient urethral sphincter function. Obstet. Gynecol. 40 (1972): 634.

83. Awad S.A., Bryniak S.R., Lowe P.J., Bruce A.W. and Twiddy D.A.S. Urethral pressure profile in female stress incontinence. J. Urol. 120 (1978): 475.

84. Henriksson L., Andersson K.E. and Ulmsten U. The urethral pressure profile in continent and stress incontinent women. Scand. J. Urol. Nephrol. 13, 5 (1979).

85. Susset J. and Plante P. Studies of female urethral pressure profile. Part II. Urethral pressure profile in female incontinence. J. Urol. 123 (1980): 70.

86. Eberhard J. and Lienhard P. Die Stressinkontinenz der Frau: Auswertung und Interpretation der Urethradruckprofile. Geburtsh. und Frauenheilh. 39 (1979): 195.

87. Lapides J., Ajemian E.P., Stewart B.H., Lichtwardt J.R. and Breakey B.A. Physiopathology of stressincontinence. Surg. Gynecol. Obstet. 111 (1960): 224.

88. Radej M., Hitrec V., Krivea O., Kovacic M., Parazajder J. and Pavletic M. Functional and tonometric investigation of bladder and urethra in patients with stress incontinence. J. Urol. 115, 551 (1976).

89. Gershon C.R. and Diokno A.C. Urodynamic evaluation of female stress urinary incontinence. J. Urol. 119 (1978): 787.

90. Godec C.J., Esho J. and Cass A.S. Correlation among cystometry, urethral pressure profilometry and pelvic floor electromyography in the evaluation of female patients with voiding dysfunction symptoms. J. Urol. 124 (1980): 678.

91. Öbrink A. and Bunne G. The margin to incontinence after three types of operation for stress incontinence. Scand. J. Urol. Nephrol. 12 (1978): 209.

92. Henriksson L. and Ulmsten U. A urodynamic evaluation of the effects of abdominal urethrocystopexy and vaginal sling urethroplasty in women with stress incontinence. Am. J. Obstet. Gynecol. 113 (1978): 78.

93. Constantinou C.E., Faysal M.H. and Govan D.E. The impact of bladder neck suspension on the mode of distribution of abdominal pressure along the female urethra. Proc. 10th Annual Meeting I.C.S., Los Angeles (1980).

94. Hilton P. and Stanton S.L. A clinical and urodynamic assessment of the Burch colposuspension for genuine stress incontinence. Brit. J. Obstet. Gynecol. 90 (1983): 934.

95. Weil A., Reyes H., Bishoff P., Rottenberg R.D. and Krauer F. Modifications of the urethral rest and stress profiles after different types of surgery for urinary stress incontinence. Brit. J. Obstet. Gynecol. 91 (1984): 46.
96. Ulmsten U., Henriksson L. and Iosif S. The unstable urethra. Am. J. Obstet. Gynecol. 144 (1982): 93.
97. Kulseng Hanssen S. Prevalence and pattern of unstable urethral pressures in one hundred seventy-four gynecologic patients referred for urodynamic investigation. Am. J. Obstet. Gynecol. 146 (1983): 893.
98. McGuire E.J. Reflex urethral instability. Brit. J. Urol. 50 (1978): 200.
99. Harrison N.W. The urethral pressure profile. Urol. Res. 4 (1976): 95.

I.4. The role of telemetry in the evaluation of incontinence

R.L. VEREECKEN & W. SANSEN

At a time when it is possible to send astronauts to the moon and to space-labs, and to follow their physiological signals with apparent ease over thousands of kilometers, it is not surprising that within our small hospitals various telemetric methods try to find their place.

Clinical biotelemetry can be defined as the diagnosis (telecontrol) and/or treatment (e.g. telestimulation) of illness from a distance involving some form of encoding or signal transposition. According to the nature of the carriers used, telemetry can be classified as radiotelemetry, storage (analogue magnetic tape, non volatile solid state memories), optical (mostly infrared, video with invisible camera), ultrasound, wired or cable (telephone), and combinations (e.g. split screen video). Radio and optical telemetry are used to their full potential if on-line data are essential but on-line monitoring carries additional responsibilities for physicians and nursing staff as it implies availability for observation purposes. Telemetry has already been introduced in various medical disciplines: in perinatal continuous care, Holter monitoring in cardiac arrhythmias and pacemaker implants for radioactivity measurements, and pressure monitoring in the gastrointestinal tract. In urology only radiotelemetry and storage techniques have been used until now.

The reasons for introducing field telemetry are dictated by the limitations of the classical laboratory investigation procedures:

a) The examinations take place in strongly standardized laboratory conditions which often imply non-physiological situations, e.g., the cystometry for incontinence is executed in the supine position, since sitting and standing up is difficult because of the numerous cable connections to the equipment; the patient is asked to suppress bladder contractions which normally he does not.

b) Provocative tests are often non-physiological and therefore may not be truly representative or even misleading, e.g. bladder filling at rates of more than 30 ml/min; electrical stimulations for describing urethral sensitivity. The normal causes of uninhibited bladder contractions for a given patient are mostly unknown.

c) The registration of phenomena is limited in time because of the investigation situation and the earning capacity (the shorter the duration, the more examinations a day can be done). However most biological parameters show physiological variations: circadian (day/night) variations, e.g., erections; monthly variations, e.g., different urethral pressures during the menstrual cycle, etc. Besides the normal biorhythms, pathological phenomena are not continuously present. Urinary incontinence is often more prominent in the afternoon than in the morning; it may occur only during walking or during horse riding or only during irregular nocturnal epileptiform attacks; urethral and bladder instability are often episodic phenomena; prolapsus may occur only at night during complete perineal relaxation.

d) The short observation periods may be influenced by fortuitous factors, e.g., intake of diuretics or variable amounts of fluid.

e) The numerous wires transmitting several signals from the patient to the recording equipment restrict his mobility: in this way a differentiation between stress and urge incontinence in conditions of normal life (walking, jumping, morning up and down, kneebends, handstands, running, push-ups), is impossible. Furthermore, the impressive equipment makes the patient anxious and in this way change his reactions.

f) The presence of several people during the examinations puts enormous psychological stress on the patients resulting in cortical inhibition; this is certainly the case in urodynamical examinations where the patient has to void at command and is afraid to lose urine on the examination table.

g) Adequate treatment administered at the precise moment of an abnormal signal (closed loop control mechanism) is impossible (e.g., biofeedback training).

h) Repeated examinations are difficult, e.g. repeated flow pressure measurements at different bladder volumes in the diagnosis of obstruction, monitoring the effects of drugs or training.

This summary of the shortcomings of classical cystometry has already led to the indications which can be summarized as follows: repeated and long term investigations of freely moving patients in their normal physical and psychological life conditions.

However telemetry is not a panacea and has its own drawbacks. In every telemetric system the interface with the subject is the main weak point: movement artefacts at the sensor site are equally transmitted as the physiological signal and only transcutaneous leads or implanted devices can exclude it. Fortunately bladder pressure changes are slower than movements or cable artefacts, which are usually strong, very fast and short events.

For radiotelemetry the extra main technical disadvantages are:
1. High cost of purchase and maintenance
2. Licence required

3. Limited frequency allocations
4. Necessity of frequent battery replacements
5. Interference from other stations and radio frequency interference
6. Signal nulls by directional radiation or standing waves.

If storage telemetry is applied [1], another difficulty is keeping a diary of patients' activities. Furthermore, the frequency response of the available portable storage systems (Oxford and Holter) are low (less than 100 Hz) which induces distortions of the EMG signals and fast pressure changes (coughing).

In every case it is strongly desirable to keep the original signal and as many parameters as possible. Unfortunately the number of available channels in telemetry is often limited.

For three years we have used the Biotel Glonner 3-channel radiotelemetric system for special urodynamical problems [2]. One channel measures the total intravesical pressure by a pressure catheter (Philips or Gaeltec) introduced either by the urethra or by direct suprapubic bladder punction with a Cystofix needle. The second channel gives the rectal pressure. Substraction of both pressures is performed at the receiver unit. The third channel is used either for detecting urine loss by the urilos napkins, or for measuring urethral pressure in urethral instability, or for sphincter EMG with cutaneous ECG or transcutaneous wire electrodes (Siemens, Lifetec), or for monitoring walking by a pressure sensor under the heel. In the case of examination for urethral instability a double balloon catheter used for radiographic detection of urethral diverticles is inserted into the bladder and fixed around the meatus; the small pressure catheter is fixed to this catheter so that the microsensor eye lies at the maximum pressure; in this way minimal dislocation of the catheter occurs. For nocturnal enuresis a separate radiotelemetric EEG system Biotel Schwarzer is supplemented: it provides EEG recording at 4–6 points and 2 EMG channels; the receiver units are connected to a 16 or 8 channel Elema Siemens ink jet recorder. The receiver unit of the Glonner telemetric system is also connected to a Philips recorder running at low speed; by means of a homemade electronic system the recorder starts running at a higher speed as soon as a signal key passes a presettled V/t level; in this way interesting phenomena can be analyzed [3] more easily. Let us discuss some examples.

Fig. 1 gives fragments of the rectal and urethral pressure curves of a 4-year-old child with urinary and faecal incontinence. At 11.00, during walking, simultaneous small increases occur in both pressures when the child was tilting toys. At 14.00 a bladder pressure increase, accompanied by urine loss precedes a rectal pressure increase provoking defecation. At 16.00 a forceful uninhibited bladder contraction provokes marked wetting. By following the curves over 2 days it became clear that uninhibited bladder contractions occur at a nearly fixed rhythm of every two hours; the real func-

52

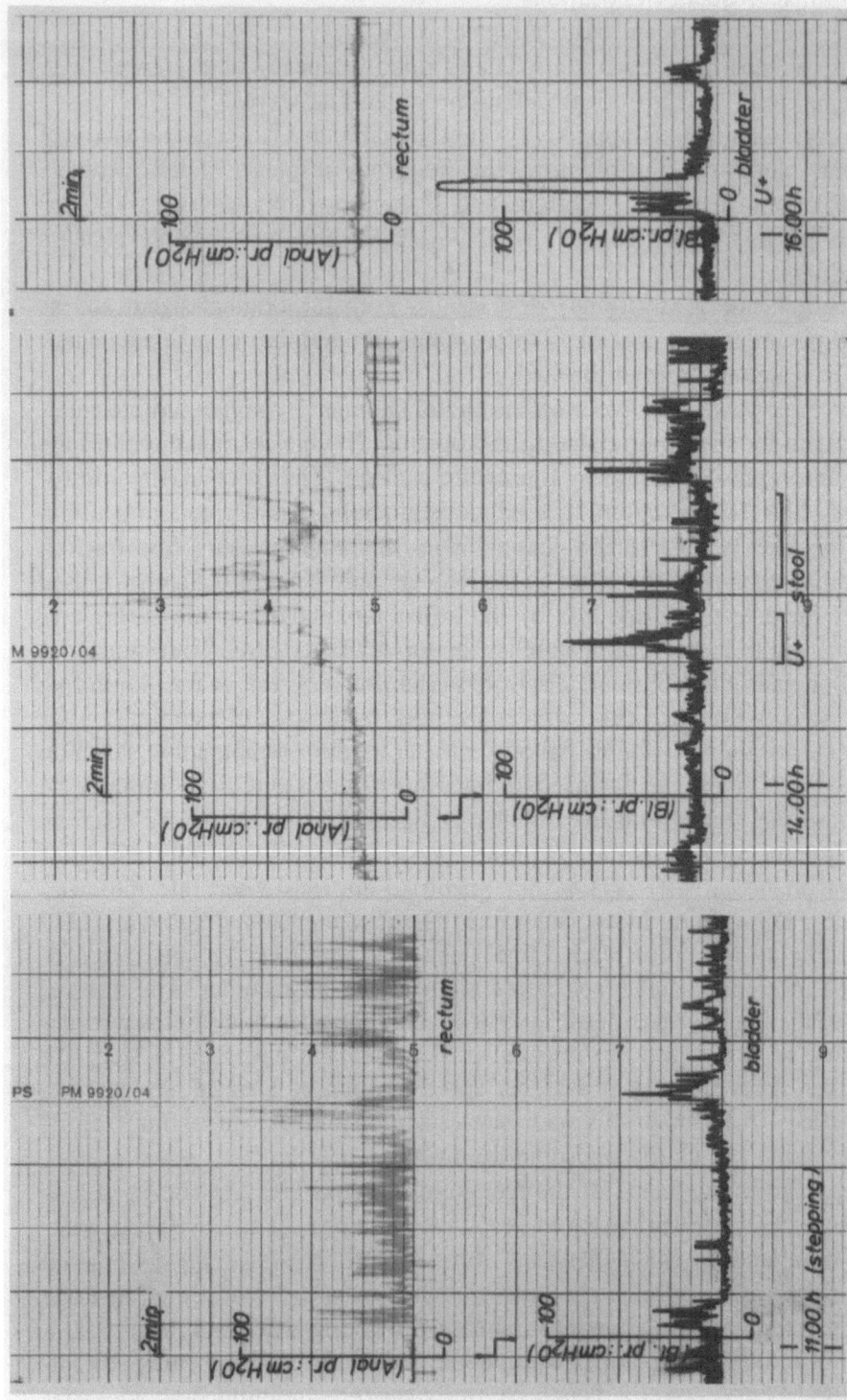

Fig. 1. Telemetry in a child with enuresis nocturna et diurna. Upper curve: rectal pressure (with some artefacts); lower curve: total bladder pressure. Fragments of curves at 11, 14 and 16 o'clock.

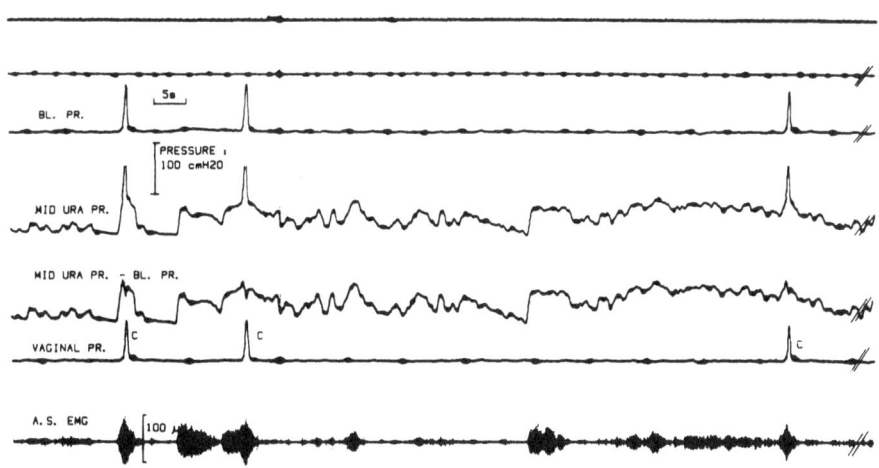

Fig. 2. 43 years old woman with urge incontinence. Total bladder, vaginal and mid-urethral pressure are radiotransmitted by the Glonner telemetric equipment. EMG of anal sphincter is radiotransmitted by the Schwarzer telemetric equipment. All parameters are recorded simultaneously on the Elema 8-channel ink recorder where also mid-urethral and bladder pressure are electronically substracted. In the fragment urethral instability is observed together with sphincter irregularities. C = cough.

tional capacity was 150 ml while during the classical cystometry voiding occurred at 70 ml bladder filling. A training programme was built up with exercises of the perineal muscles, and by putting the child on the toilet before the expected moment of bladder contraction; continence was achieved within two weeks.

In 3 patients who showed only urethral instability at the classical urodynamic examination, we observed not only pronounced urethral pressure variations at telemetric measurements during walking, but also bladder instability (Fig. 2). Thüroff also observed bladder instability without clinical evidence in normal men during sitting [4]. Irritation by the minimal movements of the transurethral catheters may be a cause of this phenomenon.

An example of a possible therapeutical link between bladder pressure and reaction is given in Fig. 3. In a paraplegic man with bladder hyperreflexia the uninhibited bladder contractions can be stopped by applying strong electrical stimulation through anal plug electrodes to the anal mucosa. Such a system can be telemonitored and even implanted as soon as problems of biocompatibility and corrosion of electronic implants are solved [5].

In conclusion, todays medical diagnosis is based on the acquisition of significant data. However, at present we think telemetry is indicated only for:

a) physiological studies, e.g. solving questions such as why some urody-

54

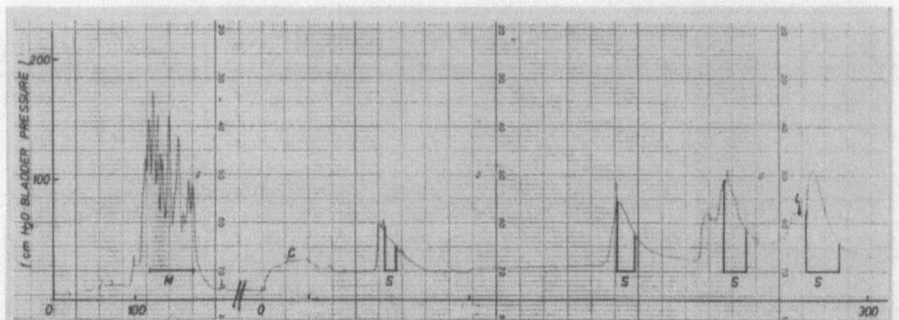

Fig. 3. Intravesical pressure in a patient with D_4 fracture. Without stimulation (left part of the curve) he voids 100 ml by an uninhibited bladder contraction. If the anus is stimulated (10 Hz, 1 msec, 100 V) at the onset of the bladder pressure increase, further bladder contraction is inhibited and no leaking occurs (right fragment of the curve). Bladder capacity afterwards is 300 ml.

namically unstable bladders do not lose urine or do not have complaints (Frewen), and drug trials.

b) a few cases where a clear discrepancy exists between history and clinical findings and the routine urodynamical examinations.

c) a few patients who underwent different therapies without success.

d) enuresis nocturna.

For these reasons I believe the technique will remain restricted to a few university centres and, as many other dramatic realisations, of limited use. On the other hand, the danger is not imaginary that by expansion of telemetry applications the doctor loses personal contact with his patient; in eliminating psychological stresses during laboratory investigations, the benefit of direct contact with the patient is also lost, and this can be worse than an incomplete diagnosis.

References

1. Bhatia N.N., Bradley W.E., Haldeman S. and Johnson B. Continuous monitoring of bladder and urethral pressures: new technique. Urology 18 (1981): 207–210.
2. Vereecken R.L., Puers B. and Das J.: Continuous telemetric monitoring of bladder function. Urol. Res. 11 (1983): 15–18.
3. Puers B., Sansen W. and Vereecken R. Development considerations of a micropower control chip and an ultraminiature hybrid for bladder pressure telemetry. Proc. 8th Internat. Symp. on Biotelemetry, Dubrovnik (1984).
4. Thüroff J.W., Jonas U., Frohenberg D., Petri E. and Hohenfellner R.: Telemetric urodynamic investigations in normal males. Urol. Int. 35 (1980): 427–434.
5. Vereecken R.L., Jacquemyn E. and Das J.: Treatment of overactive detrusor. Proc. 8th Internat. Symp. on Biotelemetry, Dubrovnik (1984).

I.5. New developments in urodynamic investigations

H. MADERSBACHER

Introduction

In 1882 two Italian physiologists, Mosso and Pellacani [1], used for the first time a rather simple type of cystometer to measure bladder pressure. During the following 100 years, but specifically during the last two decades, a variety of urodynamic techniques have been developed. Already in 1964, Scott et al. [2] described a technique allowing simultaneous recording of intravesical pressure, urinary flow rate and electromyography of the pelvic floor muscles, resp. the external urethral sphincter. But it quickly became obvious, that the X-ray-image is highly important. In 1967 Earl Miller [3] together with Frank Hinman, John Hutch, Göran Enhöring and Emil Tanagho developed a technique for simultaneous display of X-ray and physiologic data. Today we agree that this technique, nowadays called videourodynamics, is the ideal technique for a complex evaluation of lower urinary tract function.[1] New developments are focusing on the following points: measurement techniques (1), imaging techniques (2), recording techniques (3), new methods for documentation and storage (4). Furthermore, based on the progress in microelectronics, on the design of instruments (5), on how to perform urodynamic investigations (6) and on the development of new combinations of urodynamic and electrophysiologic testing (7).

Measurement techniques

With regard to measurement techniques the conventional type of external stand mounted pressure transducers is partly replaced by either external patient mounted transducers or catheter-tip transducers. The latter are strain gauges located on the catheter at the site of recording and can be made specially to suit particular applications. Advantages of microtip-transducers are the elimination of zero-error and of fluid-filled connecting lines.

---

[1] Resp. dysfunction.

56

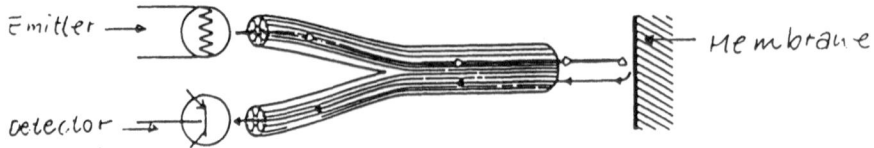

Fig. 1. Schematic drawing showing the principle of pressure recording with the use of fiber optical sensors (Kvarstein et al., 1983), for explanation see text.

The disadvantages are, that they are still expensive and some of them still relatively fragile. In comparative studies between such transducers and the conventional external fluid transducers results showed, that the implexibil-

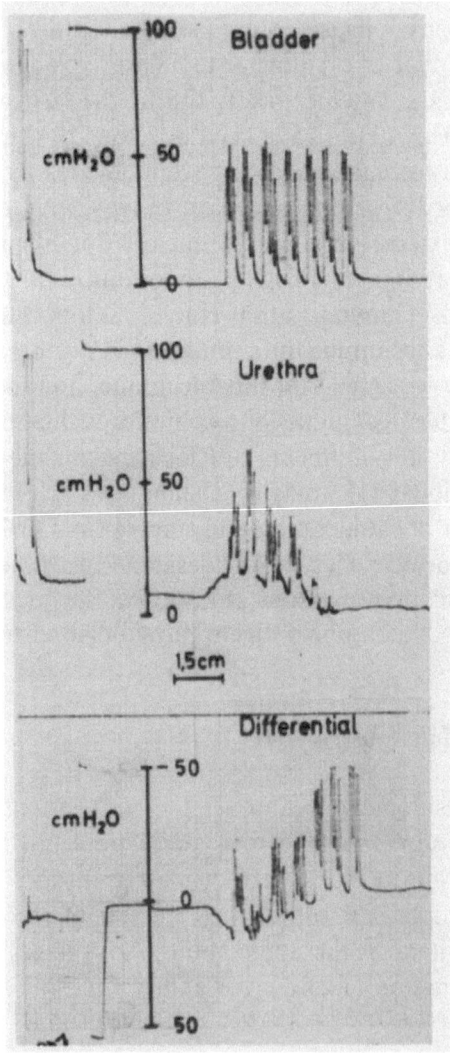

Fig. 2. Urethral-stress-profile with simultaneous recording of intravesical and intraurethral pressure using fiber light optical sensors.

ity of the catheters we are now using is such that the actual position of the sensor within the bladder does not change significantly. But one must expect that more flexible catheters which would be easier to handle could however, give rise to artefacts as position changes of the sensor within the bladder are read as pressure differences [4].

A new way of pressure recording is the use of fiber optical pressure sensors [5]. The principle of the pressure sensor consists of a bifurcated fiber optical bundle in a 7 french catheter with a pressure sensitive diaphragm of 1.6 mm diameter. One leg of this fiber bundle is connected to the light source, the other to a photo detector. The light transmitted from the light-source is coupled back into the fibers of the other leg by way of a reflecting membrane. The signal recorded in the photo-detector is dependent on the distance between the bundle and the reflecting membrane and therefore according to the pressure applied to the membrane (Fig. 1). The light received from the sensor is converted into an electrical signal in the sensor interface and displayed in units of cm. water on the front panel. Advantages of this type of sensor are a robust design and the fact that these sensors ensure a galvanic isolation of the patient from the electrical equipment.[2] Fig. 2 demonstrates a urethral-stress-profile with simultaneous intravesical and intraurethral pressure recording by this technique.

Imaging techniques

So far X-ray-monitoring of the lower urinary tract was the method of choice within video-urodynamics. The problem of radiation dosage, especially in repeated investigations, led to the use of realtime sonography combined with urodynamics, to 'sonographic urodynamics' [6, 7]. For imaging of bladder and urethra a rectal probe is used. Real time sonography is combined with CMG, EMG and UPP being recorded all together on one single monitor and on a videotape. Fig. 3 demonstrates the sonographic appearance of bladder and posterior urethra, Fig. 4 shows a combined urodynamic-sonographic study showing detrusor-external-sphincter-dyssynergia. Recently Nishizawa et al. [8] reported on the application of ultrasound-scanning and computer evaluation for urodynamics with particular emphasis on M-mode scanning. Although transrectal ultrasound provides an excellent view of the bladder and the urethra at rest, probe movement artefacts are a problem, which may create misleading bladder and urethral movement during stress or voiding. A fixed probe clamped to the bed or a chair mounted probe are two possibilities to avoid these artefacts. Recently Rich-

---

[2] Manufactured by AME – Aksjeselskapet Mikro-Elektronik, Knudsrødveien 7, 3191 Horten, Norway.

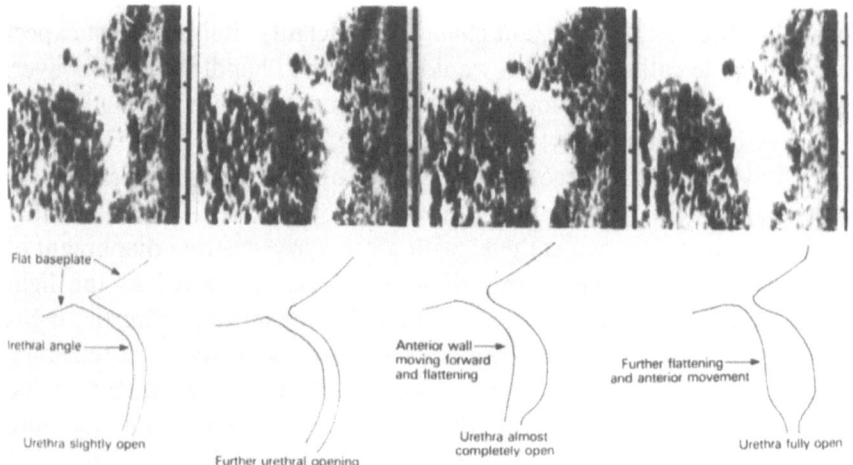

Fig. 3. Sonographic appearance of bladder and posterior urethra at the beginning and during micturition using a rectal probe for real-time sonography (reproduction with the kind permission of Dr. I. Perkash).

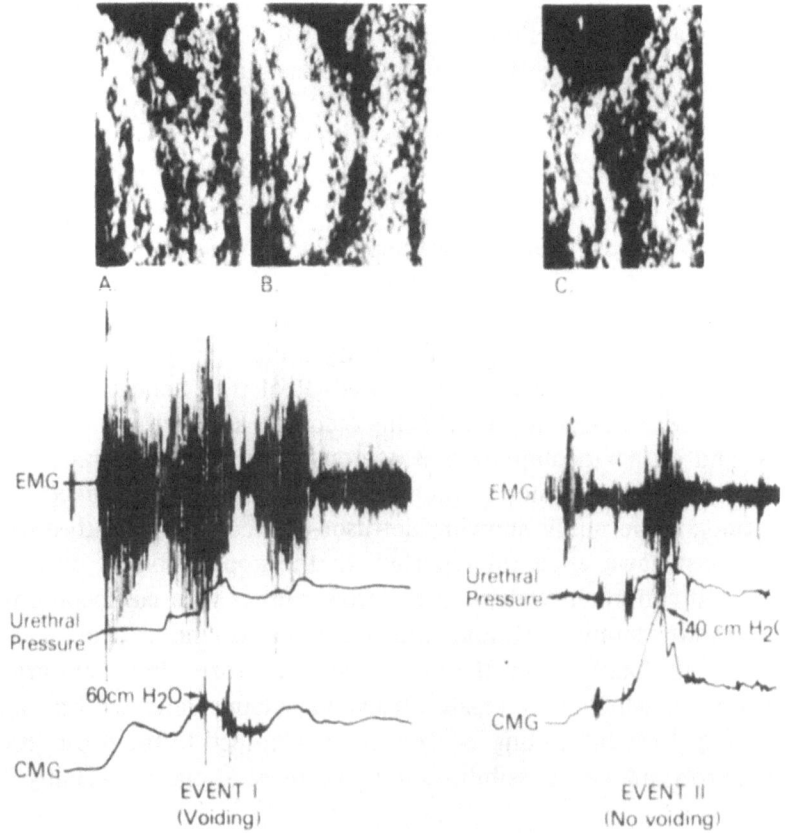

Fig. 4. A combined urodynamic-sonographic study demonstrating detrusor-sphincter ext.-dyssynergia; real time sonography is used for imaging of the bladder neck and the posterior urethra: according to the urodynamic pattern the posterior urethra is closed resp. narrow at the level of the pelvic floor. (Reproduction with kind permission of Dr. I. Perkash.)

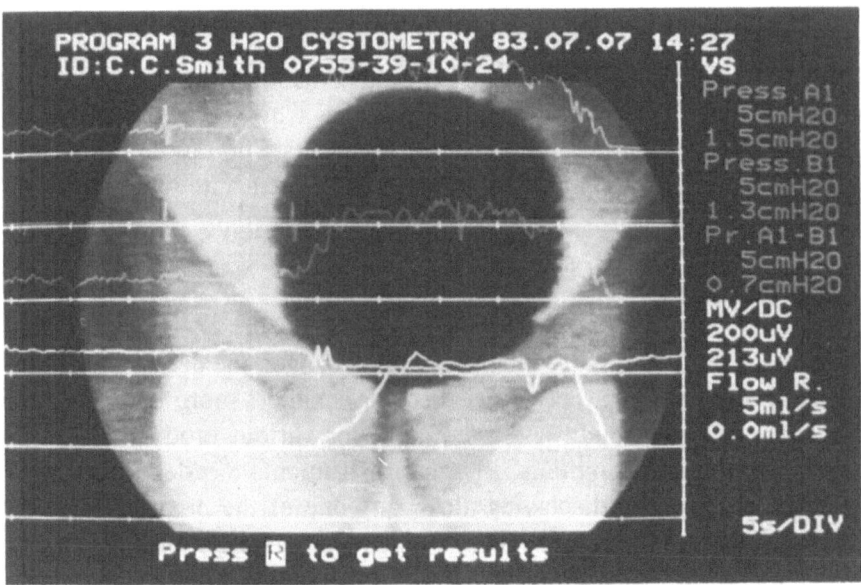

Fig. 5. Videourodynamics with simultaneous recording of intravesical, intrarectal and differential pressure (detrusor pressure), EMG of the pelvic floor and flow with graphical and digital data output superimposed on a video-X-ray image of the bladder.

mond et al. [9] described another method by superimposing pictures at rest and during movements.

Recording techniques

Computer-controlled urodynamic investigations give more data at greater speed than ever before. Fig. 5 shows a six channel of real-time-data superimposed on a high-resolution X-ray-image of the bladder presenting information on pressure, flow, EMG and volume parameters, both graphically and digitally. During the investigation, both, the X-ray picture and the urodynamic parameters can be recorded on a video cassette recorder for later reproduction and evaluation.

Documentation and storage

Computerized systems are now developed for the acquisition, analysis and storage of urodynamic data [10]. Abrams et al. [11] reported on a system by which seven parameters are measured; three pressures, using catheter mounted transducers, the filling and voiding volume, the urinary flow and electromyogramme. The signs from the transducers are passed through suitable interface electronics, using dedicated software[3] to a 16 bit microprocessor with a 10 mByte hard disc. Such a system facilitates the handling of patients files and allows rapid analysis of data from a large number of patients. A similar computer system, which collects data online during the various urodynamic investigations, is used by Kramer and Jonas [12].

Design of instruments

Sophisticated micro-computer-technology has changed the design of routine urodynamic instruments. They have become smaller, more compact and user-friendly and are digitally programmable for various urodynamic parameters in various combinations. In some instruments a video-screen provides realtime graphics, displaying all or any one of the parameters being measured. Special printers provide complete charts including procedure identification, pertinent scale values and summaries of important data (Fig. 6).

Performance of urodynamic investigations

Urodynamic monitoring has so far been done with the patient in supine, sitting or standing position. In 1984 Bradley [13] suggested that information gained from long-term cystometry differs from the results of conventional methods. The use of microtip-transducer catheters together with a telemetric system consisting of a transmitter carried by the patient on a belt and a receiver from which the signals are recorded on a tape-recorder enables us to monitor pressures as the patient is walking around, and also outside the urodynamic unit [14, 15]. The urodynamic parameters can be continuously displayed on an oscilloscope and on a low velocity strip-chart-recorder. Later on selected periods can be printed out at various paper speeds. Long term

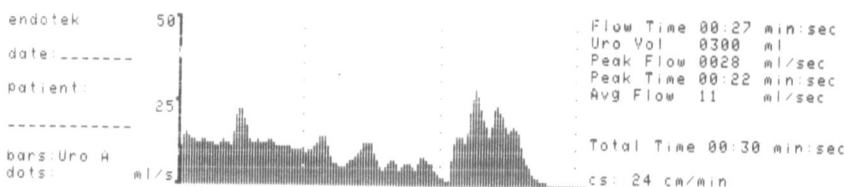

Fig. 6. Micro-computer-technology for routine urodynamic instruments: special printers provide complete charts including procedure identification, pertinent scale values and summaries for important data.

[3] Gaeltech Research, Gaeltec Ltd., Dunvegan, Isle of Skye, U.K.

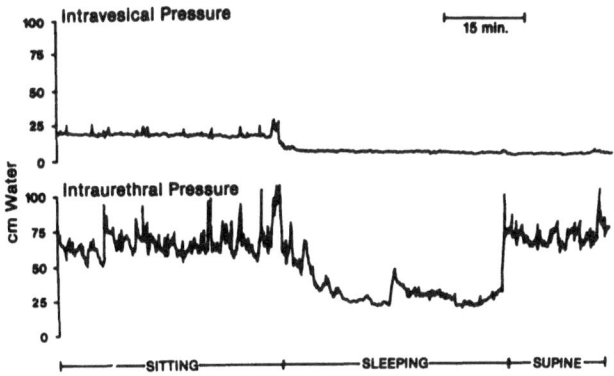

Fig. 7. Long term monitoring of urodynamic parameters gives more information about the micturition and continence phase during almost physiologic conditions: registration of intravesical and intraurethral pressure during sitting, sleeping and in supine position show a marked change of the pressure values according to the different situations.

monitoring of urodynamic parameters seems to be an appealing research tool, giving information about both the micturition- and the continence-phase during almost normal physiological conditions (Fig. 7).

A method for continuous overnight monitoring of bladder and sphincter activity was developed by Nielsen et al. [16], who investigated children with vesicoureteral reflux. The same method was used by Nørgaard et al. [17] for overnight monitoring of children with nocturnal enuresis. For this investigation longterm cystometry was combined with electroencephalographic measurements for determination of sleep stages (Fig. 8). The results so far obtained indicate that the enuretic episode seems to be a normal voiding occuring at a normal volume independent of the sleep stage.

Combined urodynamic and electrophysiologic testing

In 1977 Bradley [18] described the combination of electro-encephalography (EEG) and cystometry, stating that this provides the only method available to analyse central micturition reflex disturbances.

Katona [19] introduced the technique of stimulated urodynamic studies and has used it so far mainly on newborn myelomeningocele patients preoperatively. This study is part of a complete developmental neurological investigation including EMG, evaluation of visual and acoustic somatosensory behaviour with stimulated polygraphy, polymyography and actography of the elementary sensory motor patterns. When no bladder contraction is recorded by urodynamics, intravesical electrical stimulation is performed to activate the bladder. If EEG-recordings then show an arousal reaction simultaneously with the initial phase of bladder contraction this phenome-

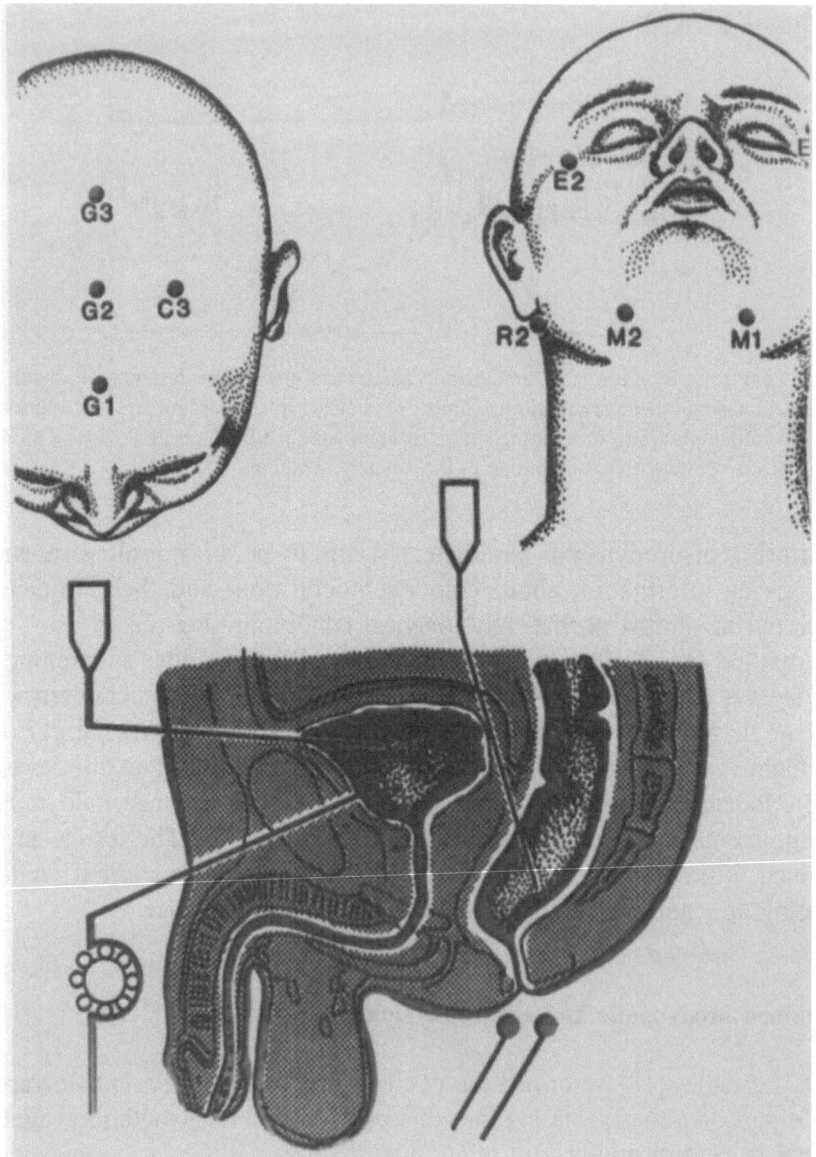

Fig. 8. The monitoring system incorporating measurements of sleep stages by EEG, EOG and submental EMG, bladder and rectal pressure registration together with the pelvic floor activity was used by Nørgaard et al. (1984) to evaluate children with nocturnal enuresis (reproduction with kind permission of Dr. Djurhuus).

non can be regarded as signs of existing vegetative afferentation. If this is present the method of transurethral electrostimulation is able to enforce damaged, but still intact neurons between bladder and cerebral micturition centers.

Haldeman et al. [20] recently described the results on spinal and cortical somatosensory evoked responses from the pudendal nerve in combination with cystometry. These tests record the somatosensory evoked responses over the spinal cord as well as cortical evoked responses on stimulation of the dorsal penile nerve together with measurements of bulbocavernosus reflex and cystometry. The same method can be used to stimulate the pelvic nerves via the posterior urethra using a catheter mounted ring electrode for stimulation.

Conclusions

The new developments described improve measurement techniques, offer alternative methods of imaging avoiding radiation, and improve recording techniques. With the help of computers quick storage of more data and easy access to the permanent files for comparative and statistical reasons will be possible. New developments in the field of microprocessing are changing the design of our urodynamic instruments. Moreover techniques using the combination of urodynamic and electrophysiologic testing will give more information on the neurophysiology and the neuropathophysiology of micturition.

References

1. Mosso M.A. and Pellacani P. Sur les fonctions de la vessie. Arch. Ital. Biol. 1 (1882): 97.
2. Scott F.B., Quesada, E.M. and Cardus D. Studies on the dynamics of micturition: observations on healthy men. J. Urol. 90 (1964): 455.
3. Miller E.R. Techniques for simultaneous display of X-ray and physiologic data. In: Boyarsky S. (ed.) The Neurogenic Bladder. The Williams and Wilkins Company, Baltimore (1967), p. 79.
4. Kramer A. Bladder pressure measurement: external or intravesical transducer position. Urodynamics Society, Proceedings, 6. Annual Symposium, May 5, 1984, New Orleans (USA) (1984).
5. Kvarstein V., Aase O., Hansen T.-E. and Doblong P. A new method with fiberoptic transducers used for simultaneous recording of intravesical and urethral pressure during physiologic filling and voiding phases. J. Urol. 130 (1983): 504.
6. Nishizawa O., Moriya J., Satoh S., Harada T. and Tsuchida S. A new video urodynamics – combined ultrasonotomographic and urodynamic monitoring. Neurourology and Urodynamics 1 (1982): 295-301.
7. Perkash J. and Friedland G.W. Transrectal sonographic urodynamics. Read at the AUA, 79. Annual Meeting, May 6-10, 1984, New Orleans. J. Urol. 131 (1984), No. 4, Part 2, p. 244 A.
8. Nishizawa O., Harada T., Satoh S., Moriya J. and Tsuchida, S. Ultrasound scanning and computer analysis for urodynamics. Proceedings, International Continence Society, 14. Annual Meeting, Innsbruck, Sept. 13-15, 1984, p. 177.

9. Richmond D., Brown, M. and Sutherst J. Measurement of bladder base movement by transrectal ultrasound scanning. Proceedings, International Continence Society, 14. Annual Meeting, Innsbruck, Sept. 13–15, 1984, p. 179.

10. Mastrigt R. van. Computer programs for urodynamics. Neurology and Urodynamics 3 (1984): 141–142.

11. Abrams P., Lewis P., Murray K. and Donald F. A computerised system for the acquisition, analysis and storage of urodynamic data. Proceedings, International Continence Society, 14. Annual Meeting, Innsbruck, Sept. 13–15, 1984, p. 176.

12. Kramer A. and Jonas U. Computer urodynamics – evaluation of practicability of on-line computing in the urodynamics laboratory. Read at the AUA – 79. Annual Meeting, May 6–10, 1984, New Orleans. J. Urol. 131 (1984), No. 4, Part 2, p. 166 A.

13. Bradley W.E. Urodynamics Society – diagnosis and management of bladder hyperreflexia – neurological basis. AUA 79. Annual Meeting, May 6–10, 1984, New Orleans, USA.

14. Vereecken R.L. The role of telemetry in the evaluation of incontinence. International Symposium 'Practical Aspects of Urinary Incontinence', Nijmegen, June 21–23, 1984.

15. Van Waalwijk Van Doorn E.S.C., Valcke A.A.P., IJsenbrandt H.P., Kimmich H.P. and Debruyne F.M.J. A miniature eight channel PCM telemetry system for objectivation of occult unstable bladder and sphincter disorders. Proceedings, International Continence Society, 14. Annual Meeting, Innsbruck, Sept. 13–15, 1984, p. 168. Buch- und Offsetdruck Plattner KG, Innsbruck, Austria.

16. Nielsen J.B., Nørgaard J.P., Schwartz S., Jorgensen T.M. and Djurhuus J.C. Continuous overnight monitoring of bladder activity in vesico-ureteral reflux patients. Neurourology and Urodynamics 3 (1984): 1–22.

17. Nørgaard J.P., Knudsen N., Hansen J.H., Nielsen J.D. and Djurhuus J.S. Overnight monitoring of children with nocturnal enuresis. Proceedings, International Continence Society, 14. Annual Meeting, Innsbruck, Sept. 13–15, 1984, p. 105.

18. Bradley W.E. Electroencephalography and bladder innervation. J. Urol., 118 (1977): 412–414.

19. Katona F., Berenyi M., Szabados P., Balazs M., Tunyogi E. and Vegh J. Early electrourodynamics and early intravesical electrotherapy. Proceedings, International Continence Society, 14. Annual Meeting, Innsbruck, Sept. 13–15, 1984, p. 35. Buch- und Offsetdruck Plattner KG, Innsbruck, Austria.

20. Haldeman S., Bradley W.E. and Bhatia N. Evoked responses from the pudendal nerve. J. Urol. 128 (1982): 974–980.

CHAPTER TWO

Genuine urinary stress incontinence

II.1. The female sphincter mechanisms and their relation to incontinence surgery

R. TURNER-WARWICK

Introduction

The introduction of objective functional studies has led to a fundamental review of the factors involved in the development of female urinary incontinence and a basic re-evaluation of the various operative procedures that have been developed for its resolution.

Basic facts

Simple video-cystography shows, unequivocally, that continence can be maintained either by the mechanism at the bladder neck or by the mid-urethral mechanism – very rarely between these levels. Every female who leaks urine involuntarily must have an incompetent mechanism at bladder neck level because normally, this is occlusive, cough proof and leak proof. Incompetence of the female bladder neck may be the result of intrinsic weakness of its mechanism; however, a normal mechanism opens automatically in association with a detrusor contraction and thus rendered incompetent by unstable detrusor behaviour.

Every female who leaks involuntarily not only has an incompetent bladder neck mechanism but also an incompetent urethral mechanism. Although it is less powerful than that of a male, a normally efficient urethral sphincter can contain intravesical pressure rises resulting from both abdominal straining and from unstable detrusor contractions (provided the maximum contraction pressure is not abnormally high) – the video-pressure 'stop-test' evidence for this is incontrovertible.

Although it is rare in the male, idiopathic weakness of the bladder neck mechanism and of the urethral mechanism is not particularly unusual in the female. Studies of nulliparous women show that 10–15 % have occasional stress leakages: however the incidence of acquired weakness after childbirth is very much higher.

Tanagho (1978) has shown that normal voiding is associated with a reflex-mediated relaxation of the bladder neck and urethral mechanisms which marginally preceed the intravesical pressure rise; there is good evidence that sphincter incompetence occasionally results from involuntary reflex relaxation, 'the unstable urethra' (James, 1979).

The anatomy of the sphincter mechanism

Contrary to some gynaecological concepts, the pelvic floor of the female anterior to the vagina contains no significant muscular element that relates closely to the urethra, either anatomically or functionally; the urological concept of a 'urogenital diaphragm' containing a bulk of muscle surrounding the distal part of the sphincter-active urethra, is as fictitious in the female as it is in the male (Turner-Warwick, 1970; Chilton & Turner-Warwick, 1981).

The bladder neck mechanism, by an extension of cholinergic smooth muscle detrusor fibres, is concentrically arranged around the internal meatus together with striated urethral muscle. The intrinsic urethral sphincter mechanism is somewhat eccentrically positioned anteriorly so that posteriorly the vaginal aspect of it is often relatively thin. Like that of the female it is composed of two layers, the inner smooth muscle and the outer striated muscle; however unlike that of the male it extends throughout the sphincter-active urethra, right up to the internal meatus to form a considerable part of the bulk of the bladder mechanism. The striated muscle element of both the female and the male urethral sphincter is composed of a high proportion of small diameter 'slow-twitch' fibres which, unlike the larger 'fast-twitch' fibres of skeletal muscles, are apparently capable of sustained contractions (Gosling, 1981).

The striated component of the urethral mechanism is under voluntary control and innervated by myelinated nerves; however whether these run with the pudendal nerves as Tanagho believes or with the pelvic nerves (Donker et al., 1976; Gosling, 1981) is currently uncertain. The function of the smooth muscle element of the urethra is very difficult to evaluate separately.

The significance of unstable detrusor behaviour and the maximum detrusor pressure (P. max. det.)

A patient's continence tends to be compromised by an involuntary contraction of the detrusor because this is not only associated with opening of the bladder neck but it raises the intravesical pressure. Consequently it is not surprising that the results of the surgical treatment of incontinence are less satisfactory when this is associated with unstable detrusor behaviour and furthermore, they are even less satisfactory when unstable contractions create abnormally high pressures (Turner-Warwick, 1979). However, in our experience, when conservative treatment of unstable stress incontinence fails (as it often does), patients with low-pressure (less than about 35 cm H_2O) unstable stress incontinence have a fair chance of improvement after a simple repositioning procedure (Turner-Warwick & Whiteside, 1982); this relates to the fact that many females with idiopathic detrusor instability do not leak because the urethral mechanism can contain the intravesical pressure rise – consequently a marginal improvement of the impaired urethral function achieved by repositioning of a prolapsed urethra, may prove sufficient.

The relationship between vaginal prolapse, vesico-urethral descent and sphincter competence

Vesico-urethral descent is best identified video-radiographically; it may or may not result in impaired function of the bladder neck and urethral bladder sphincter. Furthermore, it is important to appreciate that vesico-urethral descent does not necessarily correlate with the clinical assessment of an anterior vaginal wall laxity; a urodynamically significant descent may be associated with a vault prolapse which is difficult to evaluate clinically in the absence of lower vaginal wall laxity. The evidence accruing from the video-cystographic studies of more than 6000 females (Turner Warwick & Whiteside, 1982) confirms that many patients with severe vesico-urethral descent are continent, either at bladder neck or at urethral level, and that many patients who have no significant descent have stress leakage. Conceptually, it seems that:
1. prolapse/descent of a normally functioning bladder neck and/or urethral mechanism does not cause them to become incompetent; in fact the majority of parous women are perfectly continent inspite of an overtly visible anterior vaginal wall laxity;
2. prolapse/descent of an intrinsically weak bladder neck/urethral mechanism is commonly associated with leakage.

The urodynamic effect of operative procedures for incontinence (Fig. 1)

Most operative procedures for incontinence have more than one functional effect.

Intra-abdominal peri-urethral pressure support. When the anterior vaginal wall is directly visible at the introitus, the urethra has usually escaped from

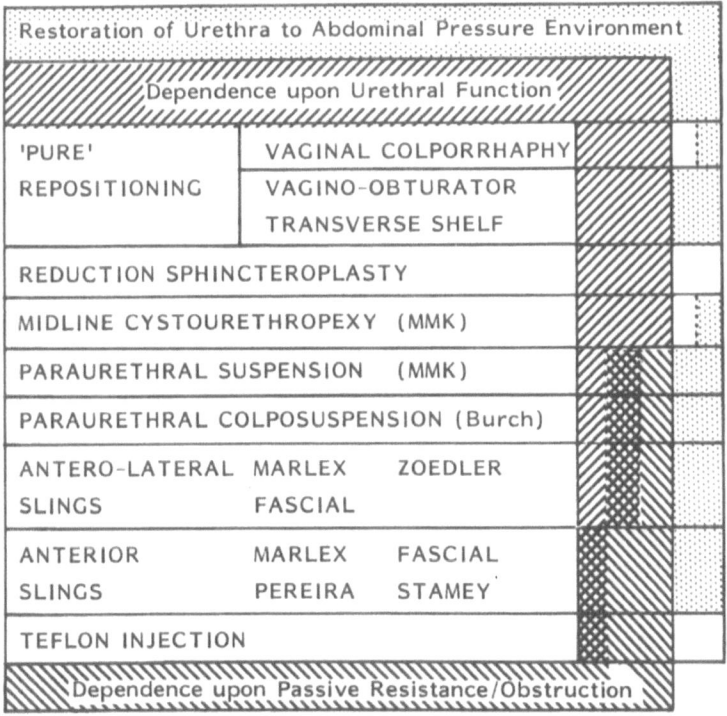

Fig. 1. The functional effect of operative procedures for incontinence.

its normal intra-abdominal pressure environment and the consequent differential abdominal-stress pressure may further compromise the competence of a sub-standard sphincter mechanism; this differential peri-urethral pressure can be demonstrated urodynamically by cough/strain urethral profilometry (Stanton, 1980) and occasionally clinically, when the isolated repair of a posterior vaginal enterocoele by colporrhaphy results in the development of stress incontinence simply due to the removal of the vaginally transmitted abdominal pressure-support of the urethra (Brown & Turner-Warwick, 1979). All effective repositioning procedures restore the urethra to the intra-abdominal pressure environment and this, itself, is sometimes sufficient to resolve stress leakage.

It is important to distinguish between the principles and the effect of the various urethral repositioning procedures, many of which introduce an element of urethral compression-obstruction, indeed some are almost entirely dependent on this; while the creation of a 'passive obstruction' may increase the leak-proof success of some procedures, it increases the incidence of complications resulting from postoperative voiding inefficiency associated with under-active detrusor function (Turner-Warwick, 1979).

'Pure' repositioning procedures

'Pure' repositioning procedures are those which do not involve any element of urethral fixation, compression or para-urethral distraction (Brown & Turner-Warwick, 1979); their success is fundamentally dependent on the consequent improvement in bladder neck or urethral function because, in spite of restoration of peri-urethral abdominal-pressure-support, even the most effective repositioning of an inert bladder neck/urethra will not restore continence unless it also creates a significant passive urethral obstruction. Furthermore, although many repositioning procedures are conceptually directed at the 'bladder neck', video-urodynamic evaluation shows that in the absence of passive obstruction, functional competence is more frequently restored at urethral sphincter level rather than at the bladder neck (Brown & Turner-Warwick, 1979).

This calls into question the whole concept of the traditional measurement of the 'posterior urethro-vesico angle' on the lateral film cystourethrogram or on a bead-chain urethrogram (long since abandoned by its author Jeffcoate, 1956; Turner-Warwick, 1979). This angle does not provide urodynamically valid information about bladder neck sphincter function or dysfunction; many patients with a poor angle are perfectly continent; restoration of a good 'vesico-urethral angle' after a simple repositioning procedure is simply a by-product of effective repositioning and does not indicate that competence has been restored to the bladder neck mechanism nor indeed, that the patient is continent.

Vaginal repositioning. Anterior colporrhaphy usually restores the peri-urethral abdominal pressure environment and may improve sphincter efficiency but, urodynamically, it cannot be regarded as a good procedure for incontinence because, however expertly it is performed, the bladder base and the urethra can be more efficiently repositioned by retropubic procedures (Brown & Turner-Warwick, 1979; Stanton, 1977).

The retropubic vagino-obturator shelf procedure. The retropubic vagino-obturator shelf procedure not only repositions the urethra and bladder neck sphincter mechanism most efficiently but leaves them free-lying in an elevated position without compromising its action and fixation, para-urethral tethering or urethral compression – furthermore secondary immobilisation of the intrinsic urethral function by retropubic healing fibrosis is positively prevented by interposing an omental pedicle graft between the back of the pubis and the urethra to ensure freedom of urethral contraction in the long term. In this procedure the lower vaginal wall is prolapsed through an incision in the para-urethral fascia on both sides and firmly anchored to the internal aspect of the obturator muscle. This procedure should not be confused with procedures commonly described as 'colposuspension' which generally includes paraurethral fascia in a higher 'sling' to Coopers ligament.

It is fundamentally important to appreciate that only the lower 4 cm of the vaginal wall relate to the support of the urethral and bladder neck. – Above this it relates to the bladder base and descent of this associated with a vault prolapse may create voiding problems, particularly when the detrusor is under-active (Farrar & Turner-Warwick, 1979). In the vagino-obturator shelf procedure the peritoneum is opened to achieve a vaginal suspension and an occlusion of the rectovaginal pouch to prevent a subsequent enterocoele.

Urethral and paraurethral suspension procedures. Many different operative procedures are described as 'Marshall-Marchetti-Krantz' or 'colposuspension'. In midline cystourethropexy the urethra and bladder neck are directly fixed to the back of the pubis; this provides no support for the back of the urethra and is inappropriate for patients with vaginal wall laxity owing to its tendency to 'tent' the bladder neck in an 'open' position, quite apart from the potential disadvantages of immobilising the urethral sphincter mechanism by this anchorage. It is worthy of note that the commonest cause of incompetence of the male bladder neck after pelvic fracture injuries is its immobilisation by surrounding haematoma fibrosis; simple lysis and a supporting omental wrap is usually sufficient to restore its competence (Turner Warwick, 1982). Colpofixation by lateral fixation of the paraurethral fascia and the vaginal vault (the Burch procedure and some varieties of the Marshall-Marchetti procedures) effectively repositions the urethra and may provide support from behind if the vaginal wall is specifically included in the supporting structures. However the anterolateral fixation of the paraurethral fascia creates additional unpredictable effects upon the urethra which may or may not improve the functional result; bilateral stretch-fixation may introduce a helpful element of partial mechanical occlusion but on the other hand the lateral tethering of the sphincter mechanism may restrict its sphincter – active occlusion.

Urethral-compression sling procedures. The more anterior the fixation of a urethral sling or hammack, the more likely it is to create a positive outlet obstruction; the Pereyra bilateral nylon-sling paraurethral suspension sutures have the advantage of simplicity, however in the Stamey variety these are positively tied to create an endoscopically verified passive occlusion of the bladder neck so that voiding problems requiring prolonged suprapubic catheter drainage are not unusual and sometimes long term self catheterisation is necessary.

Passive urethral resistance can also be augmented by the intramural injection of Teflon. Such procedures are particularly appropriate for the elderly, the unfit and for younger patients whose urethral function has proved inadequate after repositioning and reduction procedures.

Reduction sphincteroplasty. Urethral laxity associated with a large calibre urethra commonly results from over dilatation and is an occasional cause of persistent incontinence after an efficient repositioning procedure; owing to the anterior location of the bulk of the urethral sphincter mechanism, this can occasionally be resolved by a posterior reduction sphincteroplasty (Turner-Warwick, 1979).

Urodynamic effect of hysterectomy. There are no urodynamic indications for hysterectomy; it is normal for the bladder to be 'pressed upon by the uterus' and this never causes bladder dysfunction until a massive fibroid or a pregnant uterus virtually occludes the pelvic cavity. Urologic symptoms and bladder dysfunction are often made worse by hysterectomy and are always an indication for appropriate preoperative urodynamic evaluation whenever a hysterectomy is indicated for strictly gynaecological reasons (Brown & Turner-Warwick, 1979; Farrar & Turner-Warwick, 1979).

The evaluation of incontinence surgery (Fig. 2)

The essence of good clinical treatment of urinary incontinence is a satisfied patient and if a given procedure results in 70% of the patients claiming to be 'cured' and another 15% feel that their leakage has been 'improved', this may be regarded as satisfactory, however the real problem is that the technical failure rate may be considerably higher than this suggests because even the simplest objective evaluation shows that a considerable proportion of patients who claim to be dry postoperatively do, in fact, still leak (Brown & Turner-Warwick, 1979; Stanton, 1977). Thus it is no longer contributory to publish a series of cases based upon subjective clinical follow-up in support of a particular operative procedure; improvements in surgical treatment naturally stem from an analysis of the causes of failure based on objective urodynamic evaluation.

Hence the selection of patients for operative treatment of incontinence is most important. Even a clinician with long experience of objective urodynamic evaluation cannot reliably distinguish between those with 'stable detrusor' stress incontinence and those that are associated with 'unstable detrusor behaviour' on the basis of history and examination.

Investigations of patients with clinically determined 'simple stress incontinence' by provocative cystometry shows that 10–15% have unstable detrusor behaviour – for practical purposes the inclusion of these is not inappropriate, it simply means that the chances of a succesful outcome for these

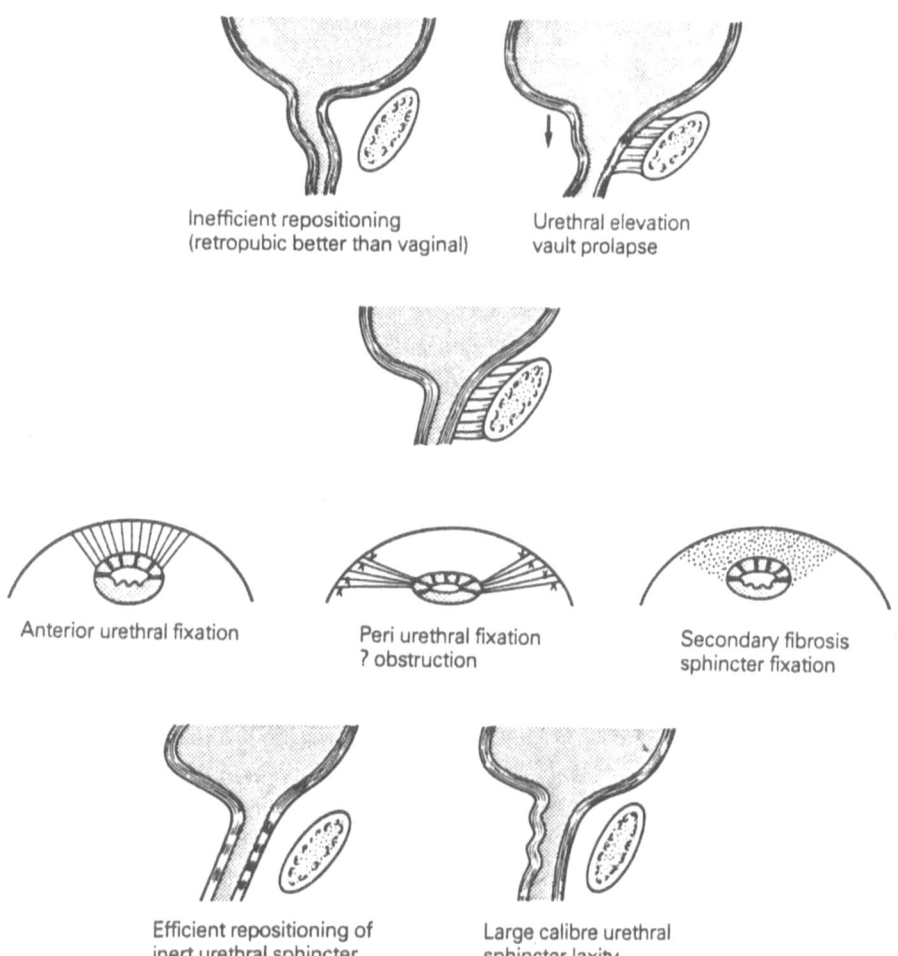

Inefficient repositioning
(retropubic better than vaginal)

Urethral elevation
vault prolapse

Anterior urethral fixation

Peri urethral fixation
? obstruction

Secondary fibrosis
sphincter fixation

Efficient repositioning of
inert urethral sphincter

Large calibre urethral
sphincter laxity

Fig. 2. Some reasons for failure of repositioning operations for urinary incontinence.

particular patients is rather less, however this may distort the results if a series is designed to accurately evaluate a particular operative procedure.

On the other hand urodynamic evaluation of patients with 'stress + urge' incontinence shows that about 1 in 5 have sensory urgency and that their stress incontinence is essentially 'stable'; although a repositioning procedure may not improve such patient's frequency and urgency, it is likely to resolve any true stress-leakage element and may occasionally improve urge-leakage. Therefore refusal to operate on a patient on the basis of a clinically determined stress-urge-incontinence may be both unkind and unjust. In the absence of objective urodynamic evaluation the rational clinical indications for an incontinence operation are the simple observation of *instantaneous* coughleak when the patient has a moderately full bladder (itself a perfectly valid urodynamic observation), together with anterior vaginal laxity. A history of associated urgency should be irrelevant provided the patient accepts that this particular symptom is unlikely to improve.

The prognostic value of the Bonney-Marshall test, to determine whether a patient's cough-leakage is controlled by digital support of the anterior vaginal wall, is very poor. The most appropriate urodynamic investigations for the preoperative evaluation of female incontinence are:

1. simple video-recorded cystourethrography to assess the vesico-urethral descent, the efficiency of the urethral sphincter mechanism and the voiding efficiency (Turner-Warwick, 1979);
2. subtracted detrusor-pressure provocation cystometry to assess detrusor behaviour during filling and voiding together with measurement of the maximum detrusor contraction pressure by interrupted voiding studies (Turner-Warwick & Whiteside, 1982).

Urethral pressure profile studies must be unusually expertly performed and precisely interpreted; otherwise they are often non-contributory or even misleading.

Conclusion

There is no doubt that the most satisfactory incontinence to treat surgically is that associated with a significant vesico-urethral vaginal prolapse and a stable detrusor that develops a volitional voiding contraction that is sustained till emptying is complete; the success rate of effective simple retropubic repositioning operations for such patients is high and the voiding complications rate low. Patients with a stable incontinence associated with relatively inefficient voiding detrusor contractions are particularly likely to develop bladder emptying problems after incontinence operations but create an element of outlet obstruction. Unstable detrusor behaviour is not necessarily a contra-indication to the surgical treatment of unstable detrusor behaviour. If the Maximum Detrusor Contraction pressure (P. det. max.) is relatively low the results may be quite acceptable; the results of treating high-pressure unstable incontinence, both surgically and pharmacologically, are very poor.

References

1. Brown A.G. and Turner-Warwick R. A urodynamic evaluation of urinary incontinence in the female and its treatment. Urol. Clin. N. America 6 (1979): 31–38.
2. Chilton C.P. and Turner-Warwick R. The relationship of the distal sphincter mechanism to the pelvic floor musculature. Esch Man Prize BAUS 1981 – Brit. J. Urol. (1981).

3. Donker P.J., Droes J.Th.P.M. and Van Ulden B.M. The anatomy of the musculature and innervation of the bladder and urethra. In: Williams D.I. and Chisholm G.D. (ed.) Scientific Foundations of Urology. 32–39 (1976).
4. Farrar D. and Turner-Warwick R. Outflow obstruction in the female. Clin. N. America 6 (1979): 217–227.
5. Gosling J.A. and Dixon J.S. Structural changes associated with obstruction of the lower urinary tract: a comparison between upper and lower systems. In: Zinner N.R. and Sterling A.M. Progress in Clinical & Biological Research – Female Incontinence. Alan Liss, N.Y., 78 (1981): 283–284.
6. James E.D. Continuous urodynamic monitoring. Urol. Clin. N. America 6 (1979): 125–135.
7. Jeffcoate T.N.A. Results of Aldridge sling operation for stress incontinence. J. Obstet. Gynaec. Brit. Emp. 63 (1956): 36–39.
8. Osborne J. Personal communication (1979).
9. Stanton S.L. Female urinary incontinence. Lloyd Luke, London (1977).
10. Tanagho E.A. The anatomy and physiology of micturition. Clin. Obstet. Gynaec. 5 (1978).
11. Turner-Warwick R. and Whiteside C.G. Bladder neck dysfunction. In: Enc. Riches (ed.) Modern Trends in Urology, Butterworth, London (1970).
12. Turner-Warwick R. Clinical problems associated with urodynamic abnormalities. First Internat. Urodynamics Symp. Aachen. In: Lutzyer W. and Melchior H. (eds.) Urodynamics. Berlin. Springer-Verlag, 237–263 (1970).
13. Turner-Warwick R. and Whiteside C.G. Clinical Urodynamics. Urol. Clin. N. America, 6 (1979): 1–293.
14. Turner-Warwick R. Urethral surgery. In: Glenn (ed) Urologic Surgery, Harper-Roe, chapter 68 (1982).
15. Turner-Warwick R. and Whiteside C.G. Scientific Foundations of Urology, 2nd. Ed. Henneman, London (1982).

II.2. The rational approach for the surgical treatment of urinary stress incontinence

B.L.R.A. COOLSAET, C. BLOK, G.E.P.M. VAN VENROOIJ &
Ph.E.V.A. VAN KERREBROECK

Introduction

The symptom urinary stress incontinence indicates the patient's statement of involuntary loss of urine when excercising physically. The rational method of treatment is the one that, based on knowledge of the pathophysiological mechanisms that cause the symptom, restores the mechanism that is responsible for continence. However, different opinions and theories have resulted in several methods of treatment some of which are rather contradictory. Certain authors deducted theories from the empirical results obtained by their methods. The problem of stress incontinence seemed already solved in the late fourties after the introduction of a simple vesicourethral suspension method by Marshall et al. [1]. Based on a theory of hypermobility and sagging of the bladder base, vesicourethral suspension resulted in success in 95 percent of the patients.

However, results of long-term follow-up studies and the further development of methods of examination, more specifically the urodynamic investigation [2], stimulated many clinicians and researchers to further improve the rational approach of the stress incontinence problem. Data obtained by these examinations indicate that there is a wide spectrum in the presentation of stress incontinence.

Indeed, the variability of the amount of urineloss, the bladder volume at which leakage occurs, the detrusor properties, the condition of the musculofascial elements supporting the bladder neck and urethra, the intrinsic bladder neck properties and the characteristics of the urethral competence mechanism, do cause a wide variety in the pathophysiological presentation.

The urodynamic definition of genuine stress incontinence: 'involuntary loss of urine when the intravesical pressure exceeds the maximum urethral pressure in the absence of detrusor activity' does not solve the problem of selection of patients for a surgical treatment since too many variables are not considered.

Pathophysiology of genuine stress incontinence

Continence in the female is maintained under stress conditions by several co-operating mechanisms. A competent bladder neck mechanism, which consists of intrinsic muscle components and extrinsic loopwise ligament structures, prevents leakage of urine from the bladder to the urethra under stress conditions.

The extrinsic suspension mechanisms may be insufficient. This results in either anterior or posterior suspension defects, but this only affects the position of the bladder neck and not its intrinsic function. The intrinsic bladder neck mechanism can be competent at all positions. Subsequently the position of the bladder neck and the urethrovesical angle, do not cause urinary stress incontinence on itself. These features become important when they coexist with other dysfunctions. As an isolated entity, changes of the position of the bladder neck and the size of the urethrotrigonal angle do not make the patient leak.

Changes in the bladder neck competence and abnormal urethrotrigonal anatomy in varies degrees may be combined with different stages of urethral insufficiency.

Urethral competence is produced by urethral sealing mechanisms which consist of mucal, mucosal and submucosal factors. Intrinsic urethral muscles and external skeletal musculature of the urogenital diaphragm contribute to passive and active closure of the urethral lumen. Sudden increase of the abdominal pressure results in an increase of the pressure in the bladder. Obviously, leakage will occur when the bladder pressure exceeds the urethral closure pressure. The relation of these two pressures depends on both the pressure level in the bladder at rest and the urethral closure pressure at rest. High detrusor pressures due to low compliance of the bladder may result in stress incontinence, also when urethral competence is only slightly insufficient.

On the other hand, insufficiency of the urethral closing forces due to incompetence of the bladder neck, bladder neck support, urethral and periurethral insufficiency, may disturb the bladder-urethral pressure equilibrium at various degrees.

Pressure increases in the urethral lumen during stress have been explaned as periurethral transmission of the abdominal pressure to the intra-abdominal proximal part of the urethra. Stress incontinence has been thought to be caused by a displacement of the proximal urethra from the intra-abdominal location. According to this theory, cure of stress incontinence is achieved by any method by which the proximal urethra is positioned to its normal intra-abdominal location. This widely accepted theory is an oversimplification of the pathophysiological changes. It is based on the finding that after successful repair, a positive pressure gradient is maintained under stress conditions. However, no one has ever demonstrated that the position of the proximal urethra changes from the subdiaphragmatical to the supra-dia-phragmatical area after surgical repair. Also the fact that after repair the retropubic space is completely closed by fibrotic tissue adherence of the bladder neck-urethral area to the pubic bone, seriously interferes with this theory.

Careful observations of preoperative, intraoperative and postoperative data strongly indicate that several changes of the bladder neck-urethral closure mechanism can occur preoperatively at different degrees and that several of the mechanisms which contribute to continence can be more or less restored depending on their dysfunction.

Most of the suspension or support operations compress the bladder neck area to a variable degree. In those patients who initially showed abnormal funneling of the bladder neck, postoperative control studies have shown that the bladder neck becomes competent after successful surgery. Closure of the bladder neck might explain increase of the functional urethral length in some of the patients.

Hypermobility of the urethral area during stress by either anterior or posterior suspension defects, enhances a decrease of the ability to build up urethral pressure during stress. This ability to produce pressure increase is combined to a variety of urethral closure mechanisms. Urethral closure pressure might increase in some after successful repair, while no statistical increase has been demonstrated. Simple urethral support, however, even without statistically significant changes of its position and without any direct interference with the sphincteric unit itself, will cure a large number of patients.

The problem of genuine stress incontinence becomes more complicated when bladder urethral pressure gradient is lost by active pressure decrease of the urethra (urethral instability). The pressure changes can be related to normal or decreased urethral closure pressure. Leakage during stress is then caused by sudden relaxation of the urethral closure mechanism.

The operative approach

Although extensive urodynamic investigation enables the clinician at this stage to differentiate genuine stress incontinence into a variety of pathophysiological entities, one can state that a support of the bladder neck-urethral area will ensure long-term continence in approximately 80 percent of the patients. The main goal of all different types of surgical repair is to restore the support of the urethra and simultaneously it is necessary to avoid funneling of the bladder neck. Although the anatomical position might be restored by this manoevre it does not appear to be the main goal.

Whatever a method is used, one should take to avoid any further damage of the already malfunctioning delicate continence mechanism. No dissection should be done in the region of the vesicourethral mechanism. It is furthermore of the greatest importance to avoid creation of bladder outlet obstruction.

Since a long-term failure rate of approximately 20 percent can be expected, techniques which interfere with the sphincteric unit itself should be avoided.

Numerous techniques have been described. Although the Marshall-Marchetti technique originally achieved good results, its use is not advisable because of the great risk of urethral fibrosis and dysfunction. Fortunately, the original technique has been adapted by Marchetti et al. in 1957 [3]. However, many clinicians continued using periurethral sutures. Krantz [4] used only a single suture on each side of the bladder neck. This technique is very similar to the Burch colposuspension [5]. The Burch colposuspension suspends the dome of the vagina to Cooper's ligament. No dissection is required. In the absence of a cystocele only one non-absorbable suture on each side of the bladder neck may be sufficient. In case of downward displacement of the bladder base, one or two more sutures are placed more laterally. A similar support is achieved by the Pereyra type [6] of operations, which has been modified by Stamey [7] and Raz [8]. All these types of procedures will cure approximately 80 percent of the patients with stress incontinence.

Why do support operations fail?

Twenty percent of non-selected patients will have either persistent or recurrent incontinence after suprabubic or vaginal support operations. This percentage will even be higher following anterior colporrhaphy. Failures or recurrences seldom occur in moderate stress urinary incontinence, but the failure rate increases in patients with more severe incontinence. The causes for failure can be single or associated with others. Some authors stated that the most frequent technical error is the failure to restore anatomy to normal. However, anatomy itself has very little to do with the continence mechanism. The bladder neck and urethral mechanism can function normally at different anatomical positions. Causes of failure are multiple.

1. The bladder. Bladder-urethra pressure equilibrium can be disturbed by increased detrusor pressures at rest. Detrusor pressure during the filling phase is kept low by a delicate mechanism composed of passive and active factors. Dysfunction of this mechanism by either passive or active components or a combination of both, results in a fast increase of the pressure during filling. The compliance of the bladder, which denotes the ratio of small change of volume to the associated change of pressure, will be low. Rather small decrease of urethral competence will be associated with urine leakage during stress, due to high detrusor pressures. The method of treatment for these patients is either pharmacological relaxation of the detrusor in case of active dysfunction, or bladder enlargement procedures.

2. The bladder neck. Failure occurs in patients who previously underwent Y-V bladder neck plasty or bladder neck resection. The bladder neck mechanism is irreversibly disturbed. Reconstruction of the bladder neck itself is utopian. In these patients the only possibility to become continent are a Young-Dees (Leadbetter) urethral elongation [9], artificial sphincter implantation [10] or sling procedures.

3. The urethral competence mechanism. Competence is realised by passive and active components. Active relaxation of the urethral wall may occur not withstanding normal urethral closure pressure. Treatment will be primarily pharmacological. Patients who do not respond to therapy could be managed by abdomino-vaginal sling or even artificial urinary sphincter implantation. When combined with a low urethral closure pressure, the primary therapy would be pharmacological followed by colposuspension. However failure rate is high and subsequent occluding sling procedures combined with self catheterisation, or artificial sphincter implantation will be required. However, the most frequent cause of failure is due to urethral fibrosis and/or urethral shortening. In these patients there is mostly severe or total urineloss. In such cases careful urodynamic investigation is required before any further attempt to secondary procedure is undertaken. The investigation of the urethral competence mechanism is difficult. Urethral pressure measurements, certainly in these fibrotic tubes, are of little value. The method of choice is the measurement of the antegrade leakage pressure by means of the sleeve catheter method [11]. When urethral leakage pressure is low, a Stamey-Raz operation can be tried. Failure rate will be important. Secondary management will have to be performed by a Young-Dees (Leadbetter), sling or artificial sphincter procedure.

4. Suture avulsion. Suture avulsion in the early stages might occur especially when absorbable sutures have been used. Unilateral avulsion will seldom interfere with the postoperative results. Bilateral avulsion will require a secondary support operation. Depending on the previously performed technique, this can be changed to a suprapubical or abdominovaginal procedure in order to avoid extensive dissection.

References

1. Marshall V.T., Marchetti A.A. and Krantz K.E. The correction of stress incontinence by simple vesicourethral suspension. Surg. Gynecol. Obstet. 88 (1949): 509.
2. Coolsaet B.L.R.A. Cystometry. In: Stanton St.L. (ed) Clinical Gynecologic Urology. Publ. the C.V. Mosby Co (1984), p. 59.
3. Marchetti A.A., Marshall V.F. and Shultis L.D. Simple vesicourethral suspension: a survey. Am. J. Obstet. Gynecol. 74 (1957): 57.
4. Krantz K. Marshall-Marchetti-Krantz procedure. In Stanton S.L. and Tanagho E.A. (eds) Surgery of female incontinence. Heidelberg, Springer Verlag.
5. Burch J.C. Urethrovaginal fixation to Cooper's ligament for correction of stress incontinence, cystocele, and prolapse. Am. J. Obstet. Gynecol. 81 (1961): 281.
6. Pereyra A.J. A simplified surgical procedure for the correction of stress incontinence in women. West. J. Surg. Obstet. Gynecol. 67 (1959): 223.
7. Stamey T.A. Endoscopic suspension of the vesical neck for urinary incontinence. Surg. Gynecol. Obstet. 136 (1973): 547.
8. Raz S. Modified bladder neck suspension for female stress incontinence. Urology 18 (1981): 82.
9. Leadbetter G.W. Jr. Surgical correction of total urinary incontinence. J. Urol. 91 (1964): 261.
10. Barrett D.M., Furlow W.L. Artificial urinary sphincter in the management of female incontinence. In: Raz S. (ed) Female Urology, Saunders Co (1983), p. 284.
11. Blok C., van Venrooij G.E.P.M. and Coolsaet B.L.R.A. Continuous quantification of urethral competence with a new tube foil sleeve catheter. J. Urology 132 (1984): 104.

II.3. A simplified technique of bladder neck suspension with tissue glue

W. DE SY, W. OOSTERLINCK & H. MINNAERT

Introduction

Why did we change our operative technique for cure of stress incontinence in women? Since many years the technique of Goebel-Stoeckel was followed using a fascial sling for bladder neck suspension. It gave excellent and long lasting results [1] but it has some major disadvantages:
1. It is a combined, abdominal and vaginal operation which cannot be classified as a minor intervention.
2. The resection of a rectal fascial strip resulted in frequent ($\pm 10\%$) hernias of the abdominal wound.
3. The most annoying problem was the postoperative urinary retention which frequently occured after removal of the bladder catheter; although of short duration in the majority of patients, it took several weeks to resolve in some of them. This was responsable for a long prolonged hospital stay and even, though seldom, for reintervention to transect the sling.

These were the major reasons to switch to the Marshall-Marchetti operation when dealing with primary cases of stress incontinence. Indeed it avoids the major disadvantages of the Goebel-Stoeckel operation.

But the sutures, especially the most distal ones, between the pubic bone and the ventral vaginal wall are often difficult to place. The stitches may tear through the periost or can provoke some disagreable bleeding from veins of the vaginal wall. These technical difficulties incited several surgeons to facilitate the original technique. One of the most simple modifications was to use tissue glue, instead of sutures, to fix the bladder neck at the pubic bones [2, 3].

Technique

The patient is positioned with spreaded legs. A catheter 14 Fr. is left in the bladder to recognize the urethra and the bladder neck. The lower abdomen

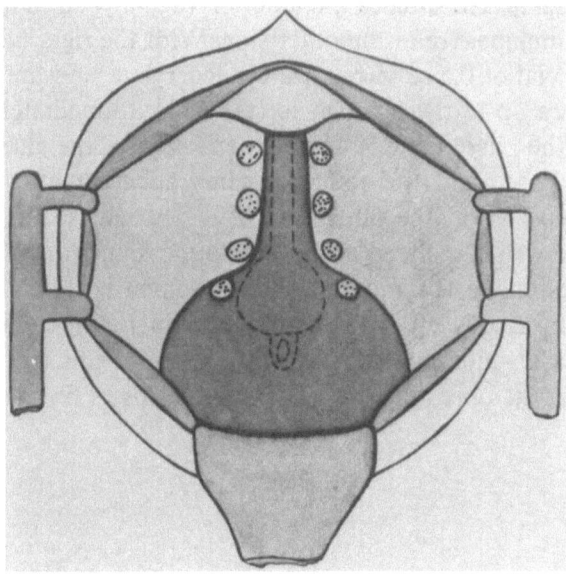

Fig. 1.

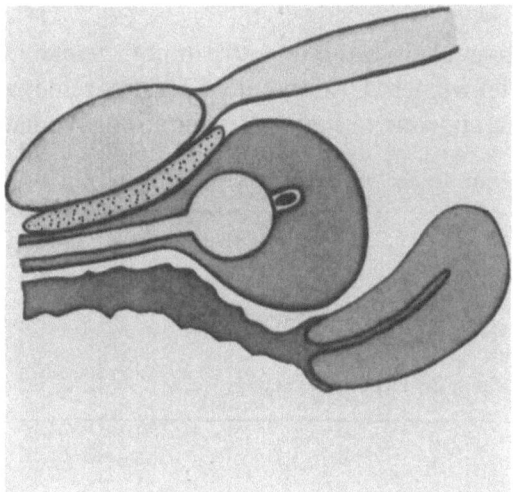

Fig. 2.

is opened at the midline or with Pfannenstiel incision. The bladder neck and ventral vaginal wall is reached retropubically by blind dissection. There are two major conditions which must be fulfilled: the areas to stick to each other must be bloodless and must be free of all fatty tissue. Indeed it will not adhere when the surfaces are not dry, and fat will tear easily afterwards even if it adheres.

In most instances the fatty tissue is pushed laterally with a tampon and its bloodvessels are coagulated. The surgeon introduces two fingers of the left hand into the vagina. He stitches the anterior vaginal wall first on one side and in a second manoeuvre at the other side. With the right hand he sprinkles one plastic vial of 0,5 cc in butyl-2 cyanoacrylate* on the vaginal wall beside the urethra up to the bladder neck (Fig. 1). Immediately the wall is pressed against the pubic bone. The polymerisation of the glue occurs very rapidly within 10 sec and the tissue remains adherent after 30 sec. The manoeuvre is repeated at the other side of the patient so the urethra and bladder neck are well suspended against the pubic bone (Fig. 2). The whole manoeuvre takes only a few minutes. The abdomen is closed as usual and the aspiration drainage is left for 24 hours. A vaginal tamponade is left for 3 days as well as a bladder catheter. We are not sure if this tamponade is an essential point of the operation but we think it helps to fix the vaginal wall upwards.

Results

The material and results are summarized in Table 1 and 2. Two of our failures were our first cases in which we omitted to dissect carefully all fatty tissue.

The postoperative complications were minor. Some wound problems were present in 7 fat women. Urinary retention after removal of the catheter occured only twice and was of very short duration. We had no perivesical

Table 1. Profile of patients treated for incontinence.

Number of patients: 63
Age: 31 y → 83 y
      mean age: 51
Previous interventions:
      hysterectomy: 30
      other operation for stress incontinence: 19

Table 2. Results of bladder neck suspension with tissue glue.

Follow-up	n	Cured	Urge incontinence	Stress incontinence
1 → 6 m	29	21	8	0
6 → 56 m	32	28	1	3
Mean: 29 m				
Lost	2			

* Histoacryl: manufactured by B. Braun-Melsungen, P.O.B. 346, D-3508 Melsungen, F.R.G.

haematomas. Postoperative hernias developed in 2 patients. A (minor) pulmonary embolism occured once in a woman suffering from recurrent phlebothrombosis.

Discussion

The use of tissue glue certainly simplifies the technique of bladder neck suspension considerably without diminishing its efficacy. It avoids the difficult sutures between the pubic bone and the anterior vaginal wall by a manoeuvre which takes no longer than a few minutes. By this way it shortens the operation time. In experienced hands it is often completely finished within half an hour.

The postoperative morbidity is low. Especially perivesical haematomas and urinary retention occurs very rarely. Nevertheless the appearance of hernia at the abdominal wound remains a problem although to a lesser extent than in techniques using a fascial sling.

It became our first choice operation for the operative cure of genuine stress incontinence in our department. We restrict the Goebel-Stoeckel operation to selected cases in which previous operations failed.

Although one can expect a slow degeneration of results with time, our experience did not indicate that this would be worser in patients treated with tissue glue than after conventional suturing.

Reintervention in the same area occured only once in our serie, without problems. Experience in other fields of surgery let expect that this will be not more hazardous than after classical suturing. Indeed histoacryl is completely absorbed after 3 to 4 months and has an excellent tissue tolerance.

References

1. Defoort R., De Sy W., Oosterlinck W. Résultats éloignés de l'opération de Michon-Goebel-Stoeckel pour la cure chirurgicale de l'incontinence d'urines à l'effort chez la femme. Ann. Urol. 5 (1971): 243–246.
2. Beer J., Thiel U. Eine einfache operative Methode zur Behandlung der funktionellen Harninkontinenz der Frau. Z. Urol. 65 (1972): 203–214.
3. Kelami A. Tissue adhesives: their use in urology. Eur. Urol. 3 (1976): 182–184.

II.4. Transurethral teflon injection for urinary stress incontinence in women
A critical evaluation after three years

J.J. MATTELAER, L. BAERT & P. DE NOLLIN

The purpose of transurethral teflon injection to cure urinary stress incontinence in women is to increase the urethral resistance to urine outflow. Although Gersuny injected glycerine around the perineal urethra to treat incontinent males it was Politano [1] who proposed teflon to treat incontinence in men after transurethral resection of the prostate and extended the technique to treat women patients. Heer [2] injected teflon into the wall of the urethra to increase its length and resistance but the technique of transurethral and periurethral injection of teflon paste was really developed in Western Europe by Sparwasser and Lampante [3, 4] in 1978 with the fabrication of specialised instrumentation by Wolf-Knittlingen and Storz-Tuttlingen. Marketing by these manufacturers certainly diffused this new technique to most urological departments but was also responsable for a subjective overevaluation!

Since 1980 we have performed 105 endoscopic periurethral teflon injections in 95 women suffering from urinary stress incontinence. Initially we were very enthusiastic [5], but after a recent review of 66 patients with a longer follow-up and a critical evaluation, our original enthusiasm has somewhat abated. Another objection to transurethral injection of teflon comes from the Mayo Clinic [14].

A recent publication on an animal-study showed that teflon particles (<50 mμ) can pass tissues and give rise to microemboli in the brain and lungs. However teflon is an inert substance and passage of teflon molecules should not be a contra-indication to its use. We have never seen any embolic complications in our own patients and no clinical study on periurethral teflon injection reports or suggests clinical emboli [4, 6–11, 13].

Technique

A 8 French gauge polyethylene catheter ending in a needle is guided through the shaft of a 22 ch. cystoscope. The needle is inserted deeply into the urethral wall about 0,5 to 1 cm below the bladder neck. With a small 1 ml dental anaesthesia syringe within a metallic sheet 2 to 3 ml of teflon is injected by a piston (Storz) in each quadrant. Personally we have never used the expensive electric pump with foot pedal (Wolf). After the periurethral teflon injection, and when the bladder is filled up with the irrigation solution, a 12 ch. suprapubic punction cystostomy catheter (Cystofix®) is introduced.

The following morning the suprapubic cystostomy catheter is clamped and the patient is allowed to void. If the patient is able to void without difficulty the catheter is pulled out in the afternoon and the patient discharged.

A urinary antiseptic is prescribed for two weeks. If the patient is unable to void, the cystostomy is reopened and reclamped again. Most injections (80%) were performed under local epidural anaesthesia.

The average hospitalisation time was 48 hours. We did not see any major complications and most patients presented minimal dysuria and stranguria for about one week. Nevertheless one case of a granulomatous tumor around the teflon paste is reported [13], and Lampante [11] reports about 3, and Schulke [13] reported 2 cases of urethra vaginal fistula after periurethral teflon injection in women.

Patients and results

A 24- to 36 months follow-up was made on 72 women whose ages varied from 15 to 90 years (mean 54.5). 28 patients (39%) presented a grade I stress incontinence, 30 patients (42%) grade II and 14 (19%) grade III. 25 (34.5%) had had previous gynaecological or urological operations. 34 patients or 47% presented some urge by history or by urodynamic evaluation. In 10 patients (13.8%) we performed a second teflon injection after failure of a first one.

Our first impression and follow-up after only 12 months was very satisfying [5]. After a few months 82.4% were cured or showed substantial improvement.

These results correlate with other publications (Table 1) based on similar short follow-up. Nevertheless, after a longer follow-up period our initial impression was not confirmed and therefore we reviewed all our patients for a critical evaluation.

72 patients were asked to reply to a list of questions and were seen personally 24–36 months after the teflon injection. During this period 2 patients had died and 4 patients were lost for follow-up. 66 patients remained for critical evaluation.

Table 2 shows that only 13 (20%) of the 66 patients were completely cured (12 after one injection; one after two injections).

Table 1. Results.

References		Patients	Follow-up	Success	Improvement	Failure
Short term follow-up success (80–95%)						
Heer [2]	1977	23	?		95%	5%
Lampante Sparwasser [3]	1979	62	1 - 22 m		92%	8%
Sparwasser Lampante [4]	1980	109	?		88%	12%
Schulman [6]	1984	56	?	70%	16%	14%
Own series [5]	1982	34	12 m		82,4%	17,6%
Schneider Rugendorff [9]	1984	25	6 m		80%	20%
Longer follow-up success (55–79%)						
Politano [15]	1982	54	6 m - 16 y		71%	29%
Thiry [7]	1983	14	3 - 24 m		71%	29%
Nienhuis [8]	1983	23	3 - 26 m	39%	22%	39%
Lampante Sparwasser Charvalakis [11]	1984	298	10 - 59 m		79%	21%
Schulke [13]	1984	50	±48 m	56%	8%	36%
Korner May [10]	1984	84	12 - 48 m		55%	45%
Own series	1984	66	24 - 36 m	20%	44%	36%

Table 2. Results of endoscopic teflon injection (follow-up 24–36 months).

		Improvement		
Number of patients	Success	> 50%	< 50%	Failure
1 injection 57	12 (21%)	15 (26%)	10 (18%)	20 (35%)
2 injections 9	1 (11%)	2 (22%)	2 (22%)	4 (44%)
Total 66	13 (20%)	17 (25,5%)	12 (18,5%)	24 (36%)
	20%	44%		36%

29 patients (44%) showed substantial improvement. Failure or only temporary improvement occured in 24 patients (36%). There was no significant statistical correlation between success or failure and the degree of incontinence. The rate of failure, however, is higher if the patient presents not only a genuine stress incontinence but also some urge incontinence. For this reason a preoperative urodynamic evaluation is important. 15 patients (22%) had an operation after failure of teflon injection (Table 3).

Table 3.

Operation	Before teflon injection	After teflon injection
Colporrhaphy	7	0
Hysterectomy	6	1
M.M.K.	5	5
Sling	1	7
Vulvectomy	1	0
Colpopromont.		
Pexie	2	1
Unknown	3	0
	25 (35%)	15 (22%)

In all these reinterventions we did not experience any difficulty or complication caused by the previous injection. A visible scar of tissue fibrosis was never observed.

Discussion

This critical review of 66 patients 2 to 3 years after the periurethral teflon injection and other longer follow-up studies shows that the long-term results [7, 8, 10, 11, 13, 15] are not as good as those published in studies with a short follow-up period [2-6, 9].

At the present time this technique may be overevaluated and our first enthusiasm may have to be toned down somewhat. The procedure however is simple and inexpensive and therefore we will continue to perform periurethral teflon injections in women with stress incontinence in the following indications:
— Very obese women.
— Older women in poor general condition.
— After failure of previous surgery.
— In younger women who want more children.
— In women who refuse any open surgery.

Comment

The main principle of this technique consists in the transurethral injection of teflon paste into the submucosal tissue of the proximal urethra. Teflon is an insert material that produces no tissue sclerosis. In order to obtain an injectable paste the fine polymer particles (< 50 mμ) of teflon – a tetrafluoro-ethylene – are mixed with 50% glycerine to a homogenic suspension. Post-

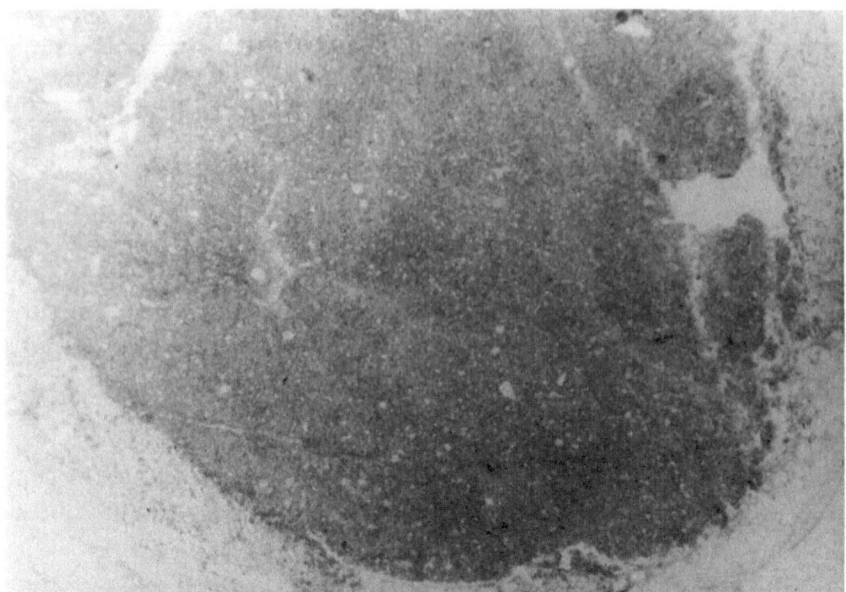

Fig. 1. A nodule of teflon particles surrounded by a foreign body giant cell reaction.

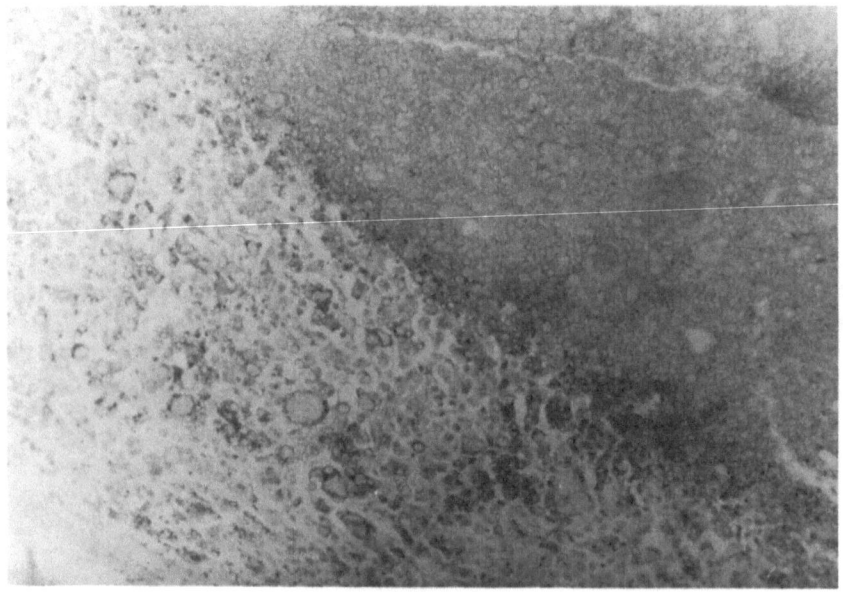

Fig. 2. Above the teflon paste – below giant cells with teflon particles.

operatively the glycerine is resorbed and the teflon particles remain in place.

Microscopically we can see a giant cell reaction around these foreign body particles (Fig. 1-2) with fibrosis of the smooth muscle fibers and a proliferation of macrophages (Fig. 3-4). This microscopic examination shows that

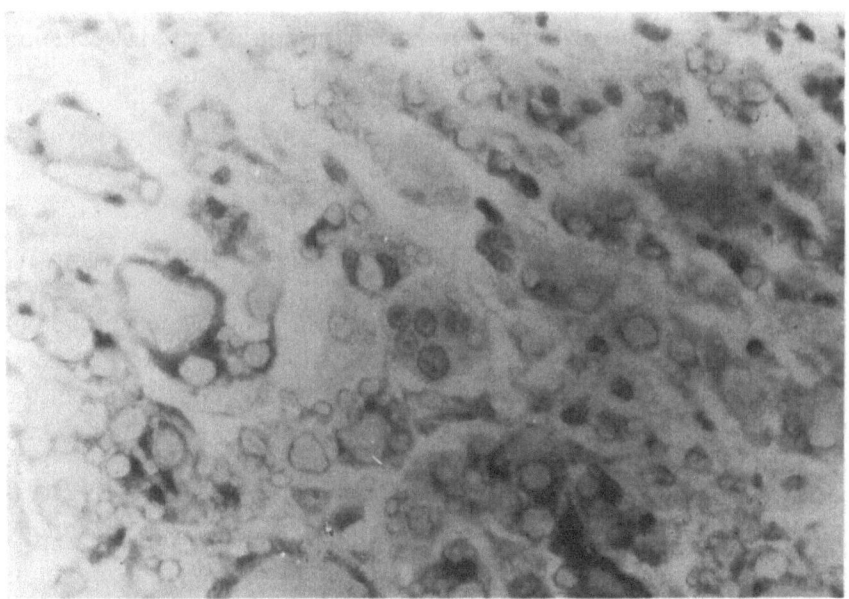

Fig. 3. Enlargement of the macrophages and giant cells with teflon inclusions.

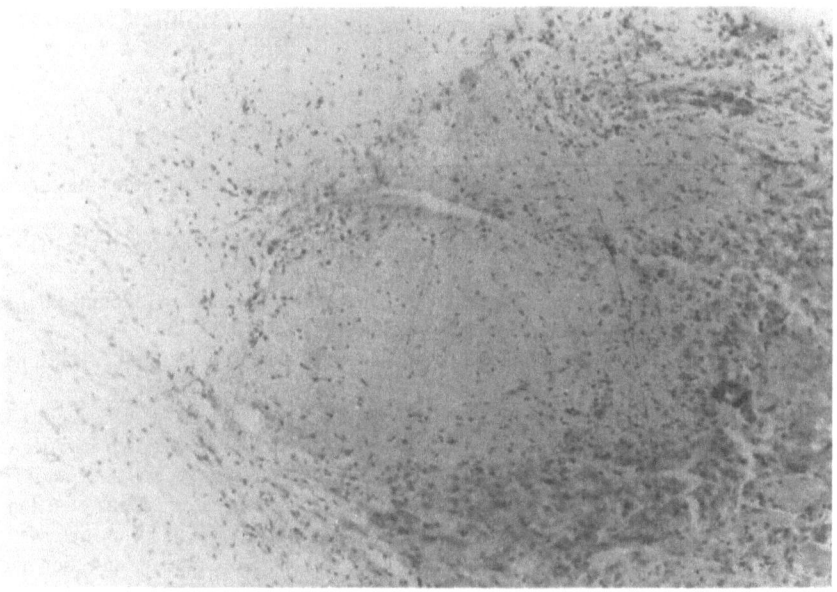

Fig. 4. Proliferation of macrophages between fibrotic groupes of smooth muscle cells.

teflon paste, although it is an inert material, still produces a slight degree of fibrosis. It also proves that microparticles can move by inclusion in giant cells (Fig. 3). This microscopic picture corresponds with the histological examinations of Behme-Wechsung on 6 cases [12].

The industry is now producing a teflon paste with large molecules in order to prevent tissue passage. It remains an open question if these larger teflon particles will not cause larger emboli instead of microemboli.

Conclusion

1. Periurethral teflon injection is one of the multiple methods available to treat urinary stress incontinence.
2. It is a technically simple, non-aggressive and inexpensive technique but the results are not as good as the open operative procedures. Preoperatively the patient should be informed objectively and honestly about the results of both procedures.
3. The technique can be repeated and does not hinder later operations. It may also be used after unsuccessful incontinence operations.
4. Although the early results of periurethral teflon injection were very satisfactory, this critical evaluation after 3 years follow-up should caution us against overoptimism.
5. Although no clinical complications of microembolisation have been reported, urologists showed the award that tissue passage is possible.

References

1. Politano V.A., Small M.P., Harper J.M. and Lynne C.M. Periurethral teflon injection for urinary incontinence. J. Urol. 111 (1974): 180–183.
2. Heer H. Die Behandlung der Harninkontinenz mit der Teflonpaste. Urol. Int. 32 (1977): 295–302.
3. Lampante L., Kaesler F.P. and Sparwasser H. Endourethrale submuköse Tefloninjektion zur Erziehlung von Harnkontinenz. Aktuelle Urologie. 10 (1979): 265–273.
4. Sparwasser H. and Lampante L. Endourethrale submuköse Tefloninjektion bei Harninkontinenz. Bericht über das 5e Klinische Wochenende Mainz, (1980): 73–74.
5. De Nollin P., Baert L. and Mattelaer J. Peri-urethrale Teflon injectie als behandeling van stress-incontinentie bij de vrouw. Resultaten na één jaar follow-up. Tijdschrift voor Geneeskunde, 39 (1983): 781–782.
6. Schulman C.C., Simon J., Wespes E. and Germeau F. Endoscopic injections of teflon to treat urinary incontinence in women. Brit. Med. J. 288 (1984): 192.
7. Thiry A.J. Traitement de l'incontinence urinaire d'effort chez la femme par injection endouréthrale de teflon. Acta Urol. Belg. 52 (1984): 274–277.
8. Nienhuis J.E. De behandeling van incontinentia urinae door submukeuze teflon injecties (Verenigingsverslag). Ned. Tijdschrift Geneeskunde. 127 (1983): 1608.
9. Schneider H.J. and Rugendorff E.W. Die Behandlung der Harninkontinenz durch endourethrale submuköse Tefloninjektion. Urologe B, 24 (1984): 73–76.
10. Korner A. and May P. Ergebnisse submuköser Tefloninjektion bei weiblicher Harninkontinenz. Urologe B. 24 (1984): 77–79.
11. Lampante L., Sparwasser H. and Charvalakis C. Behandlungergebnisse der Harninkontinenz durch endourethrale submuköse Tefloninjektion. Urologe B. 24 (1984): 80–82.

12. Behme-Wechsung D. and Luchtrath H. Morphologische Befunde nach periurethrale Teflon-injektion. Urologe B. 24 (1984): 83–87.
13. Schulke J. Komplikationen bei der transurethralen Tefloninjektion zur Behandlung der Harninkontinenz. Urologe B. 24 (1984): 88–89.
14. Malizia A.A. and Myers R.P. Migration of periurethrally injected teflon. Ann. Meet. Am. Urol. Assoc. Las Vegas, NV (1983).
15. Politano V.A. Periurethral polytetrafluoroethylene injection for urinary incontinence. J. Urol. 127 (1982): 439–442.

II.5. Burch colposuspension: method of choice?

S.L. STANTON

Introduction

Stress incontinence due to urethral sphincter incompetence and anterior vaginal wall prolapse commonly co-exist, the latter sometimes being responsible for the former. Conventionally, the anterior colporrhaphy has been the operation of choice to correct both. Over the last 30 years, there has been increased enthusiasm amongst gynaecologists and urologists for suprapubic operations to fulfil this role. Burch describes his technique of urethrovaginal suspension to Cooper's ligament in 1961 [1] and many surgeons have added their modifications since [2]. His basic concept, of a procedure which corrects urethral sphincter incompetence and anterior vaginal wall prolapse, has been vindicated by clinical experience.

Indications and contraindications

Indications. The following indications apply:
— The patient should be mentally alert and aware of the need to be dry.
— Stress incontinence due to urethral sphincter incompetence should be objectively demonstrable, with or without anterior vaginal wall prolapse.

Contraindications. The following contraindications apply:
— Success is unlikely to follow, if the bladder neck is already well elevated.
— Limitation of vaginal mobility and capacity will render it technically quite difficult to perform the operation.
— Voiding difficulty with several peak flow rates consistently below 15 ml per second, with or without a maximum voiding pressure in excess of 70 cm of water and with a residual urine of more than 200 ml, is likely to be made worse by colposuspension and should be treated before proceeding to surgery.

- Detrusor instability which has not been effectively treated conservatively. The cure of stress incontinence is always less in these circumstances and the patient should be warned that urgency and frequency may be made worse.
- The patient should preferably have completed her child bearing. If not, an elective caesarean section may be a wise suggestion, to avoid harmful effects of the vaginal delivery on the pelvic floor.

Pre-operative evaluation

Pre-operative urodynamic investigations should confirm that the MSU is sterile, urethral sphincter incompetence exists, there is no significant voiding disorder and that the bladder is stable. If there is uterine pathology (e.g. menorrhagia or uterine prolapse), an abdominal hysterectomy is performed beforehand, accompanied by a Moschowitz closure of the Pouch of Douglas if there is an enterocele. Any rectocele is corrected by a posterior repair, following the colposuspension. Both of these procedures should be performed as a rectocele and an enterocele are both made worse by colposuspension.

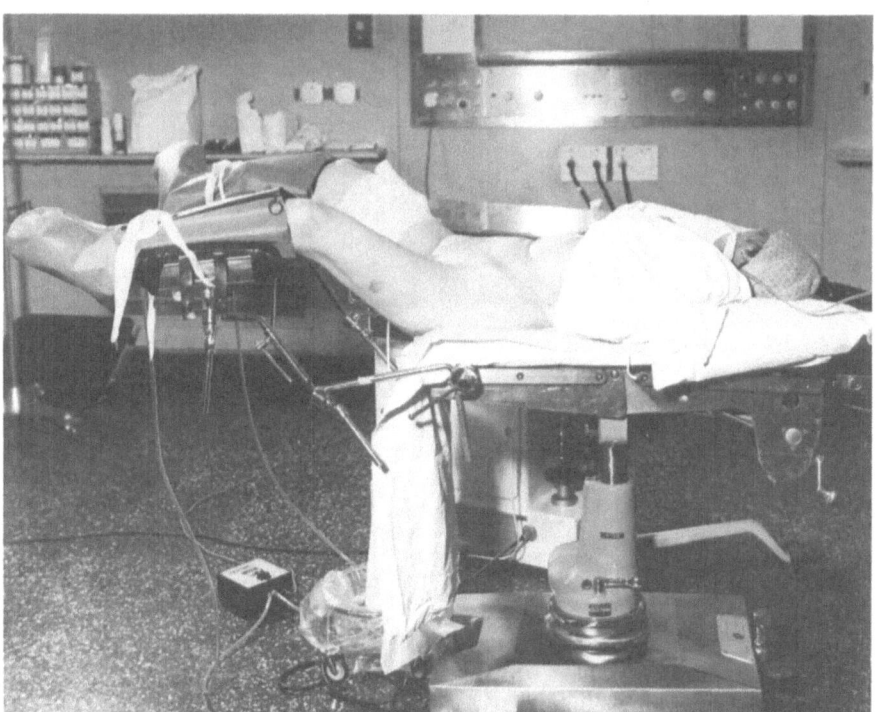

Fig. 1. Patient in horizontal lithotomy position.

96

Technique

The patient is placed in the horizontal lithotomy position, with the legs supported in Lloyd-Davies or similar stirrups (Fig. 1) and anti-thrombotic boots or stockings are worn. Both the abdomen and perineal regions are prepared and draped and a TUR drape used to cover the vulva and gain access to the vagina during the operation. A size 14 Fr Foley catheter is inserted to drain the bladder: this delineates the bladder neck and allows a suprapubic catheter to be inserted after the operation.

A low pfannenstiel incision is made, approximately 1 finger breadth above the symphysis pubis, the rectus sheath incised horizontally and the

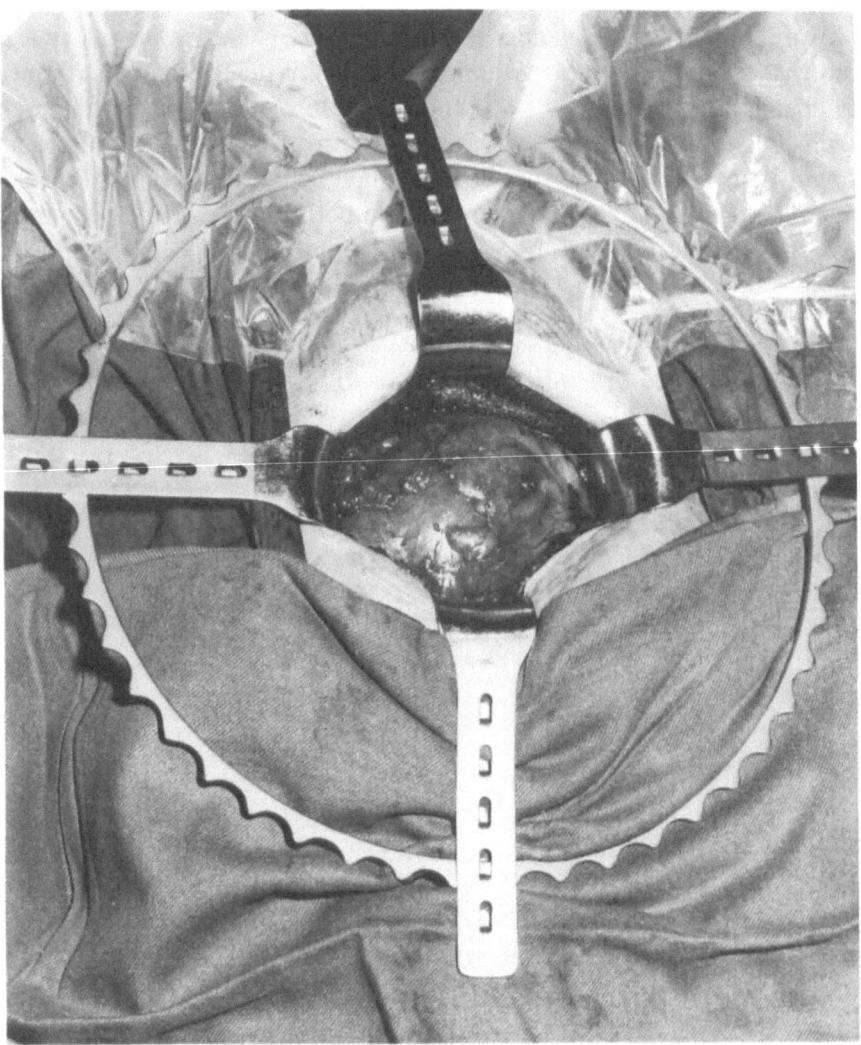

Fig. 2. Denis Brown ring retractor.

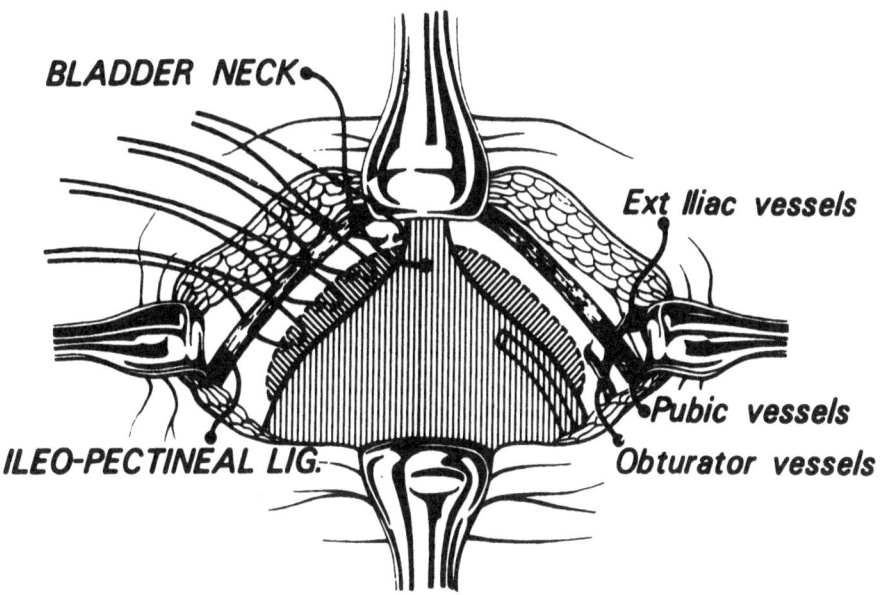

Fig. 3. Plan showing relationship of ileopectineal ligament, bladder, urethra and ureters.

bladder and urethra gently separated by a blunt dissection from the posterio-supero aspect of the symphysis. If there has been a previous lower abdominal scar, a Czerney incision is used, which incises the recti at their insertion. A four bladed Denis Brown ring retractor is used (Fig. 2). The operator inserts the forefinger of one hand into the vagina and elevates a lateral fornix. Using blunt or scissor dissection, he sweeps the bladder base medially off the underlying white paravaginal fascia. Care is taken to avoid the large perivesical veins which may be visible. The relationship of the bladder and urethra and ureters to the fascia is shown in Fig. 3. Three sutures of either an absorbable suture (number 1 polyglycolic acid e.g. Vicryl or Dexon) or unabsorbable suture (number 1 polybutylate coated polyester e.g. Ethibond) is used on either side, to anchor the paravaginal fascia to a corresponding part on the ipsilateral ileopectineal (Cooper's) ligament. A suture is placed opposite the bladder neck and two proximal (Cephalid) sutures placed alongside the bladder base. Each suture is tied in place on the paravaginal fascia before being inserted into the ileopectineal ligament. This aids haemostasis and prevents the suture seesawing through the fascia when it is tied later on. Haemostasis is also achieved by diathermy, oversewing and ultimately by elevation of paravaginal tissue.

Once all sutures are in place and haemostasis is complete, they are tied and a redivac drain is left in place. The wound is closed, the bladder is filled via the Foley catheter, and a Bonanno or similar suprapubic catheter is inserted.

Post-operative management

An accurate fluid chart should be maintained with an input of 2.5 litres a day. The patient is placed on an anti-bacterial agent e.g. Trimethoprim 200 mg bd until the catheter is removed. Regular catheter specimens of urine are sent for culture and sensitivity.

The catheter is left on free drainage for 24 hours and then clamped at 8.00 a.m. on the second day. It remains clamped for 8–10 hours and a residual urine is measured via the suprapubic catheter at the end of that time. If the patient fails to void or is in pain, the catheter is released, and reclamped the following morning. Once the evening residual urine is less than 100 ml and the patient is voiding more than 200 ml at a time, the catheter may be clamped overnight. It is removed the following morning provided neither retention nor incontinence have occurred.

The redivac drain is removed at 24–36 hours. Mobilisation is encouraged after 24 hours and if voiding normally, the patient may be discharged home by the seventh day.

The patient is asked to avoid intercourse for 2 months (because of temporary dyspareunia) and heavy lifting or any exertion which significantly raises the intra-abdominal pressure.

Complications

Intra-operative complications are not common, but they include trauma to the bladder and urethra during dissection, haemorrhage and ureteric ligation.

Post-operative complications include recurrence of incontinence, detrusor instability and voiding difficulties. Detrusor instability may occur more frequently when there has been previous bladder neck surgery. Voiding difficulties may be caused by excess elevation and diminished excursion of the bladder neck.

Results

To adequately assess continence procedures, it is necessary to use objective measures and have a follow-up extending to at least 5 years. Burch [3] followed 143 patients for varying times up to and beyond 5 years, and found satisfactory subjective improvement in 93%. We reported on 88 patients followed for 1 year [4] and found on objective testing, that an overall 87.5% were cured at one year: without previous continence surgery, this figure rose to 96%. When followed to 5 years [5], there was an overall objective cure of

78% in a smaller group of 42 patients. One explanation for the deterioration of results, is the use of polyglycolic acid suture which is absorbable, and the author now prefers the more permanent polybutylate coated polyester.

References

1. Burch J.C. Urethrovaginal fixation to Cooper's ligament for correction of stress incontinence, cystocele and prolapse. Am. J. Obstet. Gynec. 81 (1961): 281–294.
2. Hodgkinson C.P. and Stanton S.L. Retropubic urethropexy or colposuspension. 'Surgery of Female Incontinence'. Eds. Stuart L. Stanton and Emil Tanagho. Springer-Verlag, Heidelberg, 1st Edition. (1980) pp. 55–68.
3. Burch J.C. Cooper's ligament urethrovesical suspension for stress incontinence. Am. J. Obstet. Gynec. 100 (1968): 764–772.
4. Stanton S.L. and Cardozo, L. Results of colposuspension operation for incontinence and prolapse. Brit. J. Obstet. Gynaec. 86 (1979): 693–697.
5. Stanton S.L., Hertogs K., Cox C., Hilton P. and Cardozo L. Colposuspension operation for genuine stress incontinence: A 5 year study. Proceedings of the 12th Annual Meeting ICS, Leiden, (1982) pp. 94–96.

II.6. Turner-Warwick vagino-obturator shelf urethral-repositioning procedure

R. TURNER-WARWICK

The vagino-obturator shelf urethral-repositioning operation is conceptually a 'urodynamically pure' procedure [1, 2]: it not only repositions the urethral and the bladder neck sphincter mechanisms most efficiently, but leaves them free-lying in an elevated position without compromising their occlusive function by fixation, para-urethral tethering, or urethral compression; furthermore the development of secondary retropubic fibrotic adhesions is positively prevented by interposing a supple omental pedicle graft between the back of the pubis and the urethra – this not only ensures the mobility of the functional movements of the intrinsic sphincter mechanisms in the long term but ensures the circumferential transmission of intra-abdominal pressure changes to the urethra [3].

The basic principle of the procedures is that the vaginal wall is simply prolapsed through a definitive incision in the para-urethral fascia on both sides of the urethra and firmly anchored to the internal obturator muscle on either side by large-bite tissue-approximating sutures.

It is fundamentally important to appreciate that only the lower 4–5 cm of the vaginal wall relates to the urethra at the bladder neck and it is only this part that is used for the vagino-obturator shelf support: above this the anterior vaginal wall relates to the posterior bladder wall and descent of this may create voiding problems, particularly when the detrusor is under-active [4], thus the vagino-obturator shelf procedure additionally involves a transperitoneal vaginal vault suspension procedure and an occlusion of the recto-vaginal pouch to prevent a subsequent enterocoele [5].

The vagino-obturator shelf procedure can be regarded as a 'urodynamically pure' procedure, because it achieves most effective repositioning of the bladder neck and urethra in an elevated free-lying position specifically avoiding any fixation of the para-urethral fascia that might compromise the functional movements of its intrinsic sphincter mechanisms or introduce an element of urethral obstruction.

The vagino-obturator shelf procedure was originally described as a 'colpo-suspension [1], however this term has been generally adopted to include other distinctive different procedures such as the Burch suspension operation, the principle of which is distinctly different in as much as the sling-sutures which suspend the vaginal wall from Cooper's ligament anterio-laterally on the pelvic brim include para-urethral fascial fixation and commonly have to be 'bow-strung' when the tissue bites are insufficiently lax to be suture-approximated. Traction on the para-urethral fascia introduces an additional lateral tethering effect that may or may not compromise urethral sphincter function and may introduce an element of passive bladder outlet occlusion which, while it may marginally improve the leak-proof success of the procedure, may increase the incidence of postoperative voiding inefficiency.

Because the vagino-obturator shelf procedure simply repositions the urethra without any element of compression it rarely causes difficulty with voiding postoperatively and sometimes even improves a pre-existing voiding inefficiency associated with vesico-urethral descent – thus it may be particularly appropriate for the treatment of patients whose vesico-urethral descent is associated with both stress incontinence and with a significant volume of post-voiding residual urine [3].

The potential of sphincter-function impairment by retropubic tethering is readily apparent in the male after pelvic fracture injuries of the sub-prostatic urethra which almost always destroys the functional competence of the distal sphincter mechanism; in such cases the commonest cause of an associated incompetence of the only residual sphincter mechanism at the bladder neck is its tethering-open by the retraction of an extensive haematoma fibrosis surrounding it and its competence, and consequently continence can often be restored by simple lysis and replacement of the resected fibrosis by a supple omental graft. This calls to question the precept of achieving vesico-urethral repositioning by definitive retropubic cystourethropexy procedure of Marshall-Marchetti-Krantz.

The Turner-Warwick vagino-obturator shelf procedure for urethral repositioning

1. The patient is positioned on the operating table for a synchronous abdomino-vaginal approach.
2. A wide exposure of the pelvis and lower abdomen is required; a Pfannenstiel incision is quite inadequate – a suprapubic V-exposure [6] or a midline incision is appropriate: ring retraction is most effective.
3. The retropubic space is developed, the anterior wall of the lower segment of the bladder and urethra exposed and the position of the bladder neck identified with a balloon catheter in the urethra (Fig. 1A).
4. The para-urethral fascia is incised lateral to the urethra and bladder neck on both sides. No para-urethral musculature is encountered in this

102

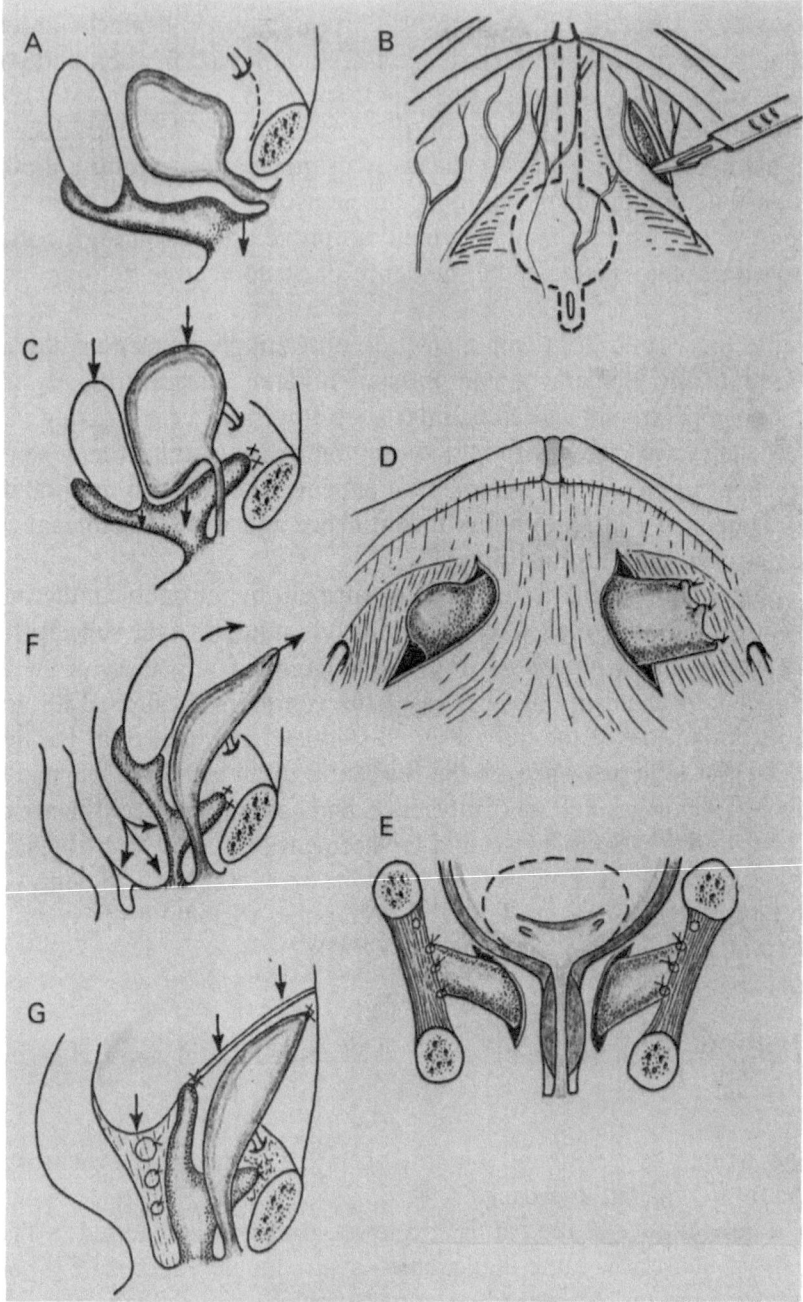

Fig. 1A-G. The Turner-Warwick vagino-obturator shelf urethral repositioning procedure (see text).

area because there is none [7]. Bleeding from the para-urethral venous plexus is primarily controlled by upward pressure by a finger in the vagina, definitive haemostasis is achieved with broad-tipped electrocoagulating forceps (Fig. 1B).

5. The long Turner-Warwick electro-coagulating scissors are particularly helpful for the development of the incision and of the para-vaginal tissue plane that enables the vaginal wall to be prolapsed through the incision to reach the inner margin of the internal obturator muscle (Fig. 1C-D).

6. The plane between the vagina and the urethra may be more difficult to develop, when there are adhesions resulting from previous surgery; in such cases the plane of scissor-dissection should be close to the finger in the vagina to avoid injury to the urethral musculature. A small perforation of the vagina wall is of no consequence. A small volume of blue dye introduced into the bladder gives early warning of the thinning of its wall in the process of separating secondary adhesions in this area.

7. The mobilised lower anterior vaginal wall is prolapsed through the retropubic para-urethral incisions and anchored to the obturator internus muscle with three or four large-bite PGA sutures (Fig. 1E). The lateral location of the obturator nerve and vessel tunnel is easy to identify and to avoid.

8. The mobility of the urethra elevated by the vagino-obturator shelf is checked to ensure that there are no residual lateral tethering adhesions.

9. A suprapubic catheter is simply inserted by pulling it into the bladder with a pair of forceps thrust through a double fold of the vault of the vagina and a simple purse-string around the opposing forceps-hole.

10. The peritoneum is open above the bladder and the bowel retracted by the deep blades of the ring retractor to expose the whole of the pelvic floor. It is sometimes necessary to relax the utero-sacral folds, or fibrosis resulting from previous pelvic surgery, to enable the vaginal vault to come foreward (Fig. 1F).

11. The vault of the vagina is elevated to ensure that there is no residual vault prolapse. This can sometimes be achieved by elevating the uterus by one of its round ligaments and suture-anchoring it to the inner surface of the anterior abdominal wall on one side (not both because this can reduce the bladder capacity by incarceration). When the uterus is insufficiently mobile to enable the anterior vaginal wall to be elevated by tractions upon it, or after a previous hysterectomy, the vaginal vault can be elevated by suturing the divided ends of both round ligaments to it directly (Fig. 1G).

12. Anterior suspension of the vaginal vault increases the exposure of the posterior vaginal wall to the intra-abdominal pelvic floor pressure and

it is generally advisable to plicate the recto-vaginal peritoneal pouch by a series of occlusive purse-string Moscovitch sutures taking care to avoid distorting the ureters with the upper sutures. Although the peritoneal approximation involved in this procedure may appear somewhat tenuous it is remarkably effective.

13. The omental apron is mobilised from the transverse colon and meso-colic mesentery and if necessary, by division of some of its left pedicle vessels [7]. The lower margin of its apron is repositioned into the retropubic space and suture-anchored there to prevent immobilisation of the V-O shelf-elevated urethral sphincter mechanisms by secondary fibrotic adhesions.

14. It is generally wise to drain the retropubic space although the lymphatic drainage of the repositioned omentum provides reasonably effective physiological drainage.

15. The urethral catheter is removed and the suprapubic catheter placed on free drainage for 4–5 days when it is trial-clamped and finally removed when measurements of the post-voiding residual urine show that the volume is acceptably small.

References

1. Turner-Warwick R. The management of bladder neck dysfunction. In: Eric Riches (ed) Modern Trends in Urology. Butterworth, London (1969).
2. Turner-Warwick R. Urethral surgery. In: J. Glenn (ed) Urologic Surgery. Harper and Roe, chapter 68 (1982).
3. Turner-Warwick R. and Whiteside C.G. Urodynamic studies and their effect upon management. In: Chisholm G.B. and Inneswilliams D. (eds) Scientific Foundation of Urology. Heineman, London (1982).
4. Farrar D. and Turner-Warwick R. In: Clinical Urodynamics. Clin. N. America 6 (1979).
5. Turner-Warwick R. The vagino-obturator shelf urethral repositioning procedure. London University, Institute of Urology, Film Library, London (1973).
6. Turner-Warwick R., Worth P.H.L., Milroy E.J.G. and Duckett J. The suprapubic V-incision. Brit. J. Urol. 46 (1974): 39–45.
7. Turner-Warwick R. Surgical access in urology. Chisholm G.B. (ed), Heineman, London (1980).

II.7. Vaginal plasty operation for stress incontinence using fascia lata substitute

L. MONTAUBAN VAN SWIJNDREGT & M. VAN GIJSEN

Introduction

After careful evaluation of a patient with stress incontinence the major problem is the choice of an adequate treatment. If conservative medical treatment fails what is then the appropriate surgical approach? After different trials of surgical interventions, we prefer the sling-operation for primary and secundary cases (patients with recurrent stress incontinence following previous surgery).

In the first period we always used the fascia of the musculus rectus, both slings were obtained by horizontal incision of the fascia after Pfannenstiel approach. This Goebel-Stoeckel method gave us very good results but we avoided sacrifying a part of the fascia, especially in patients who had a previous Pfannenstiel incision and to prevent secundary eventrations. To get round this difficulty we tried the FASCIA LATA SUBSTITUTE of Ethicon (second period). This method is simple, hospitalisation shorter and after one year we had the impression that the results were better. For several years this has been the method of choice for all our incontinent patients.

Unfortunately Ethicon discontinued production of this material and they asked us to try ZENODERM, a porcine fascia. As contrasted with autologous fascia, Zenoderm possesses more than adequate tensile strength, it is stronger, more rigid than the former but you have to adapt the tension-toleration again. The morphological similarity of porcine dermis to human collagen is preserved and presents to the host an interface of naturally orientated material (third period).

The complete urological check-up is always performed in collaboration with the urologist. If there is even a slight suspicion of infection or other urological abnormality (like bladder instability) we delay the operation and specific treatment is started.

In our opinion, the psychosomatic and neurological evaluation is very important. After scrupulous investigation we found that in about 10% of patients there were periods of neuropsychological instability with increasing incontinence. These were often in relation to the menstruation cycle, family problems or perimenopausal difficulties. Special attention was given to sportswomen complaining of incontinence during basket or volleyball games and an acceptable solution is a 'do-it-yourself' pessarium. If medical treatment with anticholinergics or estrogens or pelvic floor exercises does not result in long-standing improvement, we advise the operation.

Operation technique

The operation consists of the vagino-abdominal suprapubic approach by blunt dissection and going blindfold through the Retzius space reaching the rectus fascia. To avoid bladder injury we now perform the blunt dissection from below and also from the rectus fascia and this bidigital approach seems safer. After the introduction of the sling the bladder is filled with methylene blue to detect any possible leakage. If necessary we also execute a anterior cystocolporrhaphy and if severe relaxation of the pelvic floor is present a posterior perineorrhaphy with approaching of the levator muscle is carried out.

After the operation an indwelling catheter is left for 4 days and is pinched off every 5 hours. Parenteral antibiotics are given for 5 days and an oral urosepticum is given for 10 days after removal of the catheter.

In all peri- and postmenopausal patients the estrogen supply is imperative and we ask to continue it for the rest of their life. The dosage (oral or vaginal) depends of course on the age and menopausal problems of the patient.

Complications

In the postoperative period a slight retention is normal but if severe retention (6 cases) persists, an indwelling catheter (Ch. 20) is replaced for 3 days. In three cases the bladder was slightly injured with positive methylene blue test. The sling was readjusted by bidigital approach and in those cases we left the bladder catheter for 8 to 10 days. This complication happened twice by secundary stress incontinence operation. Two patients had a severe haemorrhage of the Retzius space so that a wicktamponade through the paraurethral spaces was necessary for two days. In two cases of irreductible retention, removal of the sling stitches on the rectus fascia was necessary but the sling was left in situ. Fortunately there were no cases with thromboembolic complications.

Results

In 60 cases the follow-up period was sufficient to evaluate the results. Distribution of the patients: average age: 45 years nullipara: 2 = 3.3%; primipara : 9 = 15%; pluripara : 49 = 81.7%.

From the 60 patients who underwent a sling procedure there were 52 primary slings and 8 patients who had had a previous stress incontinence operation. The combination of colpo-cystorrhaphy and sling was carried out in 20 cases. Two patients had a normal delivery after operation. One year after the operation very good results showed in 90% of cases; good: 5% and failure: 5%.

After three years we noticed that the very good results dropped to 85% and this was often in the postmenopausal patients who neglected to take estrogen.

Total patients: N = 70
Patients in this study: N = 60
10 Patients follow up too short (less than 1 year)
Average age: 45 years
Nullipara   2 (3,3%)
Primipara   9 (15%)
Pluripara   49 (81,7%)

Post vaginal hysterectomy	2 ×
Post abdominal hysterectomy	6 ×
Primary sling	52 ×
After former incontinence operation	8 ×
Combination with colpo-cystorrhaphy	20 ×
Anesthesia: E.D.A.	70%
Total anesthesia	30%

Results:
Very good : 90%
Good   : 5%
Failure   : 5% (2 Reinterventions)
After 3 years: Very good drops to 85% often in postmenopausal patients neglecting estrogen suppliance

---

Discussion

In spite of the opinion of some authors on the subject [2] we prefer the sling procedure for primary and secundary cases.

In our hands Kelly-, Marion- and Marshall M.K.-operations were less successful than our sling procedures. This is probably due to bigger experience with the latter operations and therefore a greater technical skill.

Beck [3] describes the results of the Marshall M.K.-operation at the University of Alberta Hospital and becomes good results in 80%. In other publications [1, 2] however he describes 88% good results with the sling procedure and 76% when cases of recurrence of incontinence due to detrusor overactivity are included. But he warns against postoperative retention and dysuria and uses this technique only in selected cases. In his monography on stress incontinence and sling operations [6] de Bruin, who followed his patients for many years, noted a success rate of 86%. Dargent [5] compares the results of three techniques in 240 patients and concludes that the sling procedures provides longer and better results. Cukier [4] reports about the same results. Non-published data by Bressel (Hamburg) and Hohenfellner (Mainz) confirm this success rate. Jarvis (University of Leeds) who now uses Zenoderm corium implants confirms that this material gives the same good results as the former fascia lata substitute Kaisary [7] uses Zenoderm with success in rectopexy. Stanton [9] presented a sling procedure with Dacron-reinforced silastic, a material that does not react with the surrounding tissues. In our material some patients presented periods of prolonged retentions, but in the literature [8-10] we found far more cases of dysuria and urge incontinence after a Burch or other procedure than in our own sling series. Fortunately we had no thrombo-embolic accidents nor major infections and the delivered patients had no postpartum recurrence.

Conclusion

This contribution to stress incontinence surgery shows that fascia lata substitute is a good material for sling operations. Therefore this technique is now our method of choice in all cases of stress incontinence.

References

1. Beck R.P., Grove D., Arnush D. and Harvey J. Recurrent urinary stress incontinence treated by fascia lata sling procedure. Am. J. O & G. 120 (1974): 613–621.
2. Beck R.P. The sling operation: gynecological and obstetrical urology. Saunders: Toronto (1978).
3. Beck R.P. Recent advances in obstetrics and gynecology. No. 13 (1979).
4. Cukier J. Les bandelettes aponévrotiques libres sous-cervicales dans la cure chirurgicale de l'incontincence des urines à l'effort chez la femme. Act. Urolog. Belgica, vol. 52 (1984): 322–325.
5. Dargent D., Mellier G. and Valentin B. (Lyon). Résultat du traitement chirurgical de l'incontinence urinaire d'effort par les techniques de Michon, Kelly et Marshall-Marchetti-Burch. Vol. 52, (1984): 297–301.
6. De Bruin A.J.J. Stress incontinentie bij de vrouw en lusoperaties. Van Gorcum's Medische bibliotheek nr. 155 Assen (1958).

7. Kaisary A., Luck R., Pendower J. Use of collagen implant for posterior rectopexy in complete rectal prolapse: preliminary communication. Journal of the Royal Society of Medicine. Volume 77, (1984): 201–203.
8. Stanton S.L. The Burch colposuspension procedure. Act. Urolog. Belgica, vol. 52, (1984): 280–282.
9. Stanton S.L. and Brindley G. A silastic sling for urinary incontinence. Proceedings of the 12th annual meeting of the Int. Cont. Society, Leiden (1982).
10. Verges et al. (Paris). Les complications de l'intervention de Burch. Act. Urolog. Belgica, vol. 52 (1984): 283–285.

CHAPTER THREE

Recurrent urinary stress incontinence

III.1. Recurrent urinary stress incontinence: evaluation and therapy

L.M. DAIRIKI SHORTLIFFE & T.A. STAMEY

Introduction

When a patient is said to have recurrent stress urinary incontinence, by definition, it means they have incontinence which occurs after apparent cure of incontinence. In many cases, the circumstances of this condition are unclear. Often it cannot be established whether the patient has incontinence which persists after treatment or whether the patient was cured of incontinence (i.e., became continent) and then has incontinence reappear. In either case, the patient has incontinence which is present after having had some form of treatment.

As others have clearly stated: 'There is no doubt that the prime operation (for stress urinary incontinence) is the initial one and that for every subsequent operation, the 'cure' rate declines more or less proportional to the number of subsequent operations' [1]. In reviewing the common operations which are currently used to correct stress urinary incontinence, we find a 5–15 percent failure rate associated with each. To deal with these failures we need to ask two questions: first, why do the failures occur, and second, what should be done about them.

Operative failure can be attributed to two causes. Either the patient was wrong for the operation or the operation went wrong. It is of paramount importance for the patient operated upon for stress urinary incontinence to have stress urinary incontinence. If the patient has detrusor incontinence caused by involuntary contractions, an acontractile detrusor, a vesicovaginal fistula, or ureteral incontinence caused by an ectopic ureter, a uretero-vaginal fistula, or urethral incontinence caused by a ureterocele, an operation designed to correct stress urinary incontinence performed under these circumstances will likely fail. On the other hand, even if the patient has stress urinary incontinence, failure may be caused by suture placement which has obstructed the urethra, inadequately elevated the urethrovesical tissues behind the pubic symphysis, or by surgical complications such as suture breakage, inability to elevate the bladder neck because of periurethral fibrosis, or early breakdown of repair related to poor tissues.

Evaluation of the patient with recurrent stress incontinence

The methods we have used to evaluate women with recurrent stress incontinence are the same as those we have used to evaluate primary stress incontinence. The patient's history of quantity and time of her urinary leakage will determine the severity of the problem for the individual, and it is particularly important to identify urgency incontinence. A history of incontinence associated with suprapubic pain, dysuria, and small bladder volumes, or nocturnal leakage alone, may cause one to consider other diagnoses, such as interstitial cystitis, or neuropathic bladder.

The physical examination is key to the identification of the woman with surgically correctable stress incontinence. Women who have such incontinence will have demonstrable stress incontinence during their examination. This usually can be established during the physical examination with only a few additional maneuvers. While the patient's history is taken she is asked to drink fluids. When she feels she must void, she voids into a measuring pan in the bathroom. Immediately after voiding she is placed in the lithotomy position and is catheterized with a 14 French urethral catheter to measure the postvoid residual urine. A specimen is taken for culture and microscopic examination. The empty barrel of a 50 ml catheter tip syringe is attached to the indwelling urethral catheter and water is run through the catheter into the patient's bladder by gravity flow until the patient says she feels comfortably full (generally 250–350 ml). The volume when the patient first senses bladder fullness, and any spontaneous detrusor contractions, manifest by sudden rises in water level during the bladder filling, are noted. While still in the lithotomy position the patient is asked to cough and she is examined for urinary leakage. If leakage is not seen in this position, the head of the table is elevated 30–45 degrees and the maneuver is repeated. If still no leakage is observed, the patient stands with her legs apart and coughs, while the observer holds the labia apart. Leakage should occur directly related to the cough without delay. A delay of a few seconds suggests that the cough has provoked a detrusor contraction which has then caused incontinence. This examination by the surgeon is important because the patient may not be able to differentiate stress incontinence from other causes of incontinence and may wrongly relate her leakage to physically stressful activity. In addition, observation of spontaneous detrusor contractions or an increased postvoid residual urine volume will identify women who may need further evaluation.

While formal urodynamic studies will determine urethral pressures and bladder dynamics, they are not the test to establish stress incontinence nor identify the patient with surgically correctable incontinence. Not only may the urodynamics urethral catheter obstruct the urethra and prevent leakage, but demonstration of bladder instability is not necessarily a contraindication to surgery. In a series of 151 women with unselected urinary incontinence in whom full urodynamic studies were performed, there were no measurements of the detrusor dynamics which differentiated women with demonstrable stress urinary incontinence from those with other kinds of incontinence [2]. And, perhaps even more interesting is that the presence of preoperative bladder instability (involuntary, unsuppressible detrusor contractions causing the loss of urine) did not predict patients who experienced postoperative difficulties with instability.

Although the lateral chain cystogram is occasionally helpful to determine the position of the bladder neck after multiple failed incontinence surgeries, in most cases this knowledge is not useful for planning further surgery, and hence, has not been performed for routine preoperative evaluation. Although earlier authors have recommended that the position of the bladder neck on the lateral chain cystogram may help plan which operation will best correct stress incontinence [3], if the corrective operation elevates the bladder neck substantially behind the pubic symphysis, these considerations may be ignored. Cystoscopy is almost never diagnostic in the evaluation of women with stress incontinence.

Therapy of recurrent stress incontinence: experience with the endoscopic suspension

If a patient was incorrectly diagnosed to have stress urinary incontinence, and was then unsuccessfully operated upon with surgery designed to correct stress urinary incontinence, this reason for operative failure should be apparent from the evaluation. If, however, a patient has genuine stress urinary incontinence even if recurrent, a procedure which reliably elevates the bladder neck behind the symphysis pubis probably will be successful in most instances. Although many modern procedures accomplish this, fibrosis and scarring in patients with recurrent stress incontinence may make surgery and suture placement difficult. Ideal surgical correction in these women should require minimal dissection around the bladder neck tissues, ensure correct suture placement at the bladder neck, and need not rely totally on the patients tissue strength alone.

Although several modern procedures fit these criteria, our experience has been with the endoscopic suspension of the bladder neck described by Stamey in 1973 [4]. This operation has been described in detail elsewhere [2, 4, 5]. It uses specially designed long needles passed from small suprapubic incisions into the periurethral tissues vaginally to place two No. 2 monofilament nylon sutures. These 2 sutures elevate the tissues on both sides of the bladder neck. Passage of the needles is guided by the surgeon with the use of the cystoscope to ensure correct placement of the sutures at the bladder neck. Dacron bolsters are used on the vaginal side of the sutures to prevent the nylon from pulling through weak tissues.

The endoscopic suspension operation has advantages over other commonly used methods designed to correct stress urinary incontinence. The need for a large, painful suprapubic incision with retraction of the rectus muscles and extensive dissection around a scarred bladder neck and retropubic region are avoided. As a result, previous pelvic fractures, previous attempts at correction of stress incontinence, obesity, or radiation fibrosis, do not necessarily increase the difficulty or morbidity of this procedure. The internal vesical neck can be easily identified with the cystoscope, which permits exact suture placement. Even with open surgical inspection of the bladder neck, the internal vesical neck cannot be identified as accurately as with the cystoscope. Moreover, using cystoscopy allows the surgeon to be certain that a suture is not placed within the bladder or uretha. Finally, dacron bolsters placed below the periurethral tissues provide additional support and strength to these tissues and help to prevent the nylon from pulling through weak tissues. This buttressing of vaginal and periurethral tissues is not possible in procedures that expose the vesical neck from the suprapubic approach alone.

The Stanford experience with endoscopic suspension of the vesical neck to correct urinary stress incontinence confirms that the operation is as successful in recurrent urinary stress incontinence as in the virginal case. In a series of 203 women who had the operation, 188 of the 203 women had had previous surgery for urinary stress incontinence. Seventy-four had had previous Marshall-Marchetti-Krantz operations. In addition, 160 of these patients had grade 2 (leakage with walking and other minimally stressful activities) or worse stress incontinence, and 41 had total incontinence. Still, of the 203 women, the majority of whom had 'recurrent stress urinary incontinence' and moderate to severe incontinence, the success rate was still 91 percent. Thirty-two of the 41 women with total incontinence were cured [6].

These studies also showed that elevation of the bladder neck was accomplished as easily in women who had had previous surgery for urinary incontinence as in those who had not. Lateral chain cystograms which show the position of the bladder base relative to the symphyseal-sacral line during straining in women who were cured of incontinence before and after operation showed a 49 mm mean elevation of the bladder base in 15 women without previous surgery and a 46 mm elevation in 19 having had previous surgery [7]. The presence or absence of a uterus played no role in the condition or treatment of the incontinence [6].

Although some authors have stated that surgery for urinary stress incontinence may be contraindicated in women who have some urgency incontinence and this may be a reason for a failed operation, data on patients at

Stanford have not supported this. In 41 women who underwent successful endoscopic suspension of the bladder neck, preoperatively 5 had marked urgency and 19 had minimal complaints of urgency; postoperatively only 1 had marked urgency and 15 had minimal urgency. The 3 patients who were not improved with the endoscopic suspension had minimal urgency incontinence preoperatively, and postoperatively one had these symptoms disappear while the other 2 had worsening of their urgency [2]. Symptoms of preoperative urgency incontinence when present with genuine stress incontinence are, therefore, not absolute contraindications to the surgical correction of urinary stress incontinence.

Conclusion

The evaluation and treatement of recurrent stress urinary incontinence should be no different from primary stress urinary incontinence, and in either case it is essential to determine if the patient has genuine and demonstable stress incontinence. Although in the majority of the patients this can be determined using careful office examination and observation alone, in some patients with confusing findings and multiple previous operations urodynamic studies may be helpful to show bladder instability. We do not feel, however, that instability in patients with demonstrable stress incontinence is necessarily a contraindication to surgical correction. Any procedure which reliably elevates the bladder neck behind the pubic symphysis will cure most women with stress incontinence, but in those women with recurrent problems and multiple previous operations, an operation which dissects the bladder neck minimally, offers good placement of the sutures at the bladder neck even if it is scarred, and provides additional support to buttress the patient's own tissues is desirable.

References

1. Hodgkinson C.P. and Stanton S.L. Retropubic urethropexy or colposuspension. In: Stanton S.L. and Tanagho E.A. (ed) Surgery of Female Incontinence, Springer-Verlag, New York, (1980) 55–68.
2. Shortliffe L.D. and Stamey T.A. Urinary incontinence in the female. In: Gittes, Perlmutter, Stamey, Walsh (eds) Campbell's Urology, 5th Edition, WB Saunders, Philadelphia (1985).
3. Green T.H. Development of a plan for the diagnosis and treatment of urinary stress incontinence. Am. J. Obst. & Gynec., 83 (1962): 632–648.
4. Stamey T.A. Endoscopic suspension of the vesical neck for urinary incontinence. Surg. Gynecol. Obstet. 136 (1973): 547–554.
5. Stamey T.A. Endoscopic suspension of the vesical neck for surgically curable urinary incontinence in the female. Monographs in Urology, 2 (1981): 65–100.

6. Stamey T.A. Endoscopic suspension of the vesical neck for urinary incontinence in females: Report on 203 consecutive patients. Ann. Surg., 192 (1980): 465–471.
7. Stamey T.A., Schaeffer A.J. and Condy M. Clinical and roentgenographic evaluation of endoscopic suspension of the vesical neck for urinary incontinence. Surg. Gynecol. Obstet., 140 (1975): 355.

III.2. The treatment of recurrent urinary stress incontinence: a urological view

H.R. HADLEY, P.E. ZIMMERN & S. RAZ

Introduction

Urinary continence in the normal female depends on the bladder's capability to accomodate increasing volumes of urine and the urethra's ability to maintain a sufficient resistance to overcome intravesical pressure. Urinary incontinence, therefore, occurs when the sphincter mechanisms of the urethra are incapable of generating enough resistance to hold urine; or the bladder is unable to accept increasing quantities of urine without a significant rise in the intravesical pressure.

In women suffering from stress urinary incontinence, the sphincteric unit (inner mucosal layer, smooth muscle, and skeletal muscle) is usually intact. Their incontinence is rarely due to an intrinsic abnormality of the urethral sphincters, but is most commonly due to the physiologic changes of the sphincter mechanisms that may be associated with the proximal urethra's descent out of its normal intraabdominal position. Because not all patients with urethral descent are incontinent, it is not entirely clear what these physiological changes are. The following are several explanations that have been proposed: (1) There is an ineffective transfer of intraabdominal pressure to the descended urethra. (2) There is inadequate urethral compression because of its hypermobility. (3) The bladder neck tends to open because it moves to the most dependent portion of the bladder. If these physiologic changes are accompanied by adequate compensation from urethral closing pressures, pelvic floor reflex contraction, etc. continence will be preserved. If compensation fails, however, the patient will suffer from stress urinary incontinence. It is the patient who has a normal intrinsic sphincteric unit, urethral descent and/or hypermobility that is most likely to be cured of their stress urinary incontinence by suspending and fixing the bladder and urethra into its normal retropubic position.

Why bladder neck suspension works

Regardless of the approach, bladder neck suspension is designed to restore and fix (without obstruction) the urethra and bladder neck into their normal intraabdominal retropubic positions. This maneuver will cure incontinence 85–95% of the time. Although the mechanism of cure is not known, there are some objective observations consistently noted in patients who have been cured by bladder neck suspension. The following is a list of these observations: (*1*) Physical examination demonstrates a well supported non-mobile urethra and bladder neck. (*2*) Cystoscopic examination demonstrates an elevated and closed bladder neck. (*3*) Lateral cystourethrogram with a urethral catheter in place demonstrates the urethra in a high fixed (non-mobile) retropubic position. A lateral cystourethrogram without a urethral catheter usually demonstrates the level of continence to be at the bladder neck. (*4*) Static urethral pressure profile (UPP) may demonstrate a return to a normal functional urethral length with or without an increase in closing pressure [1, 2]. (*5*) Dynamic urethral pressure profile may reveal a change of negative pressure gradients to positive pressure gradients [3].

As mentioned above, it is not well understood why placing the urethra back into its normal intraabdominal position cures most patients with stress urinary incontinence. We will discuss a few of the many concepts that have been proposed as an explanation for this phenomenon.

The first possible explanation is that restoration of the urethra to its normal fixed retropubic position places the urethra in a position where an increase in the intraabdominal pressure can be effectively transmitted to the urethra. During coughing or a Valsalva maneuver, therefore, the increase in intravesical pressure will be met by an equal and simultaneous increase in intraurethral pressure, thus preserving continence. A second explanation is that a bladder neck suspension places the urethra in a retropubic location where reflex pelvic floor contraction, which normally occurs during a cough or Valsalva maneuver, will be more effective in increasing the intraurethral pressure. A third explanation is that a fixed support of the urethra offers a 'backboard' on which intraabdominal pressure is exerted. Instead of the intraabdominal pressure being absorbed by downward motion of the urethra, this pressure is used to compress the urethra. In other words, after bladder neck suspension the absorption of the energy produced from an increase in the intraabdominal pressure is converted from urethral mobility to urethral compression. Another explanation may be that a bladder neck suspension moves the internal urethal orifice away from the most dependent portion of the bladder. Maximal downward forces, therefore, are no longer directed on the internal urethral orifice. Indeed, it is possible that the bladder base rotates posteriorly downward towards the newly restored and fixed bladder neck, which effectively creates a valve-like mechanism that closes off the urethra during stress [4]. Finally, restoration of the competency of the bladder neck may be a factor in the cure of stress incontinence. Preoperative radiographs typically demonstrate an open, incompetent bladder neck. After high fixation of the bladder neck and proximal urethra, the bladder neck is commonly seen to be competent on a cystogram.

No single factor can explain why a bladder neck suspension cures stress incontinence. We feel, however, that a combination of all the above mentioned factors contribute to the success of this operation.

Why bladder neck suspension fails

Unfortunately between 5–15% of women undergoing a bladder neck suspension will not be cured of their stress urinary incontinence. Failures are due to inadequate support, damage to the sphincteric unit, complications stemming from the operation, and improper operative indications. It is these operative disappointments that will be the focus of our discussion in this chapter.

Failure to restore the urethra and bladder neck in a high fixed retropubic position is the most frequent cause of continued stress urinary incontinence after bladder neck suspension. This may be due to: the inadequate mobilization of the urethra and bladder neck prior to the suspension; the improper placement of the sutures; the use of improper sutures (catgut sutures may absorb before adequate retropubic adhesions have formed); or poor tissue integrity. Treatment of these patients usually requires an additional attempt at placing the urethra in a high fixed retropubic position. Later in this chapter we will discuss in more detail the operative technique we use to treat recurrent stress urinary incontinence due to an inadequate elevation and fixation of the bladder neck.

Another technical reason for post-operative failure of bladder neck suspension is damage to the intrinsic urethral mechanisms. Multiple operations, damage to the urethra during the dissection, sutures placed too close to the urethra, and/or periurethral scarring may prevent the urethra from supplying adequate closing pressure. These patients will continue to suffer from stress urinary incontinence in spite of a well supported and fixed urethra. Damage to the intrinsic urethral mechanism is more likely to be observed in the operations that place the suspending sutures close to the urethral wall. A patient may have suffered significant damage to the urethra during a previous urethrotomy. The treatment of recurrent stress urinary incontinence due to damage of the intrinsic urethral closing mechanisms is the most challenging to the surgeon. The treatment options are to improve the closing pressure by pharmacological therapy, Polytef (Teflon) injection, urethral reconstruction, urethral fascial sling, or (rarely) artificial sphincter.

Recurrent urinary incontinence after a urethral or bladder neck operation may occur because of post-operative complications. These include: bladder instability, obstruction (with overflow), urethrovaginal, ureterovaginal or vesicovaginal fistulae, or the formation of bladder stones.

Recurrent or persistent incontinence after a bladder neck suspension that is due to improper indications are seen in patients who, in spite of a well supported undamaged urethra, suffer from post-operative urinary incontinence secondary to an overactive bladder. In retrospective studies, detrusor instability has been implicated in as many as 70% of the patients who have failed bladder neck suspension [5–8]. Cordoza and Stanton studied 92 patients with a pre-operative and a post-operative cystometrogram (CMG) and discovered that 18.5% of patients whose bladders were stable prior to a colpocystourethropexy demonstrated bladder instability on a post-operative CMG [9]. None of these patients with an unstable bladder suffered from recurrent incontinence after bladder neck suspension. Others, however, feel that detrusor instability is an uncommon cause of operative failure [10]. Although bladder instability can usually be corrected medically or by electrical stimulation, occasionally a cystolysis and/or enterocystoplasty (cecocystoplasty, ileocystoplasty, or colocystoplasty) may be required to treat the intractable bladder.

Evaluation of the patient with recurrent stress urinary incontinence

Because of the varied causes of recurrent urinary incontinence after bladder neck suspension, complete evaluation of the patient is indicated. This evaluation should include a history, physical examination, cystoscopy, radiographs of the bladder, and full urodynamic assessment. The evaluation of these patients is discussed in detail in other chapters of this text.

Treatment of recurrent stress urinary incontinence

Since most patients with recurrent stress urinary incontinence suffer from inadequate elevation and fixation of the urethra and bladder neck, we will describe first our technique for redo bladder neck suspension. This will be followed by a discussion on the different modalities of treatment we use to treat the stress incontinent patient whose bladder neck is well suspended and the bladder is stable. Finally, we will discuss briefly the treatment of the patient whose recurrent incontinence is due to an overactive bladder.

Transvaginal needle bladder neck suspension (Raz)

Our technique of transvaginal needle suspension of the bladder neck is based on the following principles: (1) An inverted 'U' incision is made in the anterior vaginal wall to allow the vaginal dissection to be lateral to the urethra and bladder neck. (2) The retropubic space is entered in order to sufficiently mobilize the urethra and bladder neck. This principle is especially important in the patient whose urethra is fixed from scarred tissue due to a previous operation(s). (3) The suspension needle is passed with fingertip control to avoid injury to the urethra or bladder. (4) The monofilament suspension sutures are anchored in full-thickness vaginal wall (excluding the epithelium). (5) The suspension sutures are placed in the vaginal wall and endopelvic fascia lateral to the bladder neck. The sutures, therefore, will not interfere with the contraction and shortening of the urethra that normally occurs during voiding. (6) Cystoscopy is done to verify adequate bladder neck elevation and to inspect for injury to the urethra, bladder or ureters. (7) In the suprapubic incision the suspension sutures are tied individually over a Teflon pledget buttress.

The night prior to surgery the patient is started on a course of parenteral antibiotics (an aminoglycoside and ampicillin) and given a Betadine douche to minimize bacterial contamination from the vaginal flora. The patient is placed in the dorsal lithotomy position and then cleansed from the umbilicus to the perineum including the vagina. A Foley catheter is inserted into the bladder and the bladder is emptied. A posterior vaginal retractor is placed in the vagina and the labia are retracted upwards with stay sutures to expose the anterior wall. Traction on the Foley catheter facilitates identification of the level of the bladder neck. A semicircular inverted 'U' incision is made in the anterior wall of the vagina (Fig. 1). The apex of the incision should cross at the level of the mid-urethra where the distinctive glistening white paraurethral fascia is identified. At the level of the bladder neck the dissection under the anterior vaginal wall is advanced laterally towards the pubic bone (Fig. 2). The retropubic space is then entered either bluntly or sharply between the pubic bone and the endopelvic fascia. A finger is inserted through this incision and gently frees the endopelvic fascia from its lateral attachments to the pubic bone (Fig. 3). If the retropubic space is entered in this plane, bleeding should not be troublesome and injury to the bladder or the ureter very unlikely. The mobilization is extended down to the level of the ischial tuberosity in order to create adequate mobility of the vaginal wall, bladder neck, and urethra. In most patients who have had a previous urethal suspension, sufficient mobility usually requires sharp dissection of the periurethral and perivaginal scar tissue. A No. 6 Mayo needle is used to secure a No. 1 Prolene suture in the vaginal wall at a point lateral to the bladder neck. The suture should include at least 3 separate passes through the whole vaginal wall excluding the epithelium so as to form a helicoidal suture line (Fig. 4). After each pass of the needle, traction should be placed on the suture to test the integrity of the tissue and to assure the surgeon that a sufficient amount of vaginal wall has been secured. The

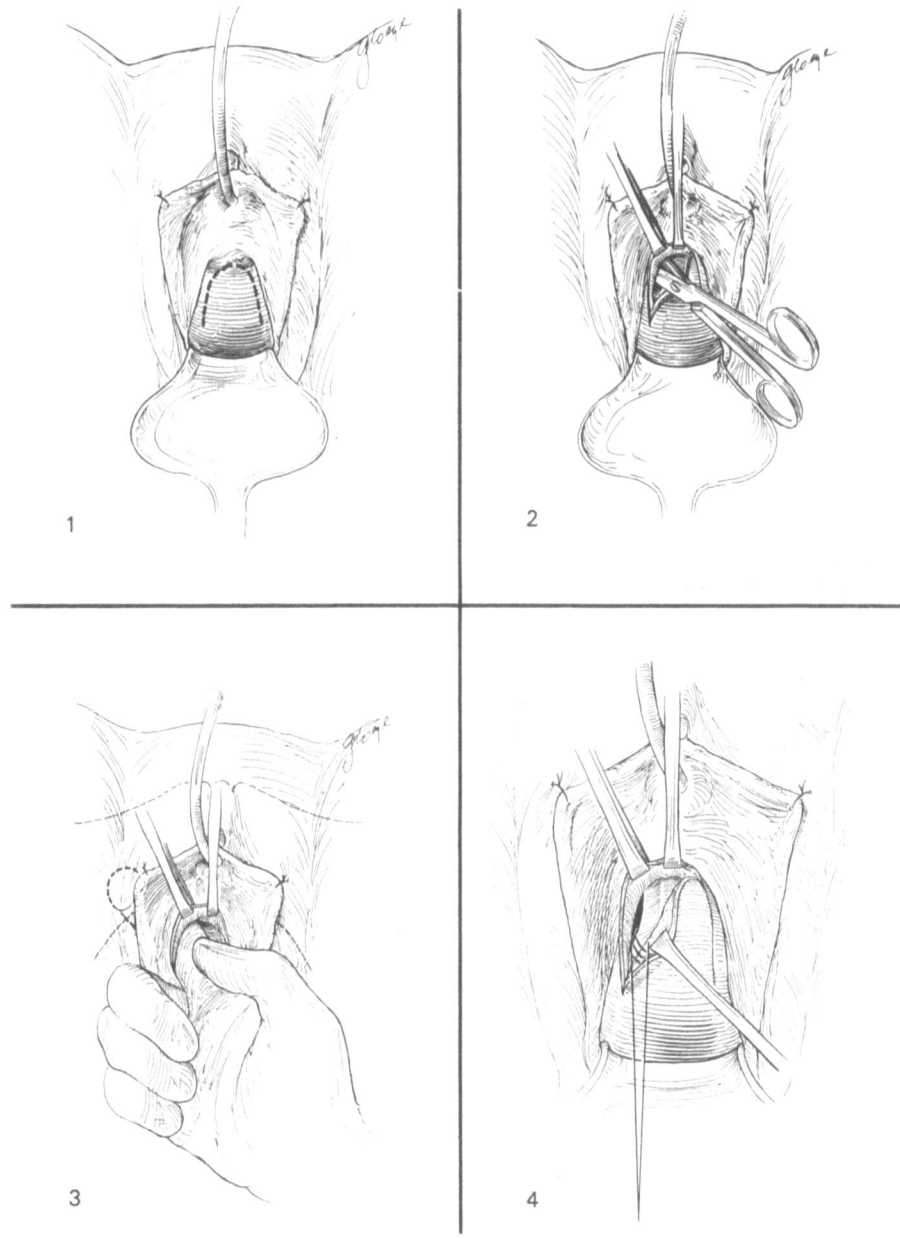

Fig. 1. The semi-circular incision in the anterior vaginal wall, which extends from the level of the bladder neck to the level of the mid-urethra.

Fig. 2. The dissection is directed laterally towards the symphysis pubis.

Fig. 3. The retropubic space is entered with the index finger.

Fig. 4. The Prolene suture is placed in the anterior vaginal wall and the endopelvic fascia.

endopelvic (pubocervical) fascia is incorporated in this continuous suture. A second suture is placed in similar fashion on the contralateral side. Through a 3 cm transverse suprapubic incision the anterior fascia of the rectus abdominus is exposed. The surgeon's finger is then placed into the retropubic space where it guides the suspension needle from the rectus fascia into the retropubic space, and out the vaginal introitus (Fig. 5). With finger guidance, penetration of the bladder by the suspension needle should not occur. The two free ends of each Prolene suture are threaded through the eye of the needle and withdrawn into the suprapubic incision (Fig. 6). The needle is passed on the contralateral side so that 4–5 cm of rectus fascia lies between the Prolene sutures in the suprapubic incision.

After the above steps have been completed, we cystoscope the patient to confirm that there has been no penetration of the bladder or urethra during the passage of the needle. Blue efflux from both ureteral orifices after intravenous indigo carmine has been given indicates no damage to the ureters. With the cystoscope withdrawn to the level of the mid-urethra, the bladder neck should elevate and close during upward traction on the Prolene sutures. Elevation of the bladder neck should not require more than minimal tension on the Prolene sutures. If considerable force is necessary to raise the bladder neck, further mobilization of the vagina is required.

The vaginal incision is then closed with a running absorbable suture. The two ends of each Prolene suture are threaded through a 2×1 Teflon pledget and then tied to each other (Fig. 7). Tying the ends of each suture over the pledget fixes the anterior vaginal wall and urethra in a high fixed retropubic position. Since each suture is secured individually, failure or breakage of one suture will not compromise the integrity of the contralateral suspension suture. Preservation of one suture commonly is sufficient for the patient to remain continent. When securing the Prolene sutures only minimal tension should be required to sufficiently raise the bladder neck (Fig. 8). If the surgeon finds that he is unable to obtain sufficient elevation of the bladder neck or if the tension required to elevate the bladder neck is excessive, then further mobilization is required. The urethra must be free from surrounding scarred tissue in order for it to be mobile enough to move easily into the retropubic space.

Because the suspension sutures of our procedure are placed in the vaginal wall lateral to the urethra, it is virtually impossible to cause permanent urinary retention by overzealous traction on the sutures. After the Prolene sutures have been secured over the Teflon pledgets, the free ends are united over the midline.

The Foley catheter and vaginal pack are removed 12 to 24 hours after the operation. Post-operatively, intravenous antibiotics are continued for 24 hours followed by a 5 day course of oral antibiotics. If the patient is unable to void she is instructed on the technique of clean intermittent self cathe-

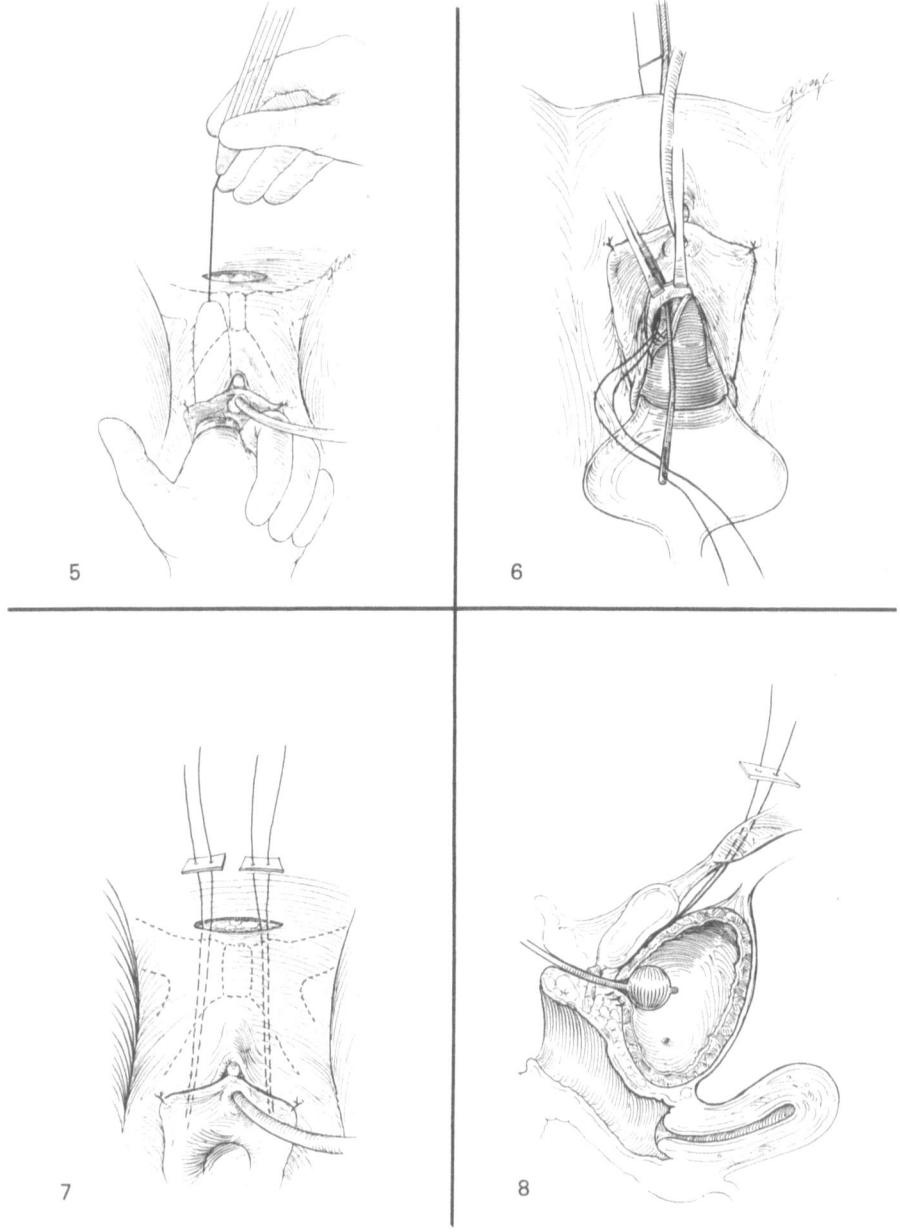

Fig. 5. With finger guidance, the suspension needle is passed into the vaginal incision.
Fig. 6. The Prolene suture is transferred from the vaginal incision to the suprapubic incision.
Fig. 7. The Prolene sutures are tied over a small Teflon pledget and then tied across the rectus fascia to each other.
Fig. 8. Lateral view of the suture fixing the bladder neck in the retropubic position.

126

terization. Hospitalization averages 3–4 days. Ninety percent of the patients are able to void without a significant residual urine within the first week after this operative procedure. The longest period of time that a patient remained on intermittent catheterization is 35 days.

In 1981, Raz reported 100 consecutive patients undergoing this technique of needle bladder neck suspension. Ninety six patients were classified as receiving an excellent result. In general, perioperative morbidity was minimal. One patient experienced significant post-operative bleeding due to anterior wall varices. Two superficial suprapubic wound infections occurred. There were no retropubic infections [11].

Recently, 52 of 55 (94%) patients who were considered failures from one or more previous operative attempts to cure stress urinary incontinence were cured after being treated with this technique. No patient suffered from a postoperative vesicovaginal or urethrovaginal fistula. The average postoperative hospital stay was three days. Approximately half of the patients experienced transient postoperative urinary retention, which required intermittent self-catheterization. The longest period of urinary retention was eight weeks [12]. A recent unpublished review by one of the authors (SR) revealed a 94% success rate in 250 patients who had undergone a transvaginal bladder neck suspension (minimum 6 months follow-up).

Treatment of recurrent stress urinary incontinence due to an incompetent intrinsic sphincter unit

Recurrent stress urinary incontinence may occur in the patient who has a well supported bladder neck and urethra but suffered significant damage to the closing mechanism of the urethra during the bladder neck suspension. This may be due to dissection of the wall of the urethra, excessive urethral manipulation, previous dilations or urethrotomies, sutures placed within the urethra, or damage to the nerve supply to the urethra. Treatment options for these patients include: (1) Polytef (Teflon) injection, (2) urethral lysis, reconstruction and resuspension, (3) urethral sling, (4) artificial urinary sphincter, or (5) continent or incontinent urinary diversion.

Paraurethral and transurethral polytef injection

Polytef (polytetrafluoroethylene, Teflon), an inert plastic, will add bulk to the urethra when injected into the urethral and paraurethral layers. In females, it is best used in patients who suffer from mild urinary incontinence due to poor urethral luminal coaptation. With the added bulk, continence may be achieved because of improved urethral coaptation and resistance.

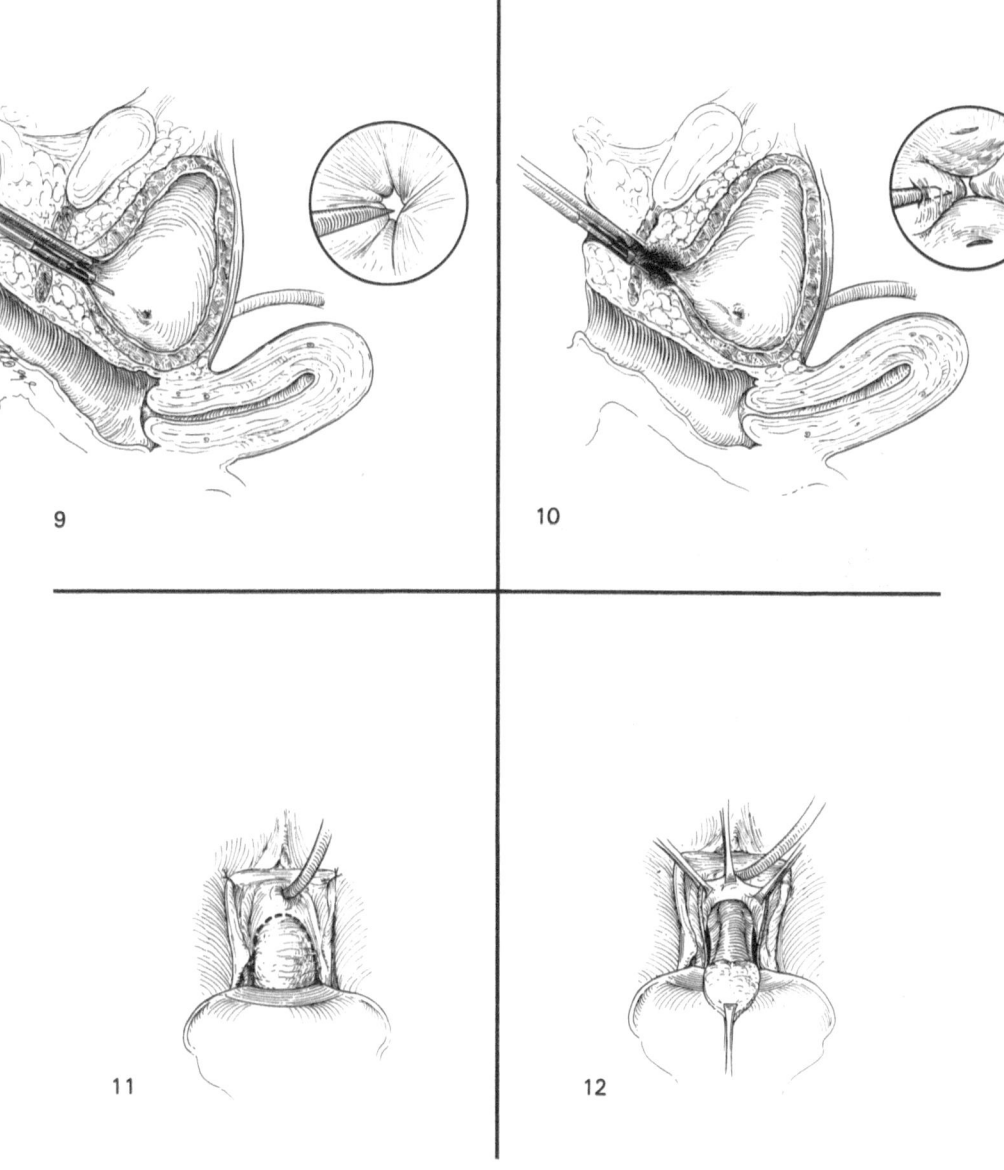

Fig. 9. illustrates the cystoscope and the cystoscopic needle that is used in transurethral injection of Polytef into the urethra.

Fig. 10. demonstrates the needle placed in the paraurethral tissue and the effect of the paraurethral Polytef injection.

Fig. 11. The semi-circular incision in the anterior vaginal wall, which extends from the level of the bladder neck to the level of the mid-urethra.

Fig. 12. The urethra is exposed from the bladder neck to just proximal to the external meatus.

Polytef may be injected transurethrally into the wall of the urethra or transperineally into the paraurethral tissues. The latter technique utilizes a 17 gauge needle 10 cm in length attached to a Lewy syringe that has been loaded with the Polytef paste. It is inserted near the external urethral meatus and advanced towards the bladder neck. Injection of the Polytef is repeated until it has been injected in the 3, 6, and 9 o'clock positions. During the injection, the urologist is observing the effects through a cystoscope to be certain that the needle has not extended beyond the bladder neck and into the bladder.

Using a cystoscope equipped with a special needle and injector, Polytef may be injected transurethrally. After the cystoscope is placed in the midurethra the needle is advanced to and then under the urethral epithelial layer. Polytef is repeatedly injected until bulk has been added to the 3, 6, 9, and 12 o'clock positions (Figs. 9, 10). The transurethral technique requires less Polytef than the paraurethral technique because it allows a more specific and accurate placement of the paste.

Between 1964-1980 Dr. Politano treated 54 females with paraurethral injections of Polytef with a 51% excellent result and 20% good result. These patients were injected an average of 1.8 times. Although many patients may remain incontinent immediately after the injection, urinary control is obtained over a period of several weeks. It is recommended, therefore, to wait from 4 to 6 months before repeating the injection [13].

Our experience with Teflon injections has included 18 cases. Of these 30% were considered to be cured, another 15% were improved. Fifty-five percent, however, were not improved and therefore classified as failures. We use Teflon injections in the high risk patient who has stress urinary incontinence and in the patient who has minimal stress urinary incontinence in spite of a well supported bladder neck and urethra after a bladder neck suspension.

This technique is attractive to the urologist because of its simplicity, the short hospitalization required, and the option for repeated injections. Although the FDA has not yeat approved Polytef for urethral use, intracordal injection of the paste has been used for many years without known complications by the otolaryngologist for the treatment of paralytic vocal dysphonia. At the 1984 meeting of the American Urological Association (New Orleans, L.A.) there was a report of experimental evidence that injected Teflon may migrate to distant organs. Whether this has a significant clinical impact remains to be seen.

Sling procedures

Since the sling procedure was first described by Goebell in 1910 [14], similar techniques have been described that aim to provide a good support to the proximal urethra in a high fixed retropubic position. Although it has been recommended by some to reserve fascial slings for the patient who has failed other types of suspension procedures, there are many medical centres throughout the world who use this technique as a primary operative maneuver for the treatment of genuine stress urinary incontinence.

Muscle, fascia, and synthetic fabrics have all been advocated. In general the muscular slings have been abandoned because of technical problems that include poor blood supply and inadequate length and bulk to provide urethral support. The synthetic materials (Marlex mesh, Mersilene strips) [15] prevailed for awhile. As foreign bodies, however, they are prone to infection and excessive scar tissue reaction [16]. Recently, most surgeons prefer to use an autologous fascial strip such as fascia lata or rectus sheath (many refs). Most sling operations involve both an abdominal and vaginal approach that require an opening of the abdomen and creation of the retropubic space. The slings lift and compress less than half of the proximal urethra.

We use fascial slings when the patient continues to have significant stress urinary incontinence despite good elevation and fixation of the bladder neck and urethra. Recently we have used a technique, which attempts to provide support over the entire length of the urethra by placing a free graft of autologous rectus fascia directly under the posterior surface of the urethra. Nonabsorbable monofilament sutures are placed on the four corners of this fascial patch and then transferred with a suspension needle to the suprapubic incision. Traction placed on these sutures will not only support and fix the urethra and bladder neck, but it may also improve the urethral closure pressure and increase the functional urethral length. The vaginal technique offers the following advantages: (1) The urethra is easily and completely mobilized. (2) There is no need to divide the rectus abdominus or rectus fascia. (3) The sling provides compression over the entire length of the urethra. The following is a description of this technique.

The patient is prepared and positioned similarily to the standard needle bladder neck suspension described earlier in this chapter. Through an inverted 'U' incision in the anterior vaginal wall, the posterior surface of the urethra is exposed from the urethrovesical angle (bladder neck) to the external meatus (Figs. 11, 12). Sufficient mobility for elevation and fixation of the bladder neck is provided by freeing the urethra and urethrovesical junction from the surrounding scarred tissue. Through a transverse suprapubic incision, a rectangular piece of rectus fascia is excised. The size will depend on the length and width of the urethra (usually about 2×4 cm). At the level of the bladder neck a helical suture of No. 1 Prolene suture is placed in the vaginal wall. This suture line is similar to the suture line placed in the vaginal wall for our bladder neck suspension as described in the preceeding

130

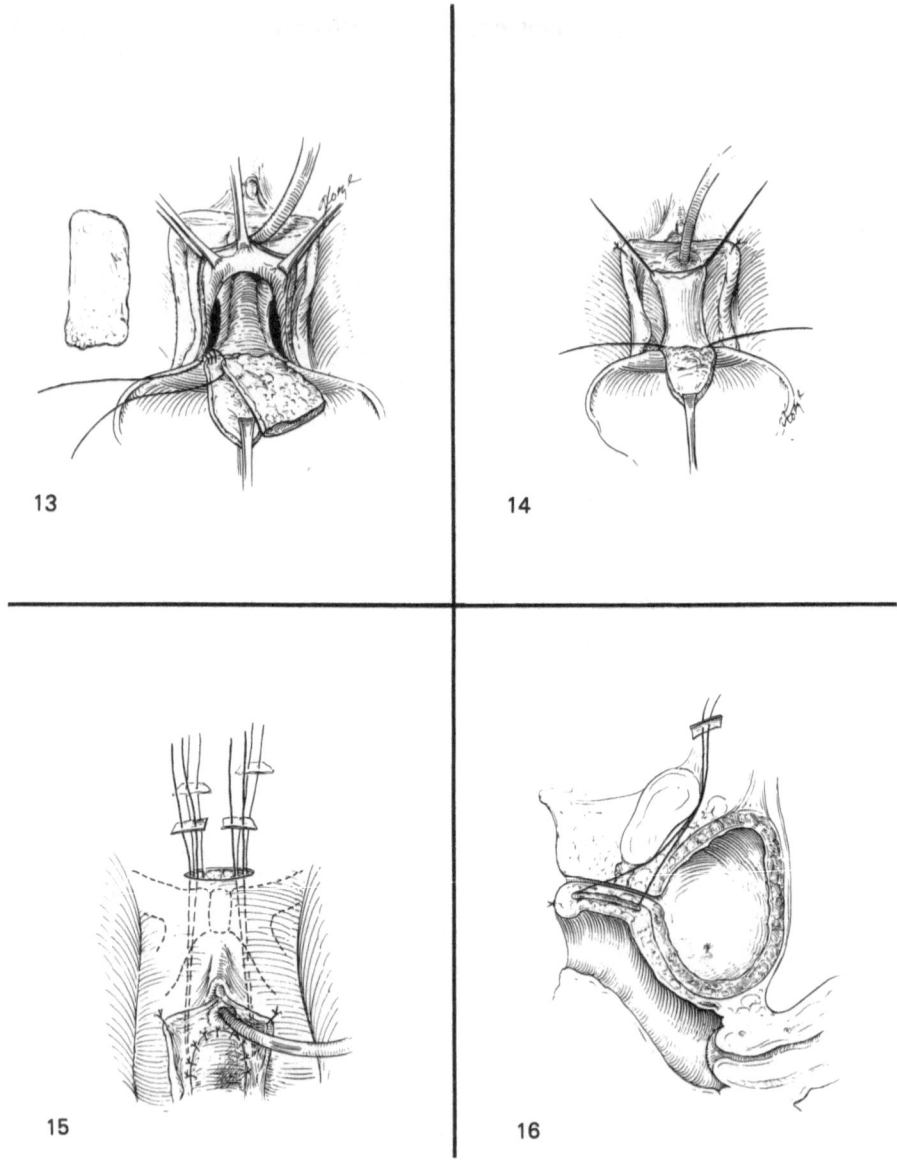

Fig. 13. The Prolene suture is placed in the anterior vaginal wall and the endopelvic fascia. One corner of the small piece of rectus fascia is anchored to this helicoidal suture line.

Fig. 14. The two distal corners of the fascial patch are attached to the periurethral fascia.

Fig. 15. The Prolene sutures are transferred from the vaginal incision to the suprapubic incision with the same needle used for the previously described bladder neck suspension. The anterior vaginal wall is closed. The Prolene sutures are tied over a small Teflon pledget and then tied across the rectus fascia to each other.

Fig. 16. Lateral view of urethral fixation and compression along its entire length.

section. The same Prolene suture is then secured to one corner of the fascial graft (Fig. 13). A similar suture is placed on the opposite side. In the distal portion of the graft two more Prolene sutures are secured to each corner. These two distal sutures are not attached to the urethra or vaginal wall (Fig. 14). Several 3-0 Dexon sutures are used to attach the lateral edges of the fascial graft to the superficial layers of the periurethral fascia to prevent migration of the graft.

By use of the suspension needle, the four Prolene suspension sutures are then withdrawn to the suprapubic incision (Fig. 15). Cystoscopy is performed to assure the surgeon that there has not been damage to the urethra, bladder or ureters. After the cystoscope is withdrawn to the mid-urethra, elevation and closure of the urethra should be noted when traction is placed on the suspension sutures. The anterior vaginal incision is closed with a running 3-0 Dexon suture. In the suprapubic incision, each Prolene suture is threaded through a 2×1 Teflon pledget (Fig. 16). This pledget acts as a buttress on which the Prolene sutures are secured. The fascial defect created by the excision of the graft is closed with interrupted sutures of 0 Dexon. The skin is closed according to the surgeon's preference.

We have used this technique in 14 patients. Because the longest follow-up is 9 months, it is too early to draw substantial conclusions about the procedure. Patients undergoing this operation have had minimal pre-operative closure pressures because of multiple urethral operations, severe urethral damage from trauma, and/or a neuropathic urethra. Because of the nature of the operation, most of our patients are in urinary retention and do intermittent self catheterization.

Urethral lysis, reconstruction and resuspension

When the patient's recurrent stress urinary incontinence is due to the periurethral scarring that 'holds open' the urethra (e.g. after a Marshall-Marchetti urethropexy), urethrolysis with reconstruction and resuspension has been used to improve urethral resistance. In the operating room, a 16-F urethral Foley catheter is inserted. Through a similar inverted 'U' incision in the anterior vaginal wall, the urethra is completely mobilized from its periurethral scarred tissue. A series vertical mattress of 3-0 Vicryl suture is placed in the attenuated periurethral fascia from the distal urethra to the bladder neck to restore the strength of the urethral wall. These sutures reinforce and approximate the weakened periurethral fascia. A second layer of Lembert type 3-0 Vicryl sutures is then placed to reinforce the approximation of the attenuated periurethal fascia. Urethroscopy is then done to exclude the possibility of intraluminal suture entry and to evaluate the degree of urethral coaptation which has been obtained. The urethra and

bladder neck are then supported with the same needle suspension as out-
lined in the previous sections of this chapter.

Artificial urinary sphincter

Another treatment option for the women whose stress urinary incontinence
is due to inadequate urethral closure pressures is to place an artificial urinary sphincter. Since Scott first introduced his inflatable anti-incontinent
device in 1973 [17] numerous modifications have been devised. Presently,
the device includes a periurethral inflatable cuff, a prevesical reservoir balloon, and a pump, which is placed in the labia majora. By compressing the
pump, fluid shifts out of the periurethral cuff into the reservoir. This
decompression of the cuff permits bladder emptying. Because of a positive
pressure gradient between the reservoir and the periurethral cuff, fluid
returns automatically to the cuff to reestablish urethral continence. To
assure complete emptying of the bladder a resistor is inserted between the
reservoir and the periurethral cuff. The return of fluid to the cuff, therefore,
will require 2–3 minutes thus allowing sufficient time for the bladder to
completely empty.

Placement of the artificial sphincter requires suprapubic exposure of the
bladder neck and the urethra. The urethra must be circumferentially mobilized for a sufficient distance in order to pass the cuff around the urethra.
Because these patients have usually had previous urethral and bladder neck
operations, this dissection is often difficult.

Because stress urinary incontinence due to inadequate urethral closure
pressure can usually be corrected by urethral reconstruction and/or autologous fascial slings, we feel the indications for the use of an artificial inflatable urinary sphincter are few. The artificial sphincter is frought with the
inherent problems associated with the placement of a foreign body and a
mechanical device with moving parts.

Continent urinary pouch

Occasionally, we are confronted with the incontinent patient whose urethra
has been damaged beyond repair. Not only is the closure pressure and the
functional urethral length inadequate in these patient's urethra, but the short
anatomical length precludes reconstruction or placement of a sling or an
artificial urinary sphincter. Urethral diversion with an indwelling urethral
catheter, a suprapubic catheter, or supravesical ureteroileal cutaneous conduit may become the only options for these unfortunate patients. The
Young-Dees, Leadbetter and Tanagho techniques of urethral reconstruction

use the bladder wall for the creation of a neourethra. The success of these procedures is variable [18–25]. Another treatment alternative is the creation of a continent valve from a segment of small bowel.

Since the bladder in these patients is usually normal and is capable of storing urine, the making of a continent pouch involves only the creation of a nipple that has enough resistance to hold urine. We have used an intussuscepted segment of small bowel that is interposed between the bladder and the abdominal wall. Self intermittent catheterization of the bladder through this nipple is required 3–4 times each day. The continent nipple is formed similarly to the afferent and efferent limbs of the Kock pouch [26]. Problems that arise from this operation are related to deintussusception and difficulty of catheterization of the nipple.

Treatment of recurrent urinary incontinence due to an overactive bladder

There is a group of patients who suffer from recurrent or persistent incontinence in spite of good support of the urethra and a normal sphincteric unit. Urodynamic evaluation will commonly demonstrate an overactive bladder. Rather than stress urinary incontinence, these patients are likely to be suffering from 'stress hyperreflexia', which is manifest by a bladder contraction that occurs immediately after coughing or a Valsalva maneuver. Most of these patients will respond to medical therapy such as Ditropan (5 mg t.i.d.) and/or imipramine 25–50 mg q.i.d.

If the more conservative methods (electrical stimulation, behavioral modification, etc.) have failed to treat the patient's incontinence that is due to an overactive bladder and has forced a significant change in her life style, the physician may then consider operative therapy. Operative options available include cystolysis, bladder transection, peripheral bladder denervation and/or augmentation enterocystoplasty.

References

1. Stanton S.L., Cardozo L., Williams J.E., Ritchie D. and Allan V. Clinical and urodynamic features of failed incontinence surgery in the female. Obstet. and Gyn., 51 (1978): 515.
2. Vanderschot E.L., Chafik M.L. and Debruyne F.M.J. Has the suprapubic suspension operation any influence on the urethral pressure profile? Br. J. Urol., 51 (1979): 140.
3. Faysal M.H., Constantinou C.E., Rother L.F. and Govan D.E. The impact of bladder neck suspension on the resting and stress urethral pressure profile: A prospective study comparing controls with incontinent patients preoperatively and postoperatively. J. of Urol., 125 (1981): 55.
4. Hertogs K. and Stanton S.L. The mechanism of successful colposuspension: a new model. Proceedings I, p. 152, read at the International Continence Society, Aachen, Germany (1983).

5. Stanton S.L., Cardozo L., Williams J.E., Ritchie D. and Allan V. Clinical and urodynamic features of failed incontinence surgery in the female. Obstet. and Gynecol., 51 (1978): 515.

6. Hodgkinson C.P. Stress urinary incontinence in the female. Surg. Obstet. and Gynecol., 120 (1965): 595.

7. Turner-Warwick R.J. Some clinical aspects of detrusor dysfunction. J. Urol., 113 (1975): 539.

8. Kaufman J.M. Urodynamics in stress urinary incontinence. J. Urol., 122 (1979): 778.

9. Cardozo L.D., Stanton S.L. and Williams J.E. Detrusor instability following surgery for genuine stress incontinence. Br. J. Urol., 51 (1979): 204.

10. McQuire E.J., Lytton B., Pepe V. and Kohorn E.I. Stress urinary incontinence. Obstet. and Gynecol., 47 (1976): 255.

11. Raz S.: Modified bladder neck suspension for female stress incontinence. Urology, 18 (1981): 82.

12. Leach G.E., O'Donnel P. and Raz S. Female Urology edited by Raz S. W.B. Saunders Co. Philadelphia, 1983, p. 267.

13. Carrion H.M. and Politano V.A. In: Raz S. (ed) Female Urology. W.B. Saunders Co., p. 293.

14. Goebell R. Zur Operativen Beseiligung der Angebarenen Incontinentia Vesicae. A. Gynak, Urol., 2 (1910): 187.

15. MacFarlane K.T. Discussion of a sling operation using Marlex polypropylene mesh for treatment of recurrent stress incontinence. Am. J. Obstet. Gynecol., 106 (1970): 376.

16. Cukier J., Mangin P., Cabane H., Ruarte A., Pascal B. Traitement de l'incontinence des urines a l'effort de la femme par soutenement du col vesical à l'aide d'un greffon aponev-rotique libre. Chirurgie, 107 (1981): 67–73.

17. Scott F.B. Treatment of urinary incontinence by implantable prosthetic sphincter. Urology, 1 (1973): 252.

18. Dees J.E. Congenital epispadias with incontinence. J. Urol., 62 (1949): 513.

19. Young, H.H. An operation for the cure of incontinence associated with epispadias. Surg. Gynecol. Obstet., 28 (1919): 84.

20. Kramer S.A. and Kelalis P.P. Assessment of urinary continence in epispadias: Review of 94 patients. J. Urol., 128 (1982): 290.

21. Toguri A.G., Churchill B.M., Schillinger J.F. and Jeffs R.D. Continence in cases of bladder exstrophy. J. Urol., 119 (1978): 538.

22. Leadbetter G.W. Surgical correction of total urinary incontinence. J. Urol., 91 (1964): 261.

23. Resnick M.I. and King L.R. Use of the Leadbetter anti-incontinence procedure in children. J. Urol., 116 (1976): 366.

24. Tanagho E.A., Smith D.R., Meyers F.H. and Fisher R. Mechanism of urinary continence. II. Technique for surgical correction of incontinence. J. Urol., 101 (1969): 305.

25. Tanagho E.A. Urethrosphincteric reconstruction for congenitally absent urethra. J. Urol., 116 (1976): 237.

26. Kock N.G., Nilson A.E., Nilsso L.O., Norlen L.J., Philipson B.M. Urinary diversion via a continent ileal reservoir: clinical results in 12 patients: J. Urol., 128 (1982): 469.

III.3. The treatment of recurrent urinary stress incontinence: a gynaecological view

I. BECK

Definitions

Patients are diagnosed as having recurrent stress incontinence when they have been cured from urinary incontinence by an operation, but became stress incontinent again after several months or years. This true recurrent stress incontinence has to be well distinguished from unsuccessfully operated cases where the stress incontinence was unchanged after operation or became even worse. In the literature this differentiation is not always made when postoperative examination is done for urinary stress incontinence six months after primary surgery.

Aetiology

1. Weakness of the connective tissue and the musculature of the pelvic floor in combination with poorly trained musculature of the urogenital diaphragma and the external urethral sphincter.
2. Increasing age after menopause is an associated factor of incontinence; it is known, that urethral pressure profile is lowering after menopause.
3. Bladder dysfunction with symptoms of motor urge incontinence, in combination with stress incontinence gives no good result of incontinence surgery.
4. Badly performed surgery with scarformation and low urethral pressure.
5. Psychosomatic disorders as cause of incontinence.

Preoperative evaluation

A detailed history and a physical examination including gynaecological pelvic examination is always necessary. Urodynamic measurements are recommended such as urethral pressure profile, determination of the urethral length, cysto-urethro-tonometry, cystometry with abdominal pressure re-

136

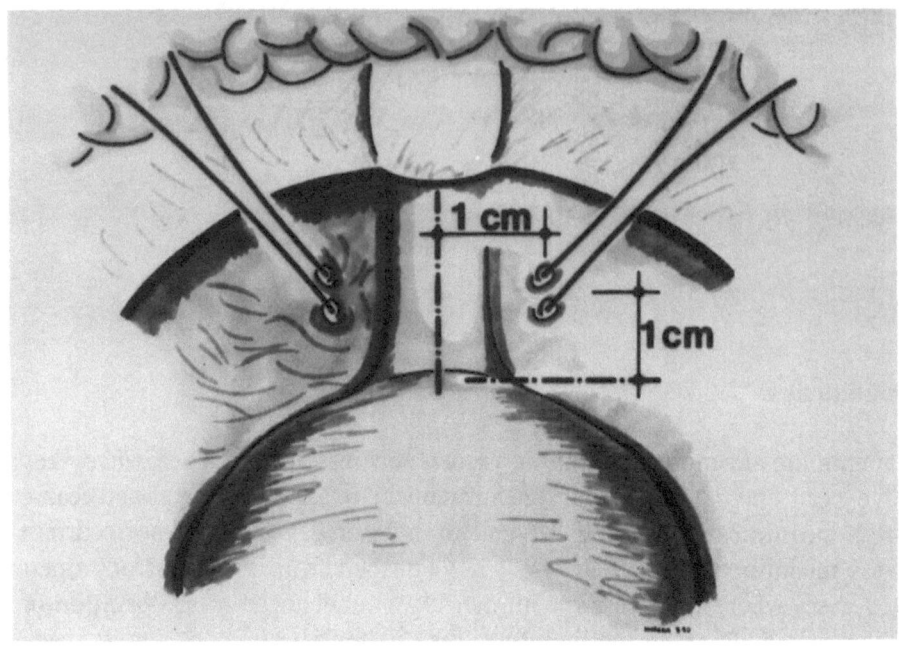

Fig. 1. Scheme colposuspension operation (from Käser, Atlas d. gyn. Op.).

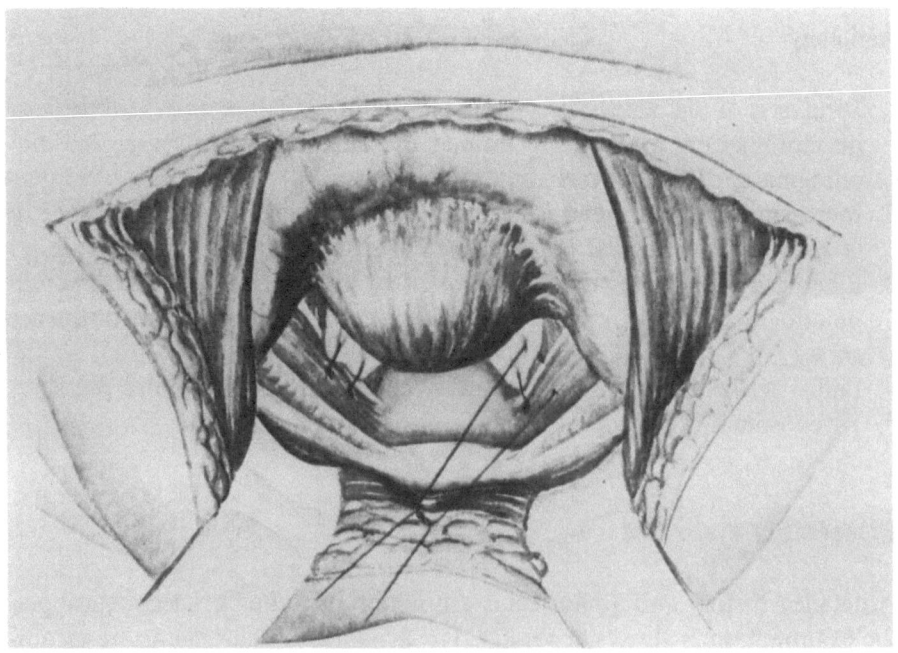

Fig. 2. Fixation of the vaginal fascia to the obturatoria fascia and the m. obturatorius internus (from Käser, Atlas d. gyn. Op.).

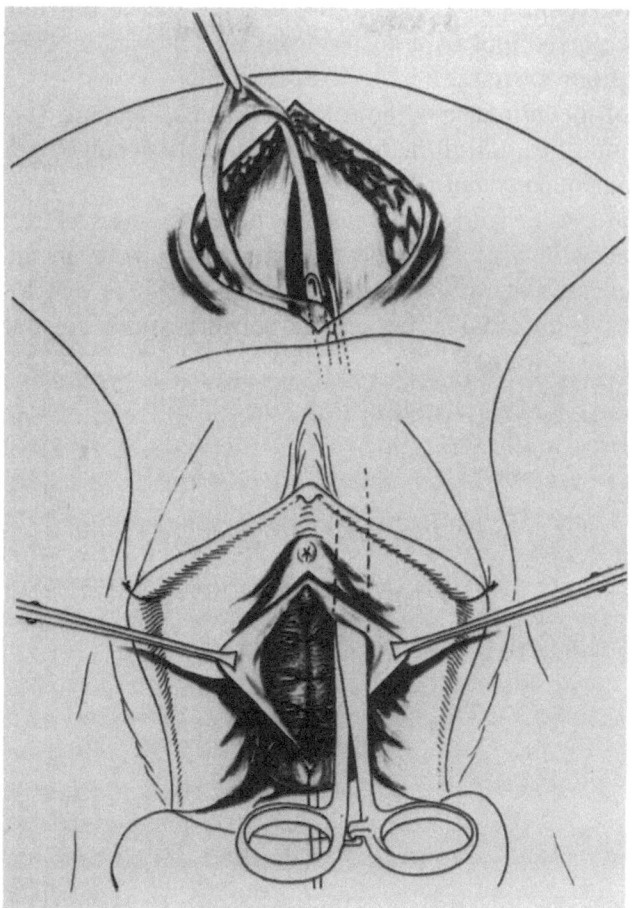

Fig. 3. Sling of the rectus fascia in combination with the colporrhaphy after Aldrige and Studdiford (from Käser, Atlas d. gyn. Op.).

cording. If the patient does not meet the criteria for true stress incontinence, further preoperative assessment tests should be considered such as X-ray evaluation, uroflow and electro-myography. In cases with suspicion of voiding dysfunction, a video-urethro-cystography with recording of the micturition process is advised.

Operative considerations

The main aim of the operative procedure is to restore the anatomic defect. Hysterectomy by itself is not an incontinence operation but helps and facilitates repair of the pelvic floor.

It is important to bring back the distal part of the urethra into the abdom-

138

inal pressure region and to restore the striated muscle function of the urethra and the pelvic floor by a posterior repair, followed by consequent physical pelvic floor exercise.

In cases of incontinence without severe vaginal descent, suprapubic suspension in modification of the Marshall-Marchetti-Krantz-operation is performed at our department (Fig. 1, 2).

A sling procedure with fascia can be chosen in cases of recurrent stress incontinence with large cystocele in combination with an anterior repair (Fig. 3) or in cases where the urethra pressure profile is very low and where other operative procedures, because of scarformations are unable to treat the urethral insufficiency.

References

1. Beck L. and Faber P. Rezidiv-Harnstressinkontinenz. In: Petri E. (ed) Gynäkologische Urologie. Thieme (1983).
2. Käser O., Iklé F.A. and Hirsch H.A. Atlas der gynäkologischen Operationen. Thieme (1983).
3. Petri E. Gynäkologische Urologie. Thieme (1983).

III.4. Recurrent urinary stress incontinence treated by fascia sling plasty: technical considerations and results

R. HOHENFELLNER & E. PETRI

Introduction

Sling operations have long occupied an established position in the treatment of severe female urinary incontinence and recidivous incontinence. While living muscle tissue was employed previously, strips made of fascia, synthetic material, or lyophilised dura are currently coming into use, simplifying the procedure considerably. The chances of curing incontinence are good, even in selected cases with a missing functional urethra or neurogenic bladder dysfunction.

Indications

The primary indication for a sling operation is severe, recurrent incontinence following one or more operations, and urodynamic proof of pure stress incontinence. The procedure should not be performed until gynaecological precautions such as hysterectomy or correction of a cystocele are taken. In selected cases with neuropathic bladder dysfunction, considerable improvement of the psychosocial status of the patient is made possible. Residual urine and an increase in uninhibited detrusor contractions are the calculated risks involved.

Pre-operative evaluation

Urine is sent for culture and sensitivity, and intravenous urography, a resting and a straining lateral cystourethrogram and voiding cystourethrogram recorded on videotape, are carried out. In addition, simultaneous recording of intravesical and intrarectal pressures, urinary flow and volume, and pelvic floor EMG are measured. Simultaneous urethral and bladder pressures are recorded with either a four channel polyvinyl chloride membrane catheter or a GAELTEC catheter tip pressure transducer withdrawn mechanically at a constant speed of 3 mm/s.

140

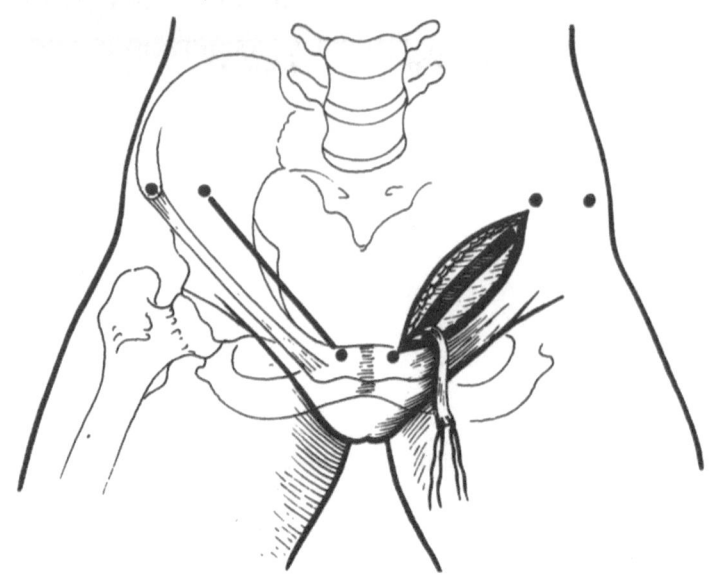

Fig. 1.

Operative technique

The patient is placed on the operating table in a lithotomy position. The legs should be movable as necessary without disturbance of sterile conditions. Both abdominal and vaginal operative fields should be disfinfected and draped before the onset of the operation.

Skin incision starts at the pubic tubercle and is directed toward a point medial to the superior iliac spine (Fig. 1). If hysterectomy is planned in the same surgical procedure, a Pfannenstiel incision is performed.

The dissection of the fascial strip from the aponeurosis of the external oblique muscle is best performed using two short, parallel preliminary incisions starting close to the pubic tubercle and two cm apart. These initial incisions are then continued to the iliac spine for a distance of about 12 cm, up to the point where the fibres of the external oblique muscle continue into the fascia (Fig. 2). The proximal end of the strip is then clamped and cut, marking each angle with a suture of a different colour to avoid contorted strips later on. The strip is then mobilised, preserving a broad attachment of the fascial strip to the pubic tubercle.

The triangular space above the tubercle, which is confirmed by the rectal sheath on the medial side and the lower part of the internal oblique muscle on the lateral side ('suprapubic trigone'), is then perforated, leading straight into the paravesical space (space of RETZIUS) (Fig. 2).

The index finger is introduced and carefully pushed downward as far as the inferior pubic artery. Instrumental manipulations within the retropubic

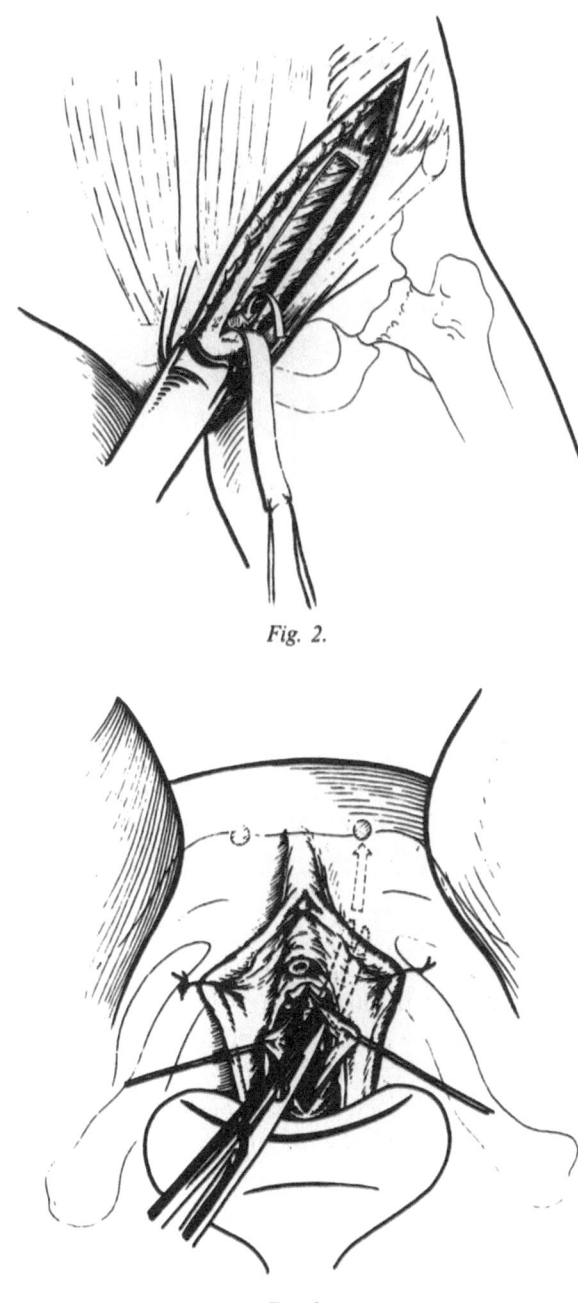

Fig. 2.

Fig. 3.

tunnel should be avoided, as they carry the danger of injury to the bladder or branches of the pudendal, obturator or epigastric vessels. It is of great importance always to use the posterior face of the os pubis as a guideline.

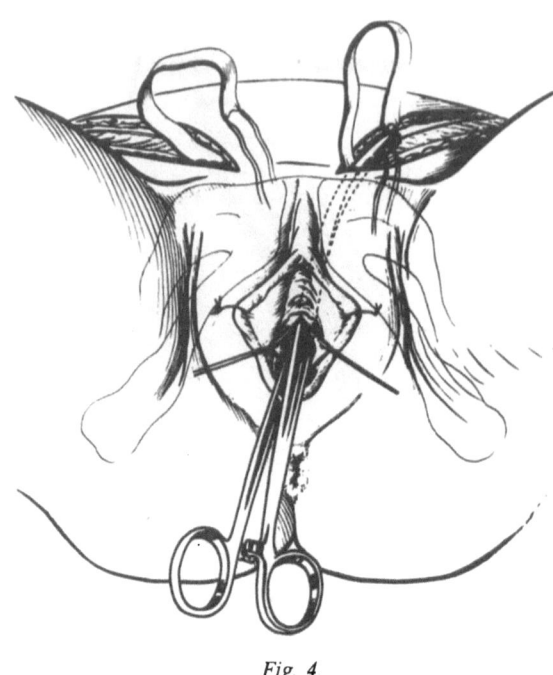

Fig. 4.

Having prepared both fascial strips as well as the retropubic tunnels, the vaginal stage of the operation is started. One assistant remains in attendance at the abdominal operative field. An anterior colpotomy is performed, exposing the urethrovesical junction and the paraurethral and paravesical spaces.

After perforation of the pelvic fascia (Fig. 3) the operator introduces the index finger into the paravesical space while the assistant at the abdominal field passes the index finger through the retropubic tunnel. Their aim should be to bring their fingers into contact by blunt dissection.

A long curved clamp is introduced through the vaginal incision. Having attached the fascial strip, the instrument is pulled downward. A rather lateral course of direction should be taken when inserting the clamp in order to bypass the urethra and bladder. Having pulled out the instrument to its full length, the fascial strip is freed and clamped. The same procedure is then performed on the contralateral side (Fig. 4). The fascial strips are approximated and united at a level close to the bladder neck. Suture is accomplished by means of fine silk or PDS and small round needles. At least three sutures should be placed to secure a firm union of the strips (Fig. 5).

Overlapping parts of the strips are then everted and sewn to the pubovesical fascia. Following resection of the vaginal edges and reconstruction of the pelvic floor, the colpotomy incision is closed. A suprapubic catheter is inserted in the bladder. Prior to closing the inguinal incisions, the vaginal

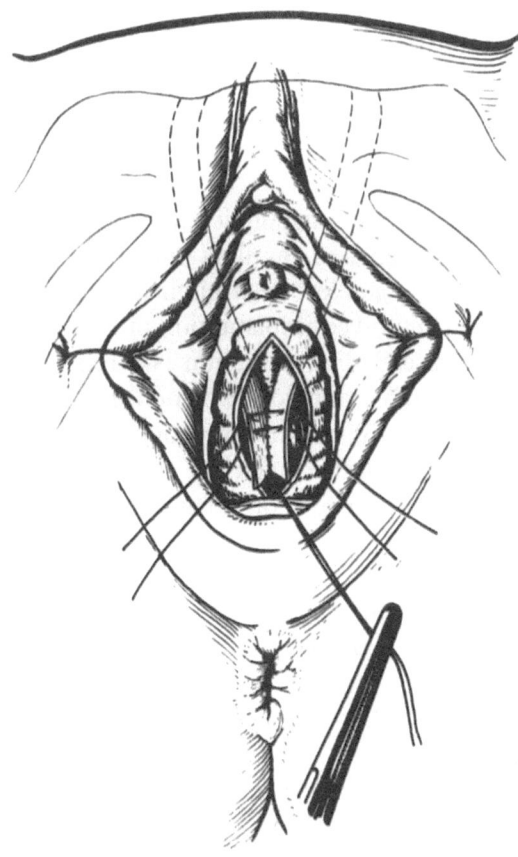

team should change gloves. Abdominal incisions are closed by interrupted sutures after having placed haemovac drains through the subcutaneous tissue, into the paravesical space.

It must be pointed out that it is not necessary to terminate the operation if an intraoperative bladder injury occurs during blunt dissection, as happens following previous suprapubic surgery (e.g. other sling procedures or Marshall-Marchetti-Krantz). The lesion is usually located retrosymphysically, and rarely requires further operative treatment.

Postoperative management

During the postoperative period patients are given prophylactic antibiotics to prevent any infection which might endanger the sling. The suprapubic catheter is removed after 10 days, if repeated measurements of residual urine are below 100 ccm. Patients with insufficient micturition are discharged with the catheter, and a control examination is done after 10–14 days.

Results

Depending on patient selection and indication, cure rates for incontinence of up to 90% have been reported for sling operations, although late results of several techniques have not yet been published. In contrast to the technically simpler and less involved implantation of one of the many modified alloplastic slings, the fascial sling operation is a relatively complex procedure. The not inconsiderable number of complications resulting from alloplastic slings referred to our clinic for correction, however, has raised some doubt as to the use of alloplastic material.

Since 1968, we have performed more than 100 inguinovaginal sling operations in our departments. The average age was 53 years, the oldest patient was 76. There were no intra- or postoperative deaths (Table 1). A total of 60% of the women had had up to ten previous incontinence operations (Table 2). In the last few years, hysterectomy was performed at the same

Table 1. Fascial sling operations (n = 106).

Mortality	n = 0
Complications	
intraoperative	n = 9 lesions of the bladder
	n = 2 bleeding
postoperative	n = 2 abdominal wound abscess
	n = 2 hernia
	n = 2 urethrovaginal fistula

Table 2. Previous treatment of incontinence.

Technique	Incontinent after treatment	Failure	Recurrence
Hysterectomy	14	9	9
Hysterectomy + vaginal repair	8	5	10
Vaginal repair	4	23	18
Sling procedure	–	2	3
Marshall-Marchetti-Krantz	–	1	4
Pessary, electrical stimulation	1	5	1
Pharmacotherapy	-	14	9
Total	30	59	54

time by a gynaecologist if it had not been done previously; he also performed an anterior and posterior repair in 12 patients with vaginal descent. In three patients, urethrovaginal fistula resulting from previous incontinence operations were closed during the sling procedure.

Continence was achieved in 84.4% of patients with urodynamic proof of pure stress incontinence in a follow-up period of up to 12 years. Differences in success-rates for primary and recurrent incontinence are demonstrated in Table 3. With increasing duration of follow-up, there was a marked increase of recurrences (Table 4, 5).

Table 3. Surgical success depending on the number of preliminary operations.

Number of previous operations	n	Continent improved (%)	Failure (%)	Recurrence (%)
0	9	78	22	—
1	41	78	19	3
2	25	80	16	4
3 up to 6	16	56	25	19
Totals	91 (86%)	75	20	5

Table 4. Long-term results.

Result	Postop.	<2 yrs.	>2 yrs.	5 yrs.
Continent	50%	86%	64%	52%
Improved	1%	9%	14%	19%
Primary retention	45%	—	4%	—
Failure	2%	—	15%	26%
Urge-incontinence	2%	5%	3%	3%
	n = 106	n = 21	n = 73	n = 63

Table 5. History in patients with surgical failure.

	n
Non-functional urethra	8
Neurologic disease	7
(e.g., MS, Myelomeningocele, epilepsy, encephalitis)	
Diabetes mellitus, hypertension	2
Radiation therapy	1

Continence was achieved in 14 of 21 specially selected patients with neuropathic bladder disturbance, some of whom had serious psychosocial conditions before the operation.

Summary

Sling procedures have found a permanent place among the operative procedures to correct incontinence in women, especially in instances of recurrent incontinence. In addition to achieving continence, it is necessary to consider such side effects as dysuria, urgency, increased amounts of residual urine and, in particular, secondary injuries to the lower urinary tract when judging the success of the operation.

References

1. Altmann P., Georgiades E., Rudelstorfer B. Zur Technik der inguinovaginalen Schlingenoperation (Modifikation nach Narik-Palmrich) und ihre Spätergebnisse. In: Verh. Ber. Dtsch. Ges. Urol. 27. Tagung. Berlin, Heidelberg, New York, Springer (1976): 213–215.
2. Anselmino K.J. Eine neue Schlingenoperation zur Behandlung der hochgradigen Urinkontinenz des Weibes. Geburtsh. Frauenheilk. 12 (1952): 277.
3. Beck R.P., Lai A.R. Results in treating 88 cases of recurrent urinary stress incontinence with the Oxford fascia lata sling procedure. Am. J. Obstet. Gynec. 142 (1982): 649–651.
4. Bracht E. Eine besondere Form der Zügelplastik. Geburth Frauenheilk. 16 (1956): 782–790.
5. Fianu S., Söderberg G. Absorbable Polyglactin Mesh for retropubic sling operations in female urinary stress incontinence. Gynec. obstet. Invest. 16 (1983): 45–50.
6. Gaudenz R. Die Bedeutung einer Zusatzoperation bei der primären operativen Behandlung einer Urethralinsuffizienz. Geburtsh. Frauenheilk. 39 (1976): 393–401.
7. Hägele D., Frühwirth O., Kriesche H., Noll C. and Berg D. Ergebnisse nach Schlingenoperation mit Tutoplast-Dura. Geburtsh. Frauenheilk. 43 (1983): 762–765.
8. Havlicek S. Schlingenoperationen mit Lyoduraband bei rezidivierender Harninkontinenz der Frau. Geburtsh. Frauenheilk. 32 (1972): 757.
9. Heidenreich J., Faber P. and Beck L. Suspension mit Lyoduraband. In: Verh. Ber. Dtsch. Ges. Urol. 27. Tagung, Springer, Berlin, Heidelberg, New York, (1976), pp. 221–222.
10. Kersey J. The gauze hammock sling operation in the treatment of stress incontinence. Brit. J. Obstet. Gynaecol. 90 (1983): 945–949.
11. Millin R. Discussion of stress incontinence in micturition. Proc. R. Soc. Med. 40 (1947): 364–367.
12. Millin T. and Read C. Stress incontinence of urine in the female. Postgrad. Med. J. 24 (1948): 3–10, 51–56.
13. Narik G. and Palmrich A.H. A simplified sling operation suitable for routine use. Am. J. Obstet. Gynec. 84 (1962): 400–405.
14. Narik G. and Palmrich A.H. Inguinovaginale Schlingenoperation zur Behandlung hochgradiger Harninkontinenz. Urologe A 4 (1965): 205–207.
15. Parker R.T., Addison W.A. and Wilson C.J. Fascia lata urethrovesical suspension for recurrent stress urinary incontinence. Am. J. Obstet. Gynec. 135 (1979): 843–852.

16. Petri E., Jonas U. and Hohenfellner R. Inguinovaginal sling operation in the treatment of female urinary incontinence. Urologe A 17 (1978): 334–337.

17. Petri E., Frohneberg D. and Thüroff J.W. Problems of loop grafts. Akt. Urol. 12 (1981): 31–33.

18. Petri E., Beckhaus I., Frohneberg D. and Thüroff J.W. Inguinovaginal fascial sling according to Narik and Palmrich-indication, problems, long-term results. Akt. Urol. 14 (1983): 286–290.

19. Sexton G.L. The risks and complications of the epiurethral suprapubic vaginal suspension for the correction of recurrent postoperative stress incontinence. Gynec. Urol. Soc., New Orleans Nov. 2–5 (1983).

20. Stoeckel W. Über die Verwendung der Musculi pyramidales bei der operativen Behandlung der Incontinentia urinae. Zentralbl. Gynaek. 41 (1917): 11–19.

21. Ullery J.C. Stress incontinence in the female. Grune & Stratton, New York (1953).

22. Wienhöwer R., Merten M. and Zoedler D. Ergebnisse urologischer Rezidiv-Inkontinenz-Operationen. In: Verh. Ber. Dtsch. Ges. Urol. 27. Tagung, Springer, Berlin, Heidelberg, New York, (1976) pp. 222–224.

23. Zoedler D. Zur operativen Behandlung der weiblichen Stressinkontinenz. Z. Urol. 54 (1961): 355–358.

24. Zoedler D. Die operative Behandlung der weiblichen Harninkontinenz mit dem Kunststoff-Netzband. Akt. Urol. 1 (1970): 28–34.

III.5. Practical aspects of vaginal sling plasty in the management of recurrent urinary stress incontinence

M. BRESSEL

Preoperative questioning

In cases of recurrent urinary stress incontinence (SUI) we have to ask ourselves: is it really a stress incontinence? What have we got to think about as far as differential diagnosis is concerned and what methods of examination are helpful in order to evaluate patients correctly?

Differential diagnosis

Regarding patients with previous surgery, we have to consider two other causes of incontinence which are first in the vesico-vaginal fistulae and secondly, incontinence produced by urge or detrusor dyssynergia. In particular in cases when due to SUI a hysterectomy and vagino plasty has been performed, one has to look for vesico-vaginal fistulae if recurrent urinary incontinence turns up. Some of these patients may have a combination of SUI and fistulae, and if these different disabilities are not found at first, this leads to confusion and failure of treatment. The second important reason for recurrent incontinence is the urge or detrusor dyssynergia. On one hand, these types of incontinence might have existed before the first operation but on the other hand they might be caused by the operation. In some cases it can be very difficult to prove a bladder instability. From the point of view to avoid failures it is better to find out if this combination exists before operating. If suspected bladder instability is recorded by cystometry, we do a test with anticholinergic drugs which are given i.v. over a period of 72 hours. In 8 hour intervals the patient receives 60 mg. N-butylscopolamine (bromide) (Buscopan®) or 1,2 mg trospiumchlorid (Spasmex®) and a 'micturition day profile' (see below) under these conditions is recorded. This profile is compared with a profile recorded without medication. If the incontinence improves we continue the test with oral medication of 15 to 30 mg trospiumchlorid (Spasmex®) every 8 hours over a period of 10 days under normal living conditions. If under these conditions, in the case of a combined incontinence an improvement occurs and a mere SUI persists, the possibility exists of combining an SUI operation with drug therapy.

Examination methods

An important aspect for diagnosis of SUI is the exact statement of patients history.

Micturition day profile. Together with complete information about the condition of micturition the patient has to write a 'micturition day profile' (time, volume, duration of miction) and also has to register when being wet or dry. Small volumes should always make us think of bladder instability. On the other hand it is well known that SUI intensifies with increasing bladder volume. In case of SUI, patients are not usually wet during the night except for nocturnal coughing paroxysms.

Cysto-urethroscopy. This method is standing at the beginning of the examination. In a combined process of getting a urine specimen and the determination of residual urine the cysto-urethroscopy gives optical information of the bladder wall especially of the bladder neck and of the urethra in addition to different bladder volumes. Finally, at a standard volume of 300 cc the instrument is removed.

Stress-test. After filling the bladder with 300 cc of warm water (about 37 °C) the patient is asked to cough forcefully in supine as well as in standing position. The urologist has to notice if the discharge of urine is simultaneous with the cough. If the urine passage lasts longer than the coughing, no real SUI exists, and a bladder instability should be considered. On the other hand all patients who did not lose any urine by this test were not considered for primary operative treatment.

We also perform the so called 'Marchetti-test' elevating the paraurethral tissue but we are not convinced of its value. In our opinion errors may very easily occur because it is often difficult to decide if the urethra has been correctly elevated or only been compressed.

Determination of residual urine. Residual urine is a bad precondition for a good result of surgery if SUI is involved, because most of the operation methods lead to a permanent increase of bladder outlet resistance.

Uroflowmetry. In my personal opinion this method is essential. It puts you in a position to make a correct prognosis, in a lot of cases before surgery. If you find a 'waterfall flow' (Fig. 1) it means a maximum flow of about 50 cc/sec, a micturition time below 15 sec and a volume more than 300 cc, you have good conditions for a successful vaginal sling plasty regarding postoperative voiding. If the flow rate is below 20 cc/sec and the micturition time above 30 sec (Fig. 2) the operative correction of SUI will not be as easy as in the first case.

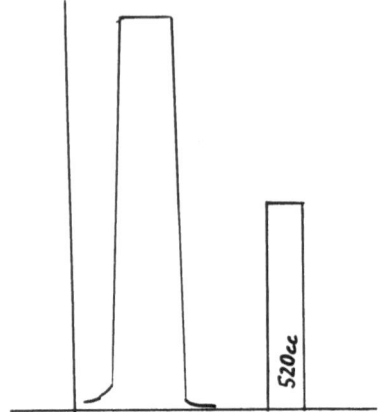

Fig. 1. A typical 'waterfall flow' in case of SUI.

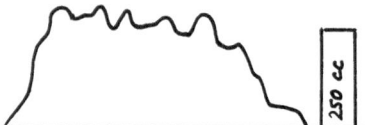

Fig. 2. Bad flow in case of SUI.

Cystometry and urethra pressure profile. On one hand there are typical results with low urethra pressure profile, shortened functional length of the urethra and pathological pressure-answer-curve in case of SUI; on the other hand there are sometimes cases with real SUI and normal urethra pressure profile. The value of this combined examination in case of SUI is due more to diagnosing detrusor instability, while the urine loss caused by stress might be recorded also by easier methods. If the combined urethra- and

Table 1. SUI examination procedure.

I	History
II	Cysto-urethroscopy, urine for analysis (microscopy, culture)
	Flow rate
	Residual urin
	I.v.p.
III	Micturition day profile
	Urodynamic measurements with X-ray
IV	Anticholinergic drug test

I + II: In the office detailed history — in one procedure cysto-urethroscopy, urine specimen for analysis, stress test, flow rate and residual urine — I.V.P.
III: Some days later the patient brings the micturition day profile and urodynamic measurements with X-ray are performed.
IV: In case of suspected bladder instability anticholinergic drug test is made.

bladder pressure measurement is done with water, contrast medium should be used and the loss of the normal posterior urethro-vesical angle is proved. If there is any doubt about real SUI as far as the history of the patient is concerned and the cystometric measurement in prone position is stable, we perform the cystometry in standing position with suprapubic pressure registration. Generally you do not need a urethra-bladder pressure measurement for diagnosing SUI if you see the coughing synchron to urine loss and if the cysto-urethroscopy is normal. The pressure measurement should be carried out in all cases of recurrent disease.

The examination procedure is summarized in Table 1.

Surgical correction methods of SUI

Nearly all operation methods of SUI, the simple plication procedures [2, 3], the urethropexy [4–6], reach their goal by augmentation of the posterior urethro-vesical angle. The 3 groups of methods are: the simple plication procedures, the urethropexies and the sling plasties.

The advocates of *urethropexy* emphasize that it is important not to elevate the urethra-bladder region directly. In all of these methods periurethral tissue or the anterior vaginal wall beside the urethra and the bladder neck are elevated in direction to the symphysis, the Cooper band or the anterior abdominal wall. Finally an elevation of the bladder neck on 6-hour position is reached whereas in some operation methods the results are proved by intraoperative urethroscopy [7, 8].

The failure of these methods relative to the recurrence rate is explained by the variations of methods which have been used by Pereyra since 1959. Together with Lebherz he performed an additional Kelly-plasty [9]. Later on dacron-tube baffles were interposed between the filament non-absorbable synthetic suspension stitch loops and the paraurethral tissue to prevent stitch penetration. Finally, the analysis of failures led to the revised Pereyra procedure using colligated pubourethral supports [8, 10].

The *sling plasties* with fascia lata strip were introduced in Germany [11] and have been used with success to date [12]. Many different techniques have been described according to different sling materials and different approaches. Aldridge [13] used a strip of the external oblique aponeurosis, Millin [14] used a strip of rectus sheath with the idea that the rectus ends of the sling are floating and not fixed to bone, so that relaxation of the abdominal wall allows micturition, whilst coughing or lifting lightens the sling and helps to occlude the neck of the bladder. Regarding the operative approach, the sling is fixed in different ways. According to the Goebell technique a free fascia strip is drawn through below the bladder neck and fixed at the anterior abdominal wall, while other authors [13] take two fascia strips fixed at the bone or the rectus muscle and the two loose ends of the fascia are adapted below the urethral vesical junction.

In agreement with Ridley [12] it is our opinion that a continuous band gives more controllable tension and less vaginal manipulation of the two loose ends of the fascia strips, as is necessary in the Aldridge technique. Furthermore we believe that the continuous band loop guarantees a more protective elevation than the adaption of the fascia strips below the bladder neck.

Instead of fascia several synthetic materials are recommended. Zoedler [15] used a nylon-mesh, Williams and Telinde [16] mersilene ribbon, Moir [17] mersilene mesh and Morgan [18] marlex mesh, to mention just a few.

We also use a sling made out of synthetic material as mentioned by Zoedler [15]. The monofile mesh ribbon material is made of polyamid-6-texture, similar to nylon.

There are many equally successful methods in the operative treatment of SUI. In the first two years after surgery nearly all authors have a high success rate, Pereyra and Lebherz [9] 94.3%, Ridley [12] 86% and Zoedler [19] 98%. While late failures with the sling procedure are very rare [12], a progressive increase in the number of failures was observed by Pereyra and Lebherz [9] with longer postoperative observation. The maximum failure rate in patients followed up to 5 years was 16% [8].

Personal operation procedure. The patient lies in lithotomy position exposing the lower abdomen and the vaginal area simultaneously. We start with the insertion of an 18F foley catheter into the urethra and the bladder and fill the balloon with 10 cc. The bladder is filled with 300 cc isotonic solution. With moderate tension the balloon is brought to the bladder neck and in front of the urethral meatus we set a sign at the catheter with a sterile ball point pen for linear urethral centimeter measurement. The catheter is taken out and the balloon is filled again with the same volume for measurement (Fig. 3). You can also use a graduated catheter, but this is more expensive. The catheter is inserted again. Between 2 stitches (catgut 2×0) at the anterior vaginal wall, a 5 cm longitudinal incision is made. The correct position of the distal stitch is approximately 2 cm behind the urethral meatus and the assistant draws this stitch to the front and anterior. The exact area for the stitches and the following incision is localized by touching the balloon of the catheter through the anterior vaginal wall. The vagina is carefully dissected to the right and left side from the urethral vesical junction. The wound edges are grasped with surgical forceps and the dissection of urethra and bladder is carried out with curved scissors (Metzenbaum), while the wound is under continuous suction. We prefer a special preparation sucker with fiberglass light for spreading the wound and elevating the urethra and

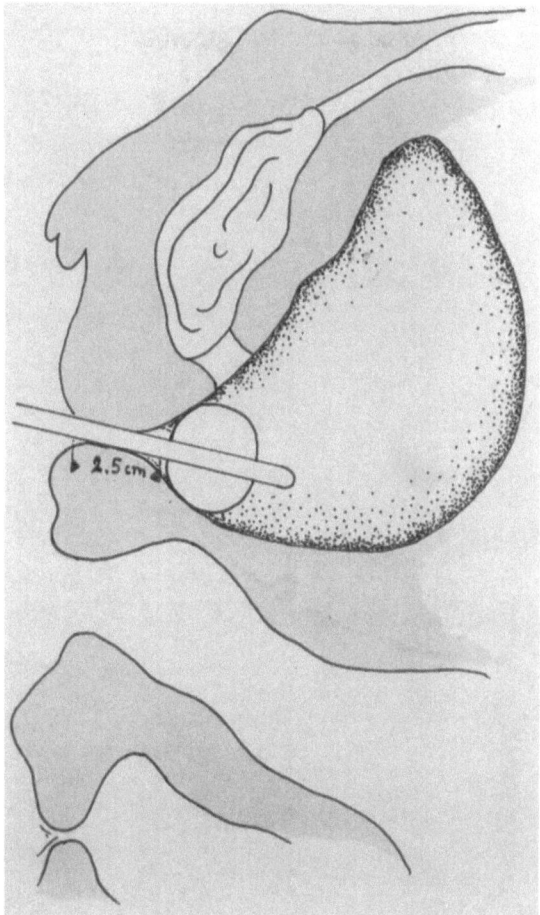

Fig. 3. The operation starts with linear measurement of the urethra.

the bladder. It is important that the curve of the scissors is directed towards the vagina and not towards the bladder. It does not matter if a hole is made in the vaginal wall by the preparation. The dissection is carefully carried out laterally until the anterior aspect of pubic rami can be felt on each side. The bladder neck is freed on both sides up to the two and ten hour position. Bleeding from veins of the diaphragm is usually controlled by pressure. Without difficulty the tip of the scissors may be pushed through the diaphragm on each side. Then the wound is tamponaged with a 7.5 × 7.5 cm sponge. Now the operative field is changed to the suprapubic area. A transverse section measuring 4 cm in length is made down to the insertion of the anterior abdominal aponeurosis in the midline at the level of the symphysis. By displacement of skin and subcutaneous tissue on each side the tuberculum pubicum is touched and immediately medial from the tuberculum the

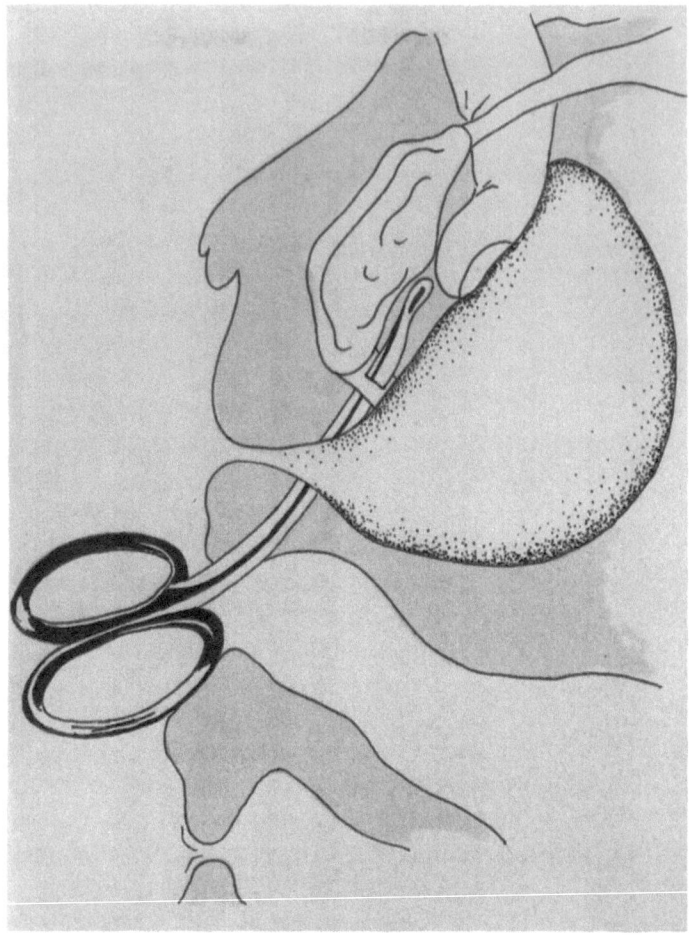

Fig. 4. The forefinger is introduced to the space of Retzius. A curved blunt forceps is brought up from the vaginal wound to the finger tip at the diaphragm.

rectus fascia and muscle are bluntly penetrated with strong short scissors. After penetrating, the tissue is spread with the scissors in the direction of the fibers far enough for the forefinger to be introduced to the space of Retzius without difficulties. The bladder is displaced away from the os pubis with the finger. While the finger tip is in position near the diaphragm we set up a curved blunt forceps in the vaginal wound the same way as the preceding dissection. The tip of the instrument is directed towards the retropubic finger tip away from the bladder. Gentle force must be used to bring forceps and finger together, especially if patients have had previous surgery (Fig. 4). Under guidance of the forefinger the tip of the forceps is brought out of the suprapubic incision and a silk or twine thread is pulled through with the forceps to the vaginal canal on both sides (Fig. 5). Lesions of bladder are

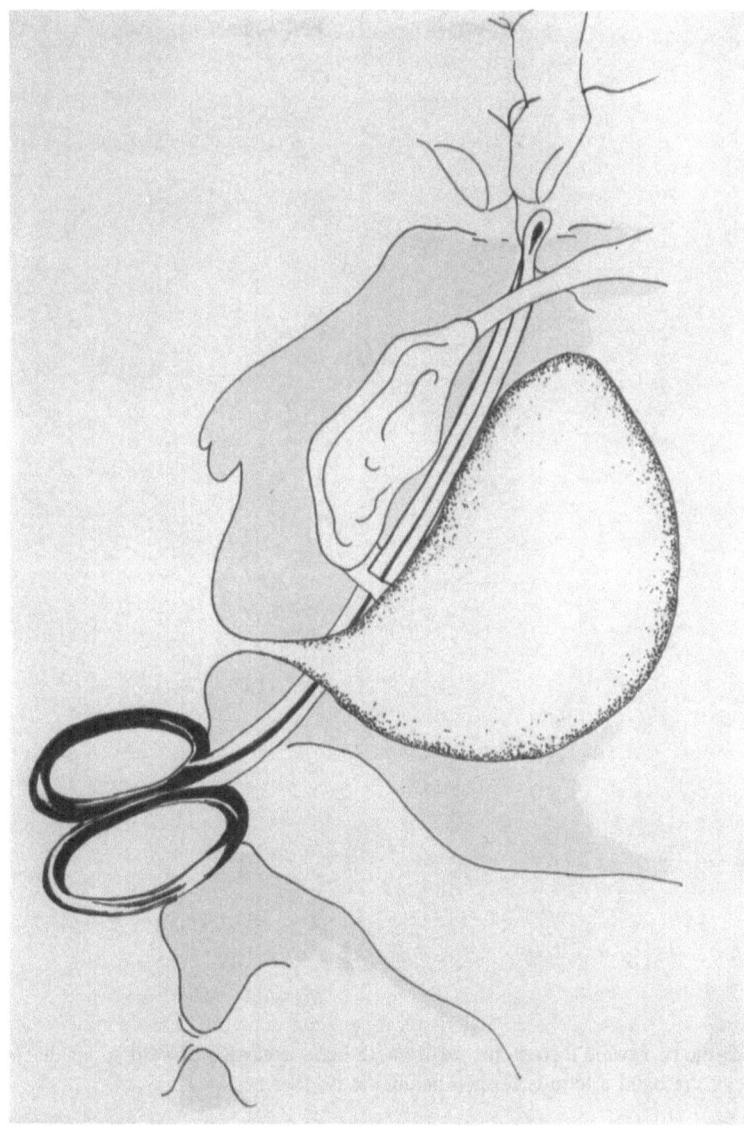

Fig. 5. A twine thread is pulled through from the suprapubic incision to the vagina.

seen by extravasation of the fluid which was put into the bladder at the start of the operation. Small lesions do not need further treatment and only the indwelling catheter is left for 10 days after surgery. Bigger lesions should be sutured. Furthermore, during the operation a control is made several times by opening the catheter to see if the bladder fluid is bloody. You can also make a check for lesions by cystoscopy, but we do not think this is necessary.

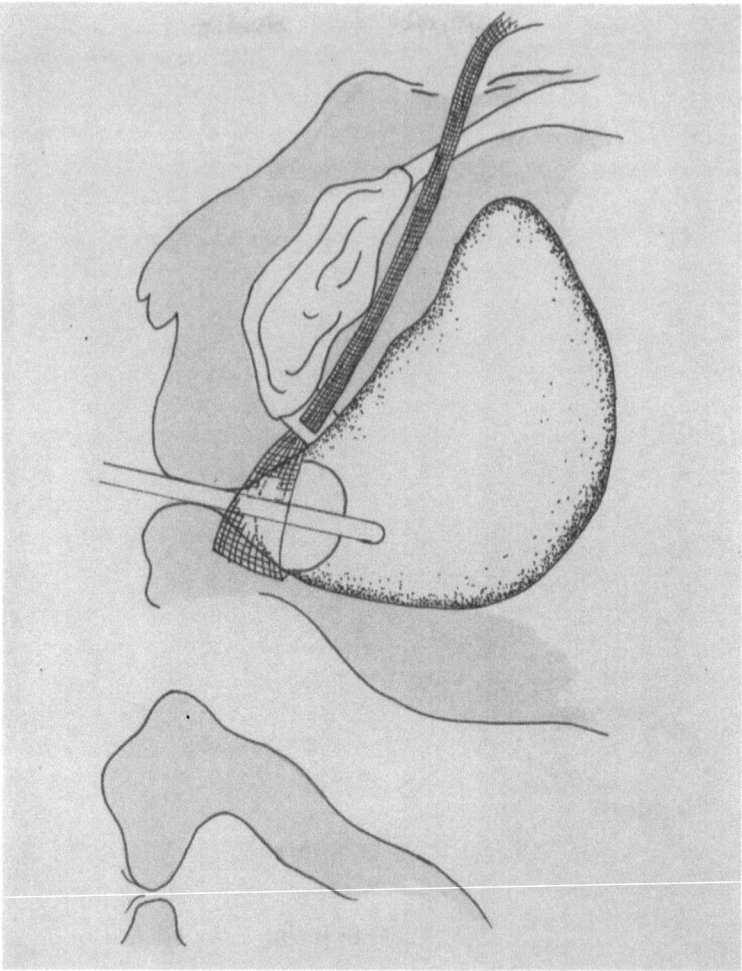

Fig. 6. With the two twine threads the nylon mesh band is carried upward so far that with the broad part of the band a loop is formed below the bladder neck.

After the vaginal ends of the twine threads are combined with the ends of the nylon mesh band, the ribbon is carried upward to a point where a loop is formed below the bladder neck (Fig. 6) with the broad part of the band. The sling should be adapted without folds (Fig. 7). If necessary the margins of the band should be fixed with one to three catgut plain sutures (4×0) to the bladder neck muscles. For the beginner it is not easy to determine the proper amount of tension to be applied to the sling. In this procedure the band should only support the bladder neck. In former times we tested the amount of tension by urethroscopy and urethra pressure profile measurement but these methods are complicated and do not give satisfactory

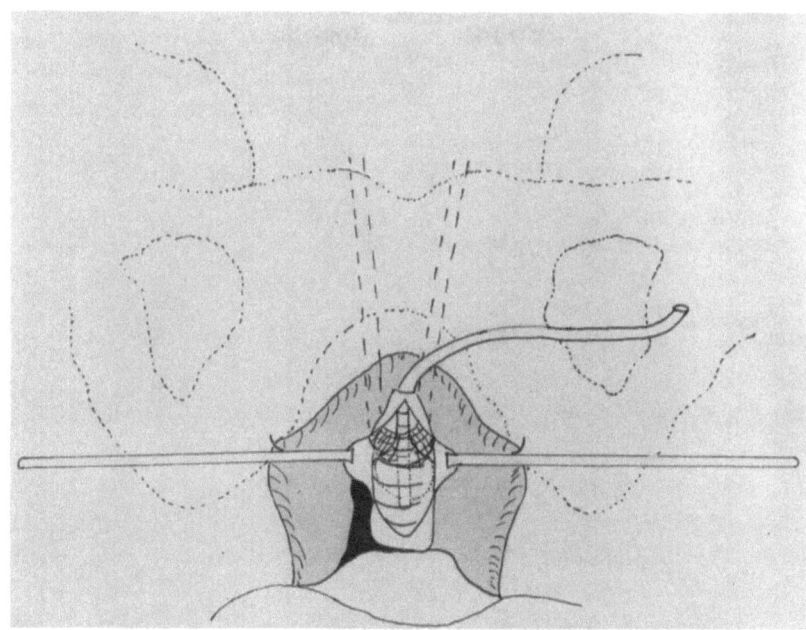

Fig. 7. The sling has to be adapted without folds.

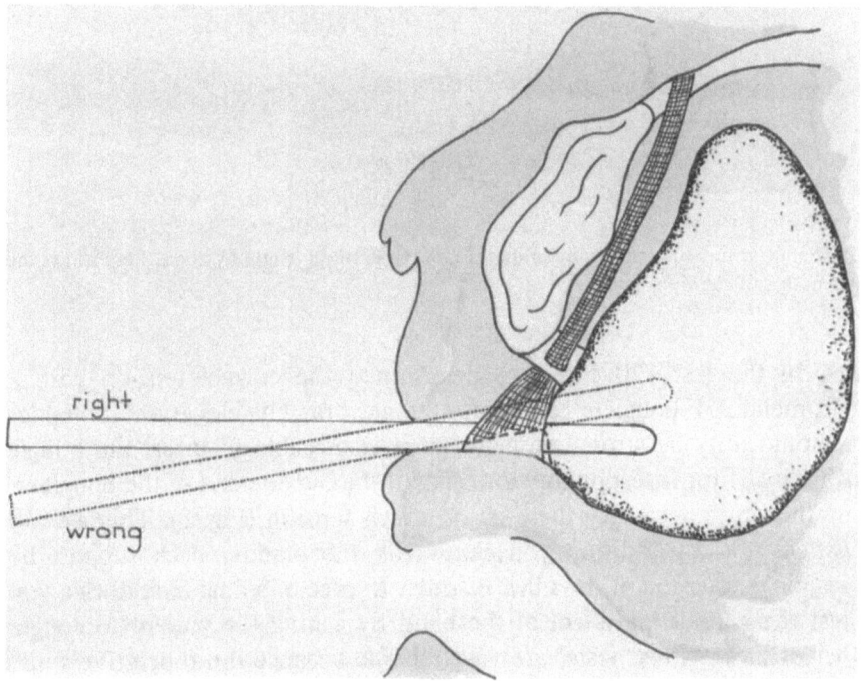

Fig. 8. The tension of the mesh band is controlled by the 'bougie test'. In case the mesh band has too much tension ('wrong') it is impossible to insert the straight metal 27F bougie horizontally.

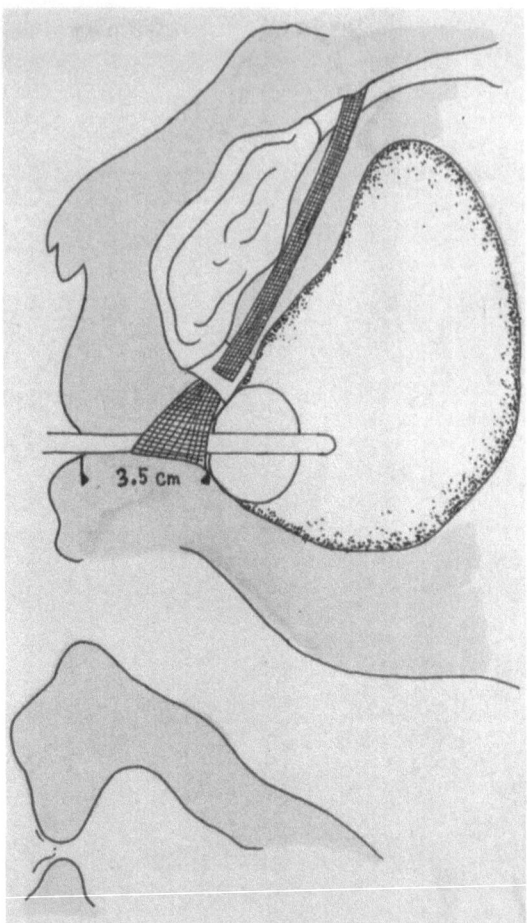

Fig. 9. The linear measurement with an increase of the urethral length by about 1 cm shows the bladder neck sufficiently supported.

results. In the last 120 cases we determined the correct tension with a straight metal 27F bougie inserted into the urethra. The elevation of bladder neck should only be strong enough that it is possible to insert the bougie horizontally. If for insertion any lowering of the outside end of the bougie or raising the tip is necessary there is too much tension (Fig. 8). This we call the *bougie test.* In addition you can verify the bladder neck support by suprapubic percussion of the filled bladder. In case of spinal anaesthesia you can test the supporting effect of the band by asking the patient to cough. Neither of these 'stress tests' are very reliable because intraoperative small loss of water is not correlated with a clinical SUI. On the other hand, if the band is too tight the patient will be unable to void freely. The *bougie test* will prevent this complication in most cases. The sling stays in the given correct position because of its mesh structure. In addition we adapt the two free ends by a dexon suture (2×0) in the subcutaneous tissue of the suprapubic wound and cut off the overlap parts.

If the bladder neck is properly supported the urethra will be lengthened. This can be registered by a repeated measurement, as already mentioned. Measurement conditions must always be the same, especially as regards filling the balloon (10 cc). Generally the increase of urethral length should be 1.0 cm (Fig. 9). The suprapubic wound is closed by subcutaneous sutures and skin clips. The vaginal wound is closed by vertical mattress sutures. We prefer monofile nylon stitches, and leave them, usually over a period of about 14 days, until the wound is healed. The vagina will be tamponaded by gauze for 36 hours. Urine drainage in a closed system has to be performed over three days. On the 4th and 5th postoperative day the catheter is plugged and the patient has to register every single bladder volume micturated. On the 6th day the catheter will be removed. For measuring the success of the operation the patient has to record the micturition day profile as done before the operation. Furthermore, the patient will be catherized for determination of residual urine, and the flow rate will be controlled again.

Complications

Most complications result from incorrect position and an inadequate tension of the sling. In those cases the sling is too far in a distal position and the bladder neck is not properly supported. No increase of urethral length can be registered, and SUI remains. If the same wrong distal position is combined with too much tension of the sling, a penetration of the urethral wall may occur. In such cases, as long as the miction is normal, the penetrated mesh can be cut with small scissors under urethroscopic control. After some weeks the urethral mucosa will close above the mesh spontaneously. If SUI still remains and the mesh is not penetrated after about 6 months a second sling procedure in correct position can be performed. However, this complication is very unusual and in one appearance occurred only once over a period of 10 years and 220 operations.

Another wrong position is the one where the sling is too far below the bottom of the bladder. In such a case the patient may have urinary incontinence produced by urge or detrusor dyssynergia, and the urethral linear measurement shows an excessive length over 4.0 to 5.0 centimeters. This abnormal distance is not the real length of the urethra. By compression of the bladder bottom the balloon of the Foley catheter used for measurement cannot reach the bladder neck. Contrary to SUI, the micturition day profile now shows very small volumes. In addition to urge incontinence SUI may continue to exist because the bladder neck is not properly supported. During the operative revision the sling should be transected so that the balloon can reach the bladder neck again and a new sling in correct position will be inserted.

In former times some infections of the suprapubic wounds occurred due to bacteria of the mersilene suture we used for adapting the ends of the nylon mesh. In such cases it was sufficient to remove the mersilene suture only as the nylon mesh did not tend to infection.

In some cases a vaginal wound dehiscence happened and the nylon mesh was uncovered. Under this condition we never noted an infection. The uncovered part of the mesh can be excised or mobilized vaginal walls can be attached to it. Since we only use monofile nylon mattress sutures for adapting the vagina a wound dehiscens very seldom turns up.

The most frequent complication is that the sling is too tight and the patient is unable to void normally. As matters stand we first put a suprapubic cystocath with a 10F silastic tube into the bladder. On the one hand the patient is able to empty the bladder in the normal way, on the other hand she can regulate the residual urine with the suprapubic catheter. If after six weeks free voiding is still impossible, the sling should be transected vaginally on one side of the bladder neck. By inserting a 27F bougie you can depress the mesh band in order to divide the band with a small scalpel or scissors. The cutting effect is sufficient when it is possible to insert the metal bougie into the urethra horizontally. This complication does not depreciate our long term results.

Conclusions

In the treatment of SUI the vaginal sling plasty has a firm place, especially in cases of recurrent disease. The disadvantages of sling plasty seen by Merrill (1975) are: infection by foreign body, mobilisation of fascial material, mobilisation of urethra with increasing iatrogenic urethral injury and finally the adjustment of the sling seems to require more surgical expertise than do other corrective procedures. In conclusion he believes that the sling procedures are usually reserved for patients who have failed previous surgery. All these points are worth mentioning. Nevertheless in our opinion some of them are inapplicable considering our method. The infection by foreign body depends upon the kind of synthetic material of the sling. As everyone knows, twisted mersilene tends to cause bacterial infection. Our experience shows that contrary to mersilene monofile nylon mesh band does not lead to infection, not even in cases of wound dehiscens with bacterial settling. We don't need fascial material. In the first place our operative procedure concerns the bladder neck so that a surgical injury of the urethra is avoidable. 'Measurement of urethra length' and 'bougie test' objectify the operative procedure in such a manner that a good result is not dependent on the surgical expertise of the urologist.

Furthermore, it is an important question whether the Pereyra procedure or the sling plasty with nylon mesh band is more reliable and easier to perform. As stated before there are some good reasons for Pereyra [8] to introduce his revised procedure. Important to this method are the posterior pillars of the pubo-urethral ligaments and the musculofascial fibers formed of the medial pillars of the pubo-coccygeus muscle which interlace with the periurethral tissues of the vesical neck. The colligated pubo-urethral ligaments supports, with the anterior musculofascial surfaces previously denuded of epithelium, when elevated retropubically by the suspensory sutures anchored to the suprapubic abdominal fascia, are held firmly against the posterior pubis. It is Pereyra's opinion that the result is that the musculofascial tissues produce fibrous union over a broad area of posterior pubic periosteum without tension between opposing surfaces. Pereyra introduced this relatively complicated revised technique because he had failures with his previous methods.

We prefer our method of sling plasty procedure rather than Pereyra's revised technique because we believe our method to be more reliable and easier to perform.

Instead of fascial sling we prefer the nylon mesh band for the following reasons:
1. No additional operation is necessary for sling acquirement.
2. The material is available any time.
3. The sling is stable, flexible and durable.
4. The excellent tissue tolerance with no tendency to bacterial infection.

Because our operation method is easy and does not last longer than 30 minutes, we use it as a primary effort for the correction of SUI and not only because other techniques have failed.

Summary

Patients with recurrent disease after operative correction of stress urinary incontinence need a special analysis. In particular vesico-vaginal fistulae and all kinds of unstable bladder have to be excluded.

The value of the various examination methods is discussed and attention drawn to the significance of the micturition-day-profile. In comparison with other methods the vaginal sling plasty with nylon mesh band is an easy operative procedure. On the basis of simple intraoperative tests, the measurement of urethra length and the bougie test which we introduced, you can carry out an exact measurable elevation of the bladder neck.

References

1. O'Conor Jr. V.J. Female urinary incontinence and vesicovaginal fistula. In: Glenn F.J. (ed) Urologic Surgery, 2nd Edition, Harper and Row Pub. Inc. Hagerstown, Maryland (1975).
2. Denos E. Note sûr une opération contre l'incontinence d'urine sur la femme. Ann. Mal. Org. Genitourin. 8 (1890): 344.
3. Kelly H.A. Incontinence of urine in women. Urol. Cutan. Rev., 17 (1913): 291.
4. Marshall V.F., Marchetti A.A. and Krantz K.E. The correction of stress incontinence by simple vesicourethral suspension. Surg. Gynaecol. Obstet. 88 (1949): 509.
5. Burch J.C. Cooper's ligament urethrovesical suspension for stress incontinence. Am. J. Obstet. Gynaecol. 100 (1968): 764.
6. Pereyra A.J. A simplified surgical procedure for the correction of stress incontinence in women. West. J. Surg. Obstet. Gynaecol. 67 (1959): 223.
7. Stamey T.A. Endoscopic suspension of the vesical neck for urinary incontinence. Surg. Gynaecol. Obstet. 136 (1973): 547.
8. Pereyra A.J. The revised Pereyra procedure using colligated pubourethral supports. In: Slate W.G. Disorders of the Female Urethra and Urinary Incontinence. The Williams and Wilkins Comp., Baltimore (1979).
9. Pereyra A.J. and Lebherz T.B. Combined urethral vesical suspension and vagino-urethroplasty for correction of urinary stress incontinence. Obstet. Gynaecol., 30 (1967): 4.
10. Pereyra A.J. and Lebherz T.B. The revised Pereyra procedure. In: Buchsbaum H.J. and Schmidt J.D. (ed) Gynaecologic and Obstetric Urology, Chapter 13, W.B. Saunders, Philadelphia (1978).
11. Goebell R. Zur operativen Beseitigung der angeborenen inkontinentia vesicae. Zentralbl. Gynaekol. 2 (1910): 187.
12. Ridley J.H. Urethral suspension using the fascia lata sling. In: Slate W.G. (ed) Disorders of the Female Urethra and Urinary Incontinence, The Williams and Wilkins Comp., Baltimore (1979).
13. Aldridge A.H. Transplantation of fascia for relief of urinary stress incontinence. Am. J. Obstet. Gynaecol. 44 (1942): 398.
14. Millin T. Discussion on stress incontinence in micturition. Proc. Sov. Soc. 40 (1947): 364.
15. Zoedler D. Zur operativen Behandlung der weiblichen Stressinkontinenz. Zeitschr. für Urologie (1961), p. 355.
16. Williams T.J. and Te Linde R.W. The sling operation for urinary incontinence using mersilene ribbon. Obstet. Gynaecol. 19 (1962): 241.
17. Moir J.C. The Gauze-Hammock operation (a modified Aldridge sling procedure). J. Obstet. Gynaecol. Brit. Cwlth. 75 (1968), I.
18. Morgan J.E. A sling operation, using Marlex Polypropylene Mesh for treatment of recurrent stress incontinence. Amer. J. Obstet. Gynaecol. 106 (1970): 369.
19. Zoedler D. Die operative Behandlung der weiblichen Harninkontinenz mit dem Kunststoff-Netz-Band. Aktuelle Urologie 1 (1970): 28.

III.6. Critical analysis of the role of surgery in the management of recurrent urinary stress incontinence

W. VERVECKEN & K. VAN CAMP

Many surgical procedures and devices have been developed and tried with varying degrees of success, including anterior colporrhaphy, suspension procedures, fascial sling, prosthetic devices and at last urinary diversion.

This wide range of methods indicates that the perfect operation does not exist. Each surgeon defends his preferred procedure according to his own experience. The cure rate varies from 60% to 85% in the first year.

As concerns women, normal continence results from the coincidence of several factors: functional urethral length, closing pressure, anatomic position of bladder neck and urethra, and the transmission of intra-abdominal pressure to the urethral wall.

The key in stress incontinence is a lack of passive transmission. Passive transmission of abdominal pressure to the intrapelvic urethra might at best balance a bladder-increase and thus maintain unchanged the resting closure pressure under stress. This pressure-transmission was found best at the bladder neck, fading gradually toward the distal urethra. Failure of this system is an indication for therapy.

The preferred treatment for recurrent stress incontinence is surgery, unless the disturbance is so mild that it causes only minor discomfort and social problems, or unless the patient is not fit to be operated owing to coexisting illness or old age.

The mild cases are sometimes corrected by exercises that strengthen the levator muscles. Pharmacologic therapy may be of some benefit.

The more serious cases need a further investigation. The basis of surgical treatment is a complete clinical, urodynamic and radiological examination.

A lot of patients are treated in different urological departments, hence the interpretation of the cases can be very difficult. The urodynamic evaluation is very important for recognizing associated illness such as unstable bladder, sphincter-dysfunction and neurological lesions.

Radiological investigations include an intravenous urography and a voiding cystography.

If one finds a transmission-failure, without other abnormalities, surgical treatment is preferred.

Otherwise one should correct first the coexistent abnormalities, and recheck after six months.

If there is no transmission-failure, but a simple sphincter-insufficiency, an endoscopic therapy is recommended. Even in recurrent urinary stress incontinence, the most used procedure is the Burch-colposuspension, as it is one of the major suprapubic procedures for the control of urinary incontinence in the female. At the same time, as it also corrects anterior vaginal wall-prolapse (cysto-urethrocele), Burch-colposuspension may now be considered as an alternative to the anterior colporrhaphy for the correction of both cysto-urethrocele and stress incontinence.

Before operation, some criteria must be fulfilled, otherwise success is not at all guaranteed.

There should be an adequate mobility and capacity of the vagina to allow elevation of the lateral vaginal fornices, no high fixation of the bladder neck, the presence of a negative urethral closure-pressure at rest. Absence of detrusor-instability and voiding-difficulty is important.

The technique is simple and an experienced surgeon will not have too many problems: it only takes a lot of time and a very careful dissection of the sclerotic tissue between bladder and symphysis.

Although the results differ from author to author, the mean success-rate with previous bladder neck-surgery is 71% at one year and 65% at five years.

The complications include trauma to the bladder; late complications are detrusor-instability and enterocele-formation. Other surgeons still use the Marshall-Marchetti-Krantz with good results. The cure rate in a first time is 80%. The better results reported in the latest papers stem partly from a far better indication. This cysto-urethropexy has been described as a highly succesful procedure for patients with primary stress incontinence. However, the possibility of obtaining good results will decrease when incontinence procedures have been done previously. Recent studies by Dr. J. Parnell show a cure rate of allmost 90% with this operation as secondary procedure for incontinence. In case the first operation consisted of vaginal procedures, the cure rate was about 10% lower, or 80%. Complications occur in 12%.

The lower cure rate in the vaginal procedure-group is probably due to the scarry-tissue that may reduce the mobility and pliability of the lower urethra, making it difficult to achieve the lengthening and fixation, required for success. Following the results, it appears that reoperation still has an excellent chance of success, approximately equal whether the first procedure was vaginal or suprapubic.

Although in our department the Burch-suspension is preferred, one cannot say that it would outweigh the other ones. Here, experience of the surgeon plays an important role. In case the sclerosis around the urethra is very tight, a perfect cervico-urethral dissection might be very dangerous and unlikely.

Therefore, it would be better to use a Stamey-Pereyra procedure or one of their modifications. And as, after previous suprapubic or vaginal operations such as slings, Burch, or M.M.K., the scartissue is often very adherent to the urethra, this operation takes also an important place in the therapy of recurrent stress incontinence.

We use a modified technique with non-absorbable materials; the urogenital diaphragm is brought superiorly to raise and to support the floor of the pelvis. This modified Pereyra-procedure gives a success-rate of 90% with very few complications. The suprapubic needle is prevented from entering the bladder or urethra by the surgeon's fingertip in the space of Retzius. Normally this procedure is quicker and more simple but can be quite difficult in case of recurrent incontinence with previous operations.

A cystoscopy afterwards excludes penetration of the sutures through the vesical wall and evaluates the correction of the vesico-urethral angle.

This technique is often preferred for treatment of very obese patients.

The above mentioned operations can be done if there exists a transmission-default.

However, in case there is only a sphincter-insufficiency, we prefer a teflon-injection. Endoscopic teflon-injection into the urethral wall is used in order to increase the urethral length and closure-pressure.

The technique has obvious advantages: short hospitalization, previous surgical interventions do not interfere with the injection, obesity does not represent a problem, as it can be repeated – if required – and does not hinder later operations, which may become necessary if teflon-therapy fails.

This is very important and a lot of surgeons consider the teflon-injection as a preferent minor procedure between surgery and conservative treatment. It is the first attempt in patients previously operated several times without success.

The cure rate is 70%. Some patients need more than one session. However, if there is no improvement after two sessions, one must consider the treatment as having failed. Nevertheless, the complications are minor.

If despite multiple operations there is a lack of success, an alternative solution exists: a number of patients with lower urinary tract-dysfunction may benefit from the implantation of an artificial sphincter. The principle is the transfer of pressure from a balloon to a cuff encording the urethra at the bladder neck level. The system operates manually by compressing a pump located in a labium majus.

The complications have been urethral erosion, leak from the prothesis and wound-infection. About 85% of the patients obtain satisfactory continence. We mention this technique as a last procedure if every other therapy has failed.

Ultimate solution in case of failure: urinary diversion or prosthetic devices.

In recurrent stress incontinence one must start at the beginning and make a total review and pay great attention to the age of the patient and previous operations. After a complete examination, eliminating all other diseases, one has to take a decision, according to ones own experience.

References

1. Burch J.C. Urethrovaginal fixation to Cooper's ligament for correction of stress incontinence, cystocele and prolapse. Am. J. Obstet. Gynaecol., 81 (1961): 281–290.
2. Dijkman and Friese. Vesical-urethral sustaining for recurrent urinary stress incontinence using the Stamey-Pereyra technique. Acta Urologica Belg., 52 (1984): 302–305.
3. Gillon G. and Stanton S.L. Long-term follow-up of surgery for urinary incontinence in elderly women. Br. J. Urol., 56, no. 5 (1984): 478–481.
4. Hald T. Artificial urinary sphincter. Boerhaave course; Second Course on surgical methods in urology (1983) 103–108.
5. Sarramon, Lher, Soulie, Courbelles, Rischmann. Recurrent stress incontinence. Therapeutic approach. Acta Urologica Belg., 52 (1984): 326–335.
6. Schulman S. Transurethral teflon-injection in the treatment of female stress incontinence. Acta Urologica Belg., 52 (1984): 269–273.
7. Stamey T.A. Endoscopic suspension of the vesical neck for urinary incontinence. Surgery, Gynaecology and Obstetrics, 136 (1973): 547–551.
8. Stanton S.L. and Cordoza L. Surgical treatment of incontinence in elderly women. Surgery, Gynaecology and Obstetrics, 150 (1980): 555–557.

CHAPTER FOUR

Incontinence and resoluting
of vaginal prolapse

IV.1. Anterior vaginal repair for urinary incontinence associated with vaginal prolapse

E. ZIMMERN, H.R. HADLEY & S. RAZ

Introduction

Classically, repair of *cystocele alone* is performed transvaginally whereas repair of *urethrocele alone* is approached transabdominally. When both problems occur simultaneously, which is quite frequent, one can consider the following options: (*1*) perform a classical transvaginal repair of the cystocele with a Kelly-Kennedy type anterior colporraphy, which is known for its high recurrence rate of postoperative incontinence (40–50%) in long term follow-ups because it leaves the urethra in a low, dependent position with very poor support, (*2*) perform a urethropexy transabdominally (Marshall-Marchetti, Burch, etc.), which certainly cures the urethrocele but is unlikely to provide a solid repair of the herniated bladder and disrupted pubocervical fascia, or (*3*) do two separate procedures, vaginal to correct the cystocele and abdominal to repair the urethrocele, which is far from being ideal for the patient. Therefore, our *proposal* for treatment of 'vaginal prolapse associated with stress urinary incontinence' is to combine both repairs of the cystocele and urethrocele by means of the same transvaginal approach, in order to not only adequately correct the cystocele but also to provide a long lasting support to the bladder neck and proximal urethra in an elevated, fixed, non-obstructed, retropubic position. Following a clinical and radiographical classification of the patients in grades of severity from I to IV, we briefly reviewed the incidence, aetiology and diagnosis of this condition. Then, we more extensively detailed the available options of treatment, with a particular emphasis on the technique of cystocele repair and modified needle bladder neck suspension that we advocate for severe cases.

Classification

Whereas cystocele represents descent of the bladder through the pubocervical fascia [8], urethrocele represents loss of support by the pubocervical fascia and the pubourethral ligaments [7]. We define cystocele both clinically and radiographically. During physical examination in the standing position with coughing and straining, grade I corresponds to a minimal descent of the bladder base. Grade II refers to the bladder base approaching the introitus. Grade III corresponds to the descent of the bladder base at the introitus. Grade IV refers to major prolapse of the bladder base outside the introitus. This subjective classification must be confirmed by objective criteria obtained radiographically. A cystocele is prolapse of the bladder base below the inferior ramus of the symphysis pubis on lateral films. The grading from I to IV refers to the amount of descent seen on spot films during straining.

We defined urethrocele as posterior deviation of the urethra which results in hypermobility that can be demonstrated during physical examination with the use of the Q-tip test. This clinical evaluation of urethrocele needs to be confirmed by radiographical findings of posterior displacement and rotation of the urethral axis more than 30 to 35 degrees from the vertical.

Urethrocele should not be confused with 'urethral prolapse', which should be reserved for 'prolapse of the mucosa at the external meatus'.

Incidence

Cystocele associated with urethrocele represents a rather commonly encountered situation both in urological and gynecological practice.

The incidence of cystourethrocele, however, is hard to evaluate. A British survey of 1000 women requiring gynecologic surgery revealed that 20% were scheduled to have repair of cystourethrocele [9] while, in the elderly, this incidence rises to 60% [10]. Stress urinary incontinence as a result of urethral sphincter incompetence is found in about 50% of patients with cystourethrocele.

Aetiology

The common causes reported in the aetiology of cystourethrocele include child delivery (prolonged and difficult labor, forceful delivery, inadequate repair of pelvic floor injuries, multiparity) and menopause (the withdrawal of estrogens weakens the pelvic floor supports of the bladder and urethra). Congenital weakness of the pelvic floor, not uncommonly associated with spina bifida or bladder exstrophy, has also been reported. Chronic cough, constipation or heavy lifting are only considered as contributing factors [7]. In our experience, the surprising number of patients that complained of cystourethrocele after a MMK operation raised some questions regarding the role of this type of abdominal bladder neck suspension in either unmasking or facilitating the appearance of a cystocele.

Diagnosis

Although it is usually a benign condition, a cystourethrocele may lead to very troublesome urinary symptoms. Patients frequently complain of: (*1*) discomfort from a mass bulging out of the vaginal introitus, (*2*) stress urinary incontinence, associated with hypermobility of the urethra or intrinsic urethral incompetence, and (*3*) obstructive symptoms with retention of urine leading to frequency, urgency, urinary tract infection, and at a later stage, overflow incontinence. In a recent review of 35 patients with severe cystourethrocele, the commonest symptom was stress incontinence (60%) whereas mixed stress and urge incontinence was only reported in 15% of the patients.

Physical examination is imperative to assess the degree of the cystocele which is noticeable on inspection. After gentle retraction of the posterior vaginal wall with a speculum, an evaluation of the degree of the cystocele during straining and coughing may be obtained. Sometimes, it may be necessary to examine the patient in the standing position and/or perform a cystourethrogram in the standing position, which objectively reproduces the physical findings.

On speculum examination, the examiner may appreciate the presence of an associated uterine descent and the hypermobility of the urethra by the Q-tip test. A Q-tip introduced into the urethra will slightly move (1–2 cm) during straining if the urethra is well supported. With loss of urethral support, however, there is a wide swing in the distal end of the Q-tip, reflecting movement within the urethra. Rectal vaginal examination evaluates the tone of the anal sphincter and, eventually, confirms the presence of a concomitant rectocele and/or enterocele.

Prior to the operation, it is important to assess continence, with a relatively full bladder. True stress incontinence should cease to be evident when the anterior vaginal wall is elevated by pressure of the tips of the examining fingers in the region of the bladder neck (Bonney's test or sign). Some patients who did not complain of urinary incontinence will demonstrate obvious leakage when the cystocele is reduced by the speculum. This was especially clear in the majority of the patients suffering from obstructive symptoms, suggesting that repair of the cystocele *alone* will produce incontinence.

Among the other preoperative investigations, it is necessary to systematically measure the residuals of urine and to obtain a mid-stream specimen for culture and sensitivity. When urinary incontinence is present, a complete urodynamic evaluation including water or gas filling cystometry, simultaneous pressure-flow study, urethral pressure profilometry, cystoscopy and voiding cystourethrogram, is also advisable prior to the surgery. These urodynamic studies help to objectively demonstrate an obstructive pattern, an incompetent sphincteric function, and/or an overactive bladder. Finally, because bilateral hydronephrosis is not uncommon, a routine IVP is recommended in cases with major cystocele (grade III to IV).

Treatment

Provided there is no urinary tract infection, outlet obstruction and/or hydronephrosis, vaginal prolapse carries very little risk for life. But its association with urinary incontinence can transform this relatively benign condition into a 'social cancer', especially in the elderly.

Conservative treatment including pads, pessaries, and hormonal treatment is considered for patients medially unfit for surgery. When surgery is contemplated, several different operations may be advocated in the treatment of cystourethrocele.

The anterior colporraphy

The basic vaginal repair was described by Kelly and Dumm in 1914 [3], then modified by Kennedy in 1937 [4]. The Kelly-Kennedy vaginal procedure continues to be widely accepted and is still the most currently performed operation.

In a recent review, Drukker examined the place of anterior colporraphy and the criteria that make it 'a procedure of choice for stress urinary incontinence associated with *moderate* cystocele' [18].

When a cystocele is present, the technique consists of an incision of the anterior vaginal wall over the extent of the prolapsed bladder. Each resulting lateral vaginal flap is freed from the underlying bladder. A row of interrupted sutures placed in the outer muscular layer of the bladder wall and the surrounding pubocervical fascia will then reinforce the bladder base posterior to the bladder neck [2].

If a cystourethrocele is present, the initial vertical incision should be carried more anteriorly to expose the proximal urethra. One or two sutures (Kelly sutures) are placed at the bladder neck to elevate and narrow it [7].

Despite many variations [10, 20] this procedure appears to have an important recurrence rate (40%–60%) of postoperative incontinence [2, 19–21]. Many surgeons believe that, whatever technique of anterior colporraphy is contemplated [1, 11, 12], it has a great chance to cure the cystocele, but it will not restore the urethra and bladder neck in an elevated, fixed, non-obstructed, retropubic position. After such an anterior vaginal repair, the urethra is left in a low dependent position, which explains why we commonly see patients after anterior colporraphy complaining of persistent or more severe stress incontinence than before the operation or appearance of stress incontinence not present preoperatively [12, 18].

The abdominal approaches

Marshall in 1949 [5] reintroduced the abdominal approach and presented evidence that his technique of suspension gave better long term results than the vaginal approach. It certainly is effective in curing stress urinary incontinence, but this approach does not allow to repair the herniation of the bladder through the pubocervical fascia. Also, the placement of periurethral stitches may result in an organic urethral obstruction as demonstrated in some patients with post-operative obstructive symptoms.

Stanton et al. in 1976 [7] using the Burch colposuspension with fixation of the paraurethral and paravesical tissues to Cooper's (ileopectineal) ligament [6, 19], confirmed that abdominal operations could be successfully performed to cure stress incontinence as well as cystocele without any potential damage to the urethra.

Needle urethral-vesical suspension procedures

By 1981, Kohorn's opinion that 'the gynecologist needs to recognize that adequate elevation of the bladder neck cannot be achieved vaginally, and the urologist needs to recognize that a cystocele or urethrocele cannot be repaired by a retropubic approach' reflected the existing problem [13]. The Kelly-Kennedy technique certainly gives satisfactory results in cystocele repair, but it provides a less than ideal support to the bladder neck and proximal urethra [18, 22]. This technique can be nowadays efficiently replaced by some newer techniques of transvaginal needle bladder neck suspension. Therefore, even if cystocele can be repaired abdominally, we feel that the same transvaginal approach can combine the advantages of cystocele repair with a good operation to cure the urethrocele.

Since Dr. Pereyra's first description of needle bladder neck suspension in 1959, different techniques have been reported [14-16]. In 1981, we described our modification which utilizes the anterior vaginal wall lateral to the bladder neck for the support of the urethra and bladder neck. Other advantages include: (1) the deeply placed and solidly anchored sutures in the vaginal wall and the endopelvic fascia in a position lateral to the bladder neck and proximal urethra, (2) the passage of the needle under finger-tip guidance to avoid bladder entry, (3) the confirmation by cystoscopy that there has been no damage to the bladder, urethra or ureters, and that the quality of the support provided to the bladder neck is adequate, and (4) the tying of the sutures individually first in order to preserve continence by the intact contralateral side if one suture line fails. Lateral placement of the sutures allows adequate elevation of the bladder neck and proximal urethra without damage to the intrinsic sphincter mechanisms and prevents over-zealous traction on these sutures from causing permanent urinary retention and/or bladder instability [23]. During a 2 to 4 year follow-up of 100 consecutive patients, we reported a 96% success rate in the cure of stress urinary incontinence [17]. More recently, an unpublished review of 250 patients followed from 1978 to 1982 revealed a similar success rate.

Operative technique

For *mild* cystoceles (grade I to II), we use a modification of the technique reported for the treatment of stress urinary incontinence without prolapse [17]. The major differences are that: (1) each side of the inverted 'U' incision is extended more posteriorly, and (2) the sutures are anchored not only at the level of the bladder neck but also at a lower level extending towards the cardinal ligaments to support the bladder base as well as the bladder neck.

The technique to repair *larger cystoceles* (grade III to IV) is described below.

On the night before and the morning of the operation, the patient is given intravenous antibiotics (aminoglycoside and ampicillin) and 2 Betadine® (povidone iodine) douches in order to reduce vaginal pathogens. After general or spinal anesthesia is induced, the patient is placed in the dorsal lithotomy position. After a weighted retractor is placed in the vagina, the labia are retracted laterally with stay sutures. A Foley catheter is inserted. Normal saline is injected into the anterior vaginal wall to facilitate the dissection of the underlying perivesical fascia from the perivaginal fascia. A vertical midline incision is made in the anterior vaginal wall, which extends from the area of the bladder neck to the posterior edge of the cystocele (Fig. 1). In case of an associated enterocele, the incision will extend more posteriorly.

The dissection is carried laterally in this avascular plane so as to free the herniated part of the bladder from the anterior vaginal wall. The pubocervical fascia is thin medially and becomes thicker laterally towards the levator ani muscles (Fig. 2). Posteriorly the dissection will reach the peritoneal fold. If an enterocele is present, it is imperative at that stage to open the peritoneal sac and to repair it.

174

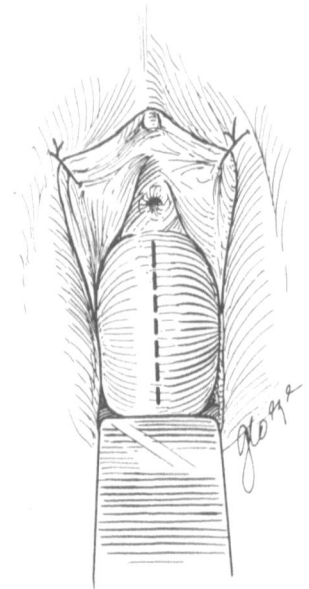

Fig. 1. Midline vaginal incision.

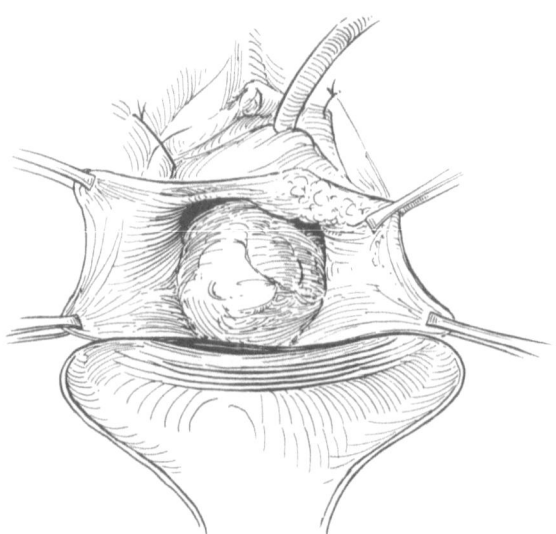

Fig. 2. Careful dissection of the cystocele from the vaginal wall on both sides.

After adequate mobilization of the herniated part of the bladder, a gauze is placed to reduce and to protect the bladder during the next step of the operation: the needle suspension of the bladder neck. At the level of the bladder neck but very lateral to it and the urethra, the retropubic space is entered on each side by bluntly or sharply dividing the endopelvic fascia.

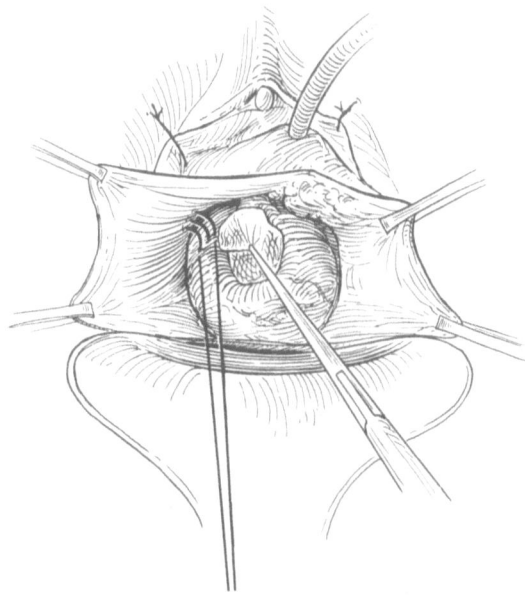

Fig. 3. #1 Prolene sutures are placed in a helicoidal fashion on each side. They secure the endopelvic fascia to the vaginal wall excluding the vaginal mucosa.

All adherent tissue is dissected free from the posterior aspect of the symphysis pubis to further define the retropubic space.

At the level of the bladder neck although distant from it, a #1 Prolene suture on a #6 Mayo needle is passed in a helicoidal fashion so as to adequately secure at least three strong 'bites' of both the medial aspect of the endopelvic fascia and the full thickness of the vaginal wall, excluding the vaginal epithelium (Fig. 3). A similar suture is placed on the opposite side at the level of the bladder neck. A 2–3 cm incision is made in the suprapubic area, just above the symphysis pubis. A blunt needle is passed bilaterally under finger-tip control through the retropubic space and into the vaginal area. Both ends of the ipsilateral anchoring suture are threaded through the eye of the needle. The needle is then withdrawn thereby transferring the suture from the vagina to the suprapubic position. After the contralateral suture is transferred in a similar fashion, upward traction on these sutures provides adequate support to return and maintain the urethra and bladder neck in a high normal retropubic position.

To repair the cystocele, 2/0 Dexon® figure-of-eight sutures are placed to approximate the lateral edges of the pubocervical fascia (Fig. 4). After indigo carmine is administered intravenously, cystoscopy is performed to confirm that blue emits from each ureteral orifice, that no sutures have entered the bladder or the urethra, and that the bladder neck is well supported.

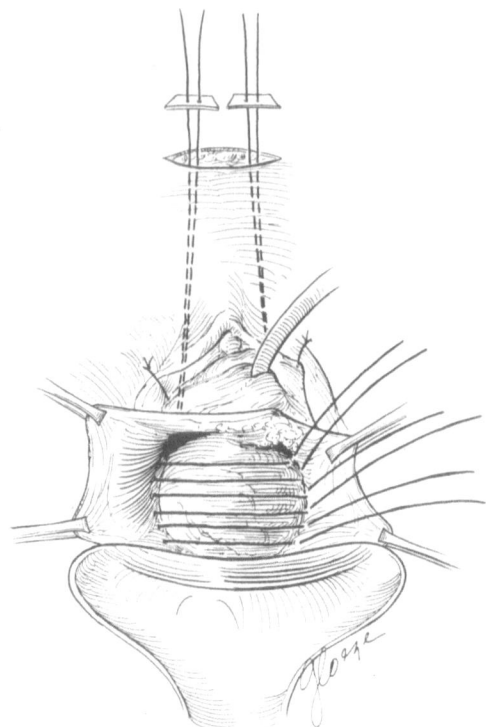

Fig. 4. The space below the bladder base is reinforced by approximating the pubocervical fascia using figure-of-eight sutures placed in the levator ani muscles and lateral vaginal wall.

The excess vaginal wall is trimmed and the vaginal incision is closed with a running 3/0 Dexon® suture. If indicated after the cystocele repair, other procedures including rectocele repair (posterior colporraphy) and/or operative repair of uterine prolapse must be done at that stage. On each side, the two ends of each Prolene suture are threaded through and then tied over a 2×1 cm Teflon pledget (Fig. 5). Then the distal ends of each suture are united over the midline with multiple knots (Fig. 6). A pack with antibiotics cream is placed in the vagina. The skin is closed with a subcuticular running suture of 3/0 Dexon® (Dexon®: polyglycolic acid).

Postoperative care

The patient is allowed a regular diet and ambulates the first day after the operation. Prophylactic antibiotics are usually given for a few days postoperatively. The vaginal packing and the Foley catheter are removed on the first postoperative day. The patient is immediately started on a program of

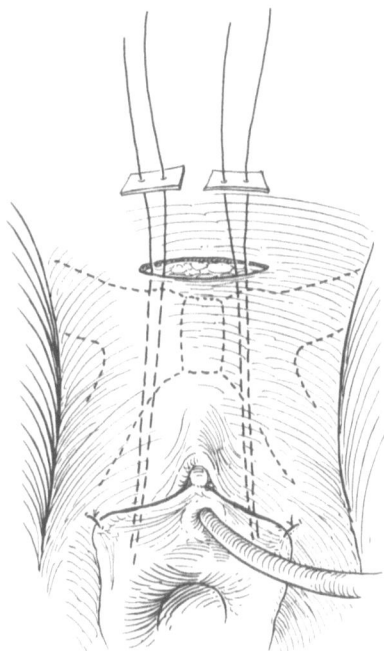

Fig. 5. The suprapubic Prolene sutures are threaded through a Teflon pledget before being tied over it. This allows tension to be exerted on a larger surface.

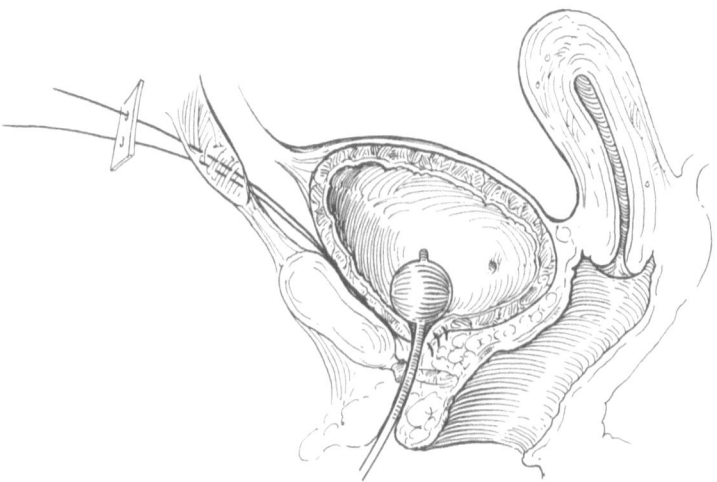

Fig. 6. Lateral view of the pelvis after cystocele repair and Pereyra-Raz bladder neck suspension.

intermittent self catheterization. If the patient is able to void (50 % after 24 hours), we discharge her the next day. If she is still in retention, we allow her to return home as soon as she learns how to perform intermittent self catheterization. The length of hospital stay ranges from 3 to 10 days with a mean of 4 days.

Indications

Our indications for surgery are patients with *symptomatic* cystocele and urethrocele, including mainly discomfort from a mass protruding out of the vagina, stress urinary incontinence and obstructive symptoms. Since bladder neck suspension *alone* is not adequate to repair a large cystocele as previously explained, we repair the cystocele transvaginally, as classically described, and, concomitantly, repair the urethrocele by means of our modified needle bladder neck suspension.

Results

We recently reviewed 35 patients with severe cystourethrocele (grade III to IV) followed for 6 to 48 months with a mean follow-up of 21 months. During the immediate follow-up there were no complications of fistula, bleeding or bladder penetration.

Cure of cystourethrocele was achieved in 34 patients after one surgery. Our only failure has been reoperated with the exact same procedure and remains cured 3 years later. Among the patients who had pre-operative stress urinary incontinence, 19 over 20 (95%) were cured by the operative repair of the urethrocele. We have 4 patients in permanent urinary retention (2 with myelomeningocele, 2 with a large bladder capacity due to a decompensated acontractile bladder which was present pre-operatively) who were doing and continue to do clean intermittent self catheterization, but are cured of incontinence.

Four patients with only urge incontinence were cured of this symptom by the operation. Among 11 patients with frequency and urgency pre-operatively, only 2 (18%) had persistence of these symptoms and they responded well to pharmacological therapy. Appearance of other prolapses not present at the time of the initial surgery was noticed in six patients who underwent a second operation, 2 for uterine prolapse, 2 for enterocele, and 2 for rectocele.

Conclusion

We have presented our experience of the anterior vaginal approach in the repair of vaginal prolapse associated with urinary incontinence, with a particular emphasis on classical cystocele repair combined with our modified bladder neck suspension for the treatment of severe cystourethrocele (grade III to IV). Our results in 35 patients with the latter condition followed from 6 to 48 months showed an excellent cure rate for cystourethrocele, a 95% cure rate for patients with pre-operative stress urinary incontinence and no late appearance of incontinence not present prior to the surgery. Our series did not show any immediate or delayed post-operative complications.

The vaginal approach has numerous advantages including: good exposure, minimal bleeding, no need to open the abdomen, possible repair of associated uterine prolapse, rectocele and/or enterocele, short procedure, and simple post-operative convalescence. Compared to the abdominal approach, it seems to give similar or maybe better long term results, and should, therefore, be recognized as part of the urological armamentarium for the treatment of anterior vaginal prolapse associated with urinary incontinence.

References

1. Delaere K.P.J., Moonen W.A., Debruyne F.M.J., Michiels H.G.E. and Renders G.A.M. Anterior vaginal repair, cause of troublesome voiding disorder. Eur. Urol. 5 (1979): 190–194.
2. Green T.H Jr. Vaginal repair. In: Stanton S.L., Tanagho E.A. Surgery of female incontinence. Springer-Verlag, Berlin, Heidelberg, New York, Publishers, chapt. 3 (1980), pp. 31–39.
3. Kelly H.A., Dumm W.M. Urinary incontinence in women without manifest injury to the bladder. Surgery, Gynecology and Obstetrics, 18 (1914): 444–450.
4. Kennedy W.T. Incontinence of urine in the female, the urethral sphincter mechanism, damage function, and restoration of control. American Journal of Obstetrics and Gynecology, 34 (1937): 576–589.
5. Marshall V.F., Marchetti A. and Krantz K.E. The correction of stress incontinence by simple vesico-urethral suspension. Surgery, Gynecology and Obstetrics, 88 (1949): 509–518.
6. Stanton S.L., Williams J.E. and Ritchie D. The colposuspension operation for urinary incontinence. British Journal of Obstetrics and Gynecology, 83 (1976): 890–895.
7. Stanton S.L. Vaginal prolapse. In: Raz S. (ed) Female Urology. W.B. Saunders Company, Chapt. 13 (1983), pp. 229–240.
8. Reiffenstuhl G. and Platzer W. Atlas of Vaginal Surgery. Vol. 1. Edited by Friedmann E.A., W.B. Saunders Company (1975).
9. Stallworthy J.A. Prolapse: aetiology, diagnosis and treatment. Parts I and II. Br. Med. J., 1 (1971): 499–539.
10. Pacey K. Pathology and repair of genital prolapse. J. Obstet. Gynaecol. Brit. Emp., 56 (1949): 1–14.
11. Gibson G.B. The repair of genital prolapse. Am. J. Obst. & Gynec. Dec., (1959), p. 1275–1284.
12. Nichols D.H., Randall C.L. In: Baltimore, Williams and Wilkins (eds) Vaginal surgery. (1976) pp. 31–43.
13. Kornhorn E.I. Disorders of pelvic architecture: Uterine prolapse, Cystocele, Urethrocele,

Rectocele, Enterocele. In: McGuire E. (ed) Urinary Incontinence. Grune & Statton, Inc., chapt. 2 (1981): 29–36.

14. Pereyra A.J. A simplified surgical procedure for the correction of stress incontinence in women. West J. Surg., 67 (1959): 223.

15. Stamey T.A. Cystoscopic suspension of the vesical neck for urinary incontinence. Surg. Gynecol. Obstet., 136 (1973): 547.

16. Cobb O.E. and Ragde H. Correction of female stress incontinence. J. Urol., 20 (1978): 418.

17. Raz S. Modified bladder neck suspension for female stress incontinence. Urology, 18 (1981): 82.

18. Drukker B.H. Anterior colporraphy. In: Buschbaum and Schmidt (eds) Gynecologic & Obstetric Urology. W.B. Saunders Co., Philadelphia (1978).

19. Burch J.C. Urethro-vaginal fixation to Cooper's ligament for correction of stress incontinence. Am. J. Obstet. Gynecol., 100 (1961): 768.

20. Ingelman-Sundberg A. Operative technique in stress incontinence of urine in the female. Nord. Med., 32 (1946): 2297.

21. Ross R.A. and Singleton H.M. Vaginal prolapse and stress urinary incontinence. W. Va. Med. J., 65 (1969): 77–79.

22. Stanton S.L., Hilton P., Norton C., Cardozo L. Clinical and urodynamic effects of anterior colporraphy and vaginal hysterectomy for prolapse with and without incontinence. Br. J. Obstet. Gynecol., 89 (1982): 459–463.

23. McGuire E., Savastano J. Stress incontinence and bladder instability. Proceedings of the Urodynamics Society. Sixth Symposium, New Orleans, Louisiana, USA, p. 43 (1984).

IV.2. Anterior colporrhaphy for urinary incontinence associated with vaginal prolapse: a gynaecological view

J. JANSSENS, F.M. KAUER & M.C. de JONGE

Introductory remarks

One should realize that also in case of a coexisting prolapse of vaginal walls and/or uterus the symptoms of stress incontinence can be caused by: (1) sphincter insufficiency, (2) bladder instability, (3) mixed type urinary incontinence (sphincter insufficiency as well as bladder instability), and (4) overflow incontinence.

Prolapse of vaginal walls and/or uterus can cause sphincter insufficiency through: (1) deficient transmission of intraperitoneal pressure because the descended bladder neck lies beneath the 'pelvic transmission sphere', and (2) an increased tension, provoked by the cystocele, on the vesical-urethral junction in case of lowered urethral tone (vesicalisation).

Prolapse of vaginal walls and/or uterus can cause m. detrusor instability through: (1) anatomical change of the bladder – cystocele formation and rotation of the bladder – causing irritability of the bladder, manifesting itself in frequency, urgency, urge incontinence and also the symptom stress incontinence caused by the stimulus of the strain on the inner bladder wall due to coughing etc., or even independent of coughing etc., only caused by walking or standing in an upright position, and (2) provoking m. detrusor contraction secondary to leakage of a small portion of urine in stress situations in only the proximal funnelled part of the urethra, the so called 'stress induced bladder instability'.

Prolapse of vaginal walls and/or uterus can cause dripping out of a cystocele when the patient is standing up after 'completed' micturition because: (1) the content of the cystocele is then evacuated like the water pouring out of a bottle held oblique, and (2) there exists – extremely infrequently – a stenosis due to pinching of the bladder neck via extreme rotation of the bladder and thus ischuria paradoxa.

As in urinary incontinence not associated with prolapse, the patient has to be examined thoroughly – including uroflowmetry, endoscopy, urethrocystotonometry and in still unclear cases also videocystourethrography.

In view of the therapeutic approach to urinary incontinence associated with prolapse it is important to know about: (1) the pathogenesis of urinary incontinence: what kind of incontinence exists? a) sphincter insuffiency, b) bladder instability, c) mixed type urinary incontinence or d) overflow incontinence and (2) the passage potency of the urethra, in case of stenosis, dilatation or meatomy, has to be considered.

One should try to ascertain: (1) the length of the urethra – whether it is shortened, elevated, stretched, narrowed or lengthened, (2) the configuration of the urethrovesical junction; in case of funnelling elevation, stretching and lengthening of the urethra as well as bladder neck plication should be added, producing some narrowing and increased smooth muscle bulk of the bladder outlet and lessening its tendency to funnel, and (3) the evacuation power of the m. detrusor vesicae; when the bladder contractility is diminished one should guard against effecting too much narrowing and creating a too strong urethra resistance. This can be done by plication of the bladder outlet, not too strong in order to avoid the danger of retentio urinae and an overflow situation.

In case of exclusively or predominantly sphincter insufficiency or 'equally' mixed urinary incontinence associated with such a moderate prolapse of the anterior wall of the vagina that by performing the elevation test complete stretching of the urethra and correction of the cystocele can be obtained, a colposuspension operation according to Burch should be the method of choice. (1) In case of relaxation of the vagina outlet and rectocele *it is urgently necessary* to combine the colposuspension operation with a colpoperineoplastic repair; (2) If descensus of the uterus exists *it is urgent* that the colposuspension operation is combined with an abdominally performed hysterectomy (except when preservation of child bearing capacity is desired: then primarily a Manchester plastic repair should be done).

In case of exclusively or predominantly sphincter insufficiency or equally mixed type urinary incontinence associated with a prolapse of the anterior vaginal wall that cannot be corrected by a colposuspension operation according to Burch, a colporrhaphy anterior and colpoperineoplastic repair should be done. Execution of a colpoperineoplastic repair should be done almost routinely because strengthening of the posterior fibres of the levator ani muscle is beneficial for several reasons. It prevents the ballooned vagina from functioning as an air chamber, which would result in a lower transmission of the intra abdominal pressure on the urethra in stress situations; it gives a better upholding of the uterus (or – if not present – the vaginal vault) and by strengthening the parurethrium via radiation of fibres of the levator muscle in it the patient can restrain the power of intraperitoneal pressure better. The colporrhaphy anterior and colpoperineoplastic repair should be combined with a vaginal hysterectomy or amputation of the portio according to Manchester procedure in case of prolapse of the uterus (the latter when preservation of child bearing capacity is desired).

In case of exclusively or predominantly detrusor instability associated with every size of prolapse of the vagina walls (and possibly also of the uterus) an anterior colporrhaphy and colpoperineoplastic repair should be performed, restricting oneself concerning the narrowing and strengthening of the bladder neck in order to prevent retention of the urine (combination with vaginally performed hysterectomy or amputation of the portio should be done as stated above).

In case of bladder instability secondary to leakage of a small portion of urine in stress situations in only the proximal funnel part of the urethra and a positive effect of the 'Coolsaet manoevre',* one should generally perform a suspension operation according to Burch, except when the cystocele is so large that it cannot be replaced totally by the elevation test; in that case a vaginal operation should be performed.

Remarks

In literature there is difference of opinion about the execution of a suspension operation in addition to anterior colporrhaphy (and colpoperineoplastic repair). The possible modifications are:
— a Stamey-Pereyra suspension
— a colposuspension according to Burch
— a urethrovesical suspension according to Marshall-Marchetti-Krantz
— a sling operation.
Concerning the Stamey-Pereyra method, several authors have stated that the results obtained by this method are in the long run just as good as those obtained with a standard anterior colporrhaphy and urethral plication only. The high suspension at the time of surgery is no longer present 6–8 months postsurgically, as mentioned by Drucker [1] and documented by Christ et al. [2]: in 72 percent of his patients after delayed postoperative cystourethrography.

We agree with Stanton et al. [3, 4], that is is difficult to assess objectively the results reported by several more optimistic authors as there is no mention of any attempt to differentiate these cases in the aetiology of the urinary incontinence. Frequently the number of patients is too small, the observation period is too short and the methods of investigation of success, improvement or failure are questionable. We do not advocate the Stamey-Pereyra procedure additional to an anterior colporrhaphy.

---

* Coolsaet claims that prevention of bladder instability caused by leakage as described by performing the elevation test, is a signal that abdominally executed suspension operation methods will have great succes.

Concerning other suspension methods: in general we do not combine anterior colporrhaphy with other suspension methods, except in case of very severe sphincter insufficiency with very low transmission rate and inability to achieve sufficient elevation of the bladder neck by the vaginal route only. Because vaginal and abdominal operations executed at the same time are fairly traumatic and frequently followed by postoperative complications, we prefer to perform the vaginal procedure only, knowing that in approximately 30% of the cases recurrent stress incontinence will appear in the future, requiring a suspension procedure, which is then usually highly successful (90%).

References

1. Drucker B.H. Discussion to: The Pereyra procedure. Am. J. Obstet. Gynaecol. 125, 3 (1976): 346–352.
2. Christ T. et al.: Urethrovesical needle suspension: Postoperative loss of vesical neck support demonstrated by chain cystography. Obstet. Gynaecol. 34 (1969): 489.
3. Stanton S.L. et al. The colposuspension operation for urinary incontinence. Br. J. Obstet. and Gynaecol. 83 (1976): 890–895.
4. Stanton S.L. Female urinary incontinence. Lloyd-Luke L.T.D., London (1977).

IV.3. The surgical possibilities and limitations of the vaginal approach

L. BECK

Vaginal prolapse is the result of an inherent weakness of the vaginal supporting structures, such as the uterosacral ligament and the lower portion of the cardinal ligament. Other contributory factors are trauma from child birth, obesity, postmenopausal atrophy, unsuccessful healing of the supporting structures following abdominal or vaginal hysterectomy and others. In cases of vaginal prolapse we have to differentiate:

1. vaginal prolapse mainly with a cystocele
2. prolapse of the uterus or, if the uterus is removed, vaginal vault prolapse
3. vaginal prolapse mainly due to a rectocele and/or in combination with an enterocele.

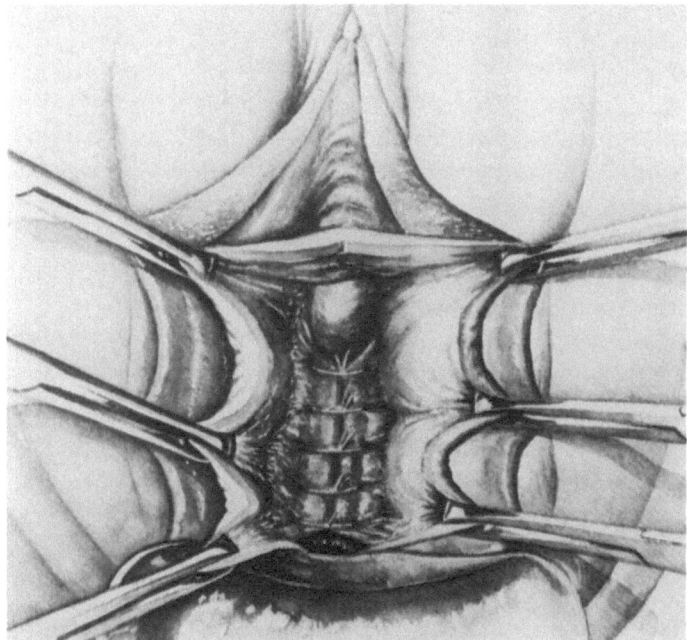

Fig. 1. Anterior colporrhaphy (from Käser, Atlas d. gyn. Op.).

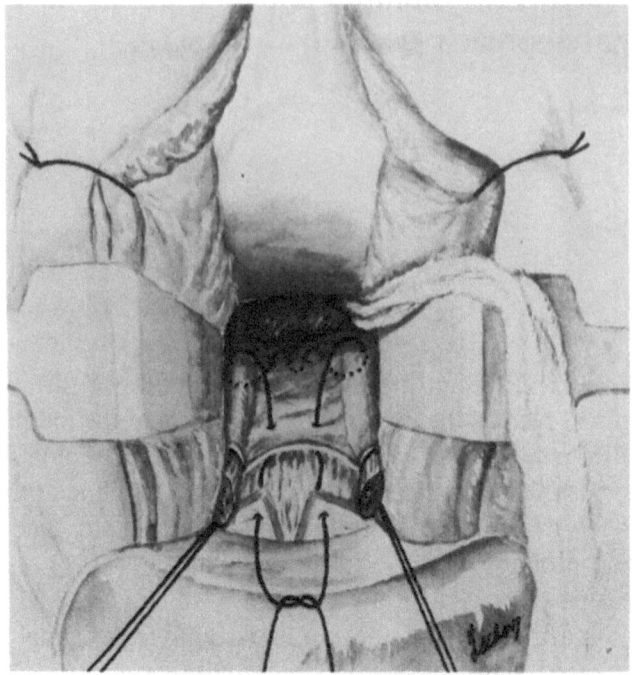

Fig. 2. Culdo-plastic after MacCall bringing together the sacro-utero ligaments with the peritoneum and the vagina wall (from Käser, Atlas d. gyn. Op.).

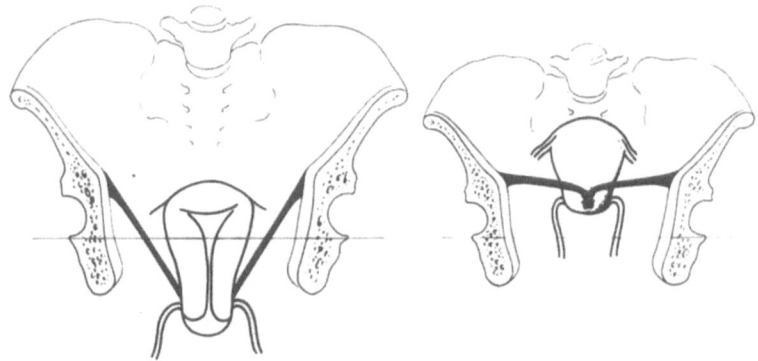

Fig. 3. The principle of the Manchester-Operation (from Käser, Atlas d. gyn. Op.).

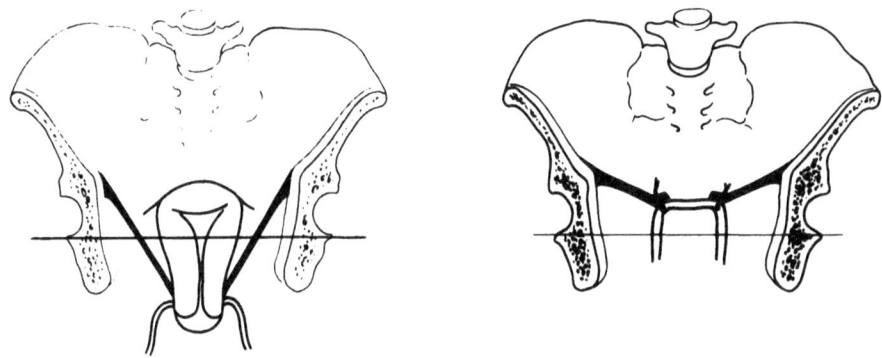

Fig. 4. Principle of the prolapse hysterectomy (from Käser, Atlas d. gyn. Op.).

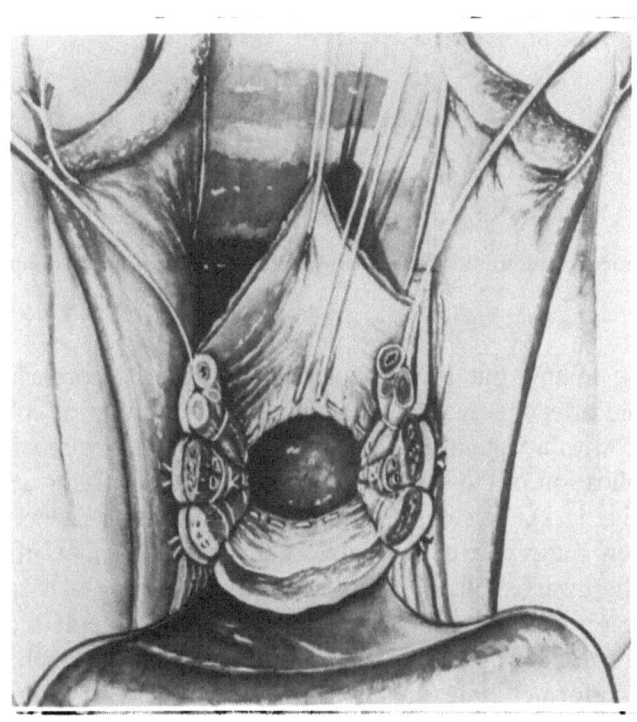

Fig. 5. High peritoneal closure after the Mayo-Ward technique (from Käser, Atlas d. gyn. Op.).

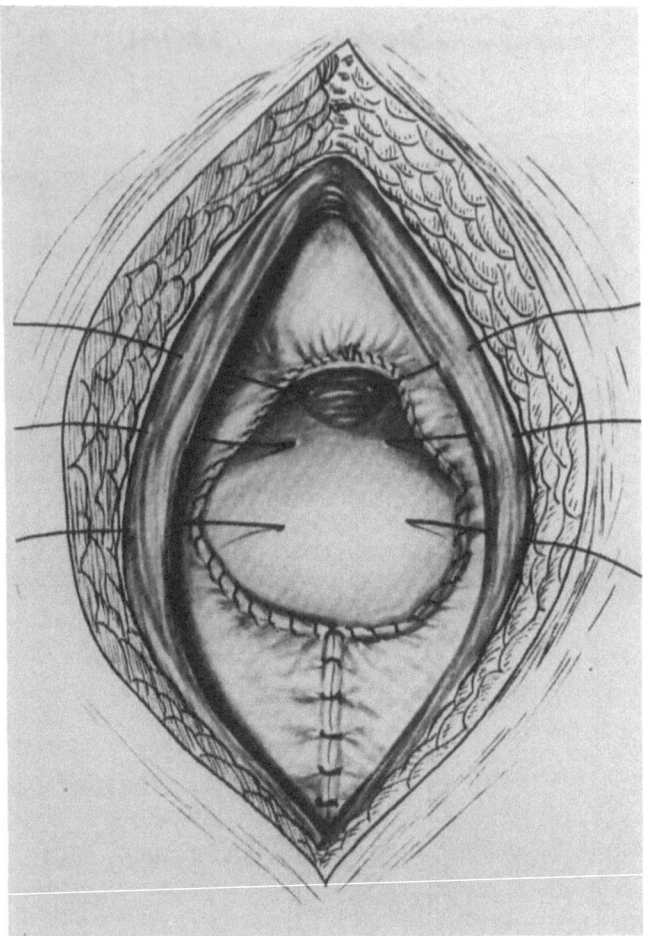

Fig. 6. Exohysteropexy with fixation of the uterus to the mm. recti (Kocher) (from Käser, Atlas d. gyn. Op.).

1. In prolapse mainly due to a cystocele the standard approach is, in our experience and after the gynecological literature, the anterior colporrhaphy in connection with a vaginal hysterectomy, and a posterior repair, if necessary with a plication of the uterosacral ligament (culdo-plastic after McCall or Käser) (Fig. 1, 2). The hysterectomy is not an incontinence operation itself, however, the repair of the pelvic floor is much more efficient after performing the hysterectomy.

In special cases of a predominant cystocele where the uterus should not be removed and pregnancy is out of question the Fothergill-Manchester-Operation can be performed (Fig. 3). Hereby, part of the cervix is amputated and the cardinal ligaments are sutured in front of the remaining cervix, elevating the uterus in a favourable condition. This is followed by a repair of the

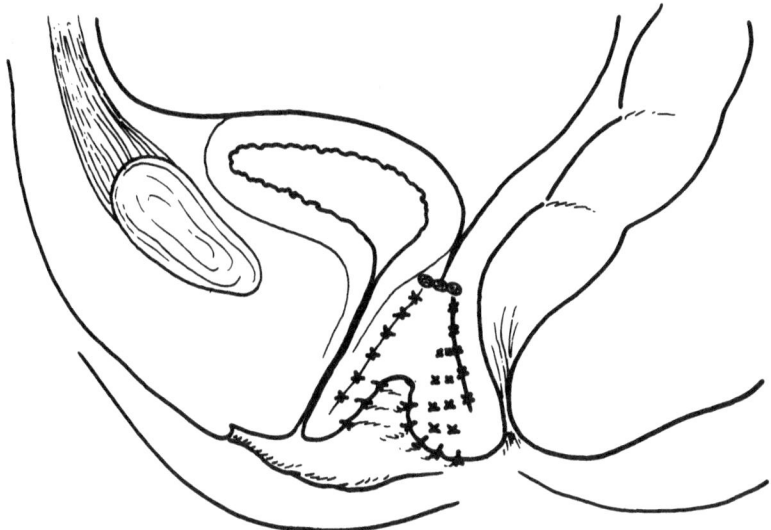

Fig. 7. Scheme of the closure of the vagina after hysterectomy and colpectomy (from Käser, Atlas d. gyn. Op.).

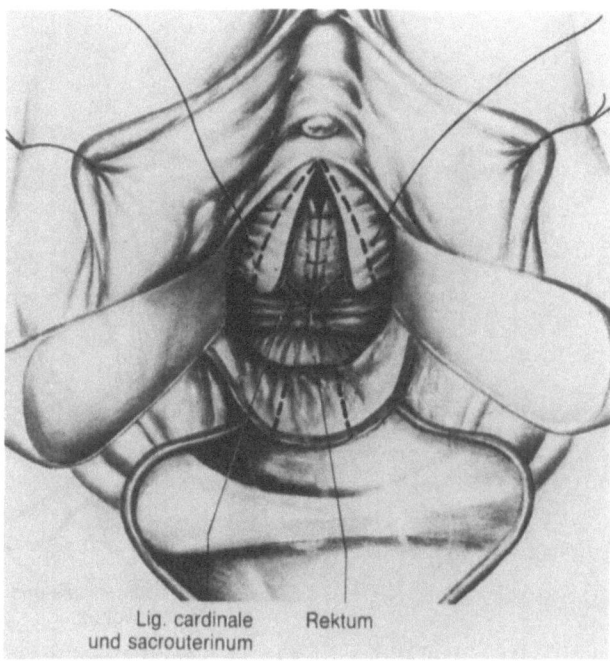

Fig. 8a. Colpoperineoplasty after prolapse of the vaginal vault.

190

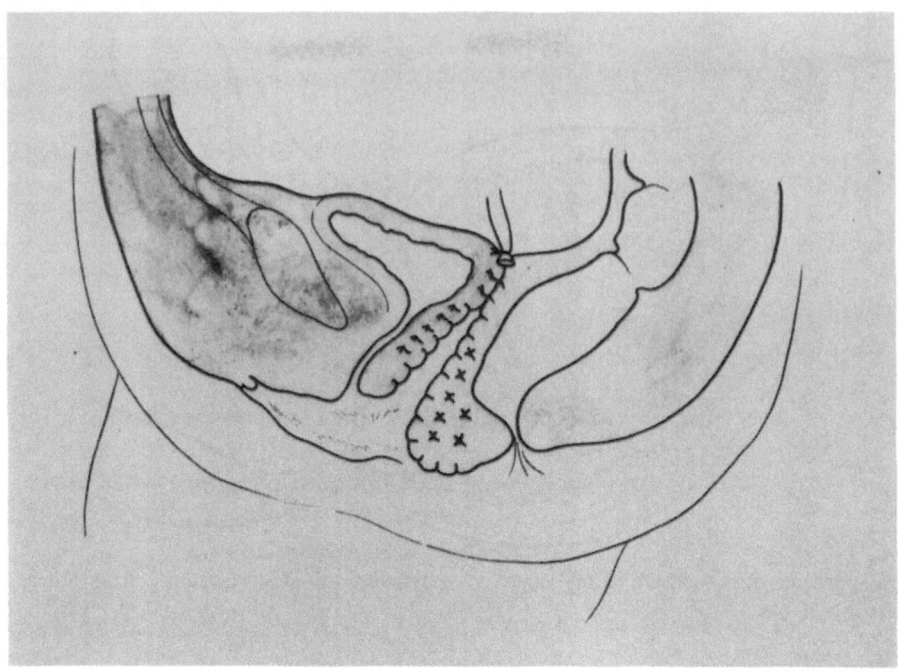

Fig. 8b. Scheme of the operation (from Käser, Atlas d. gyn. Op.).

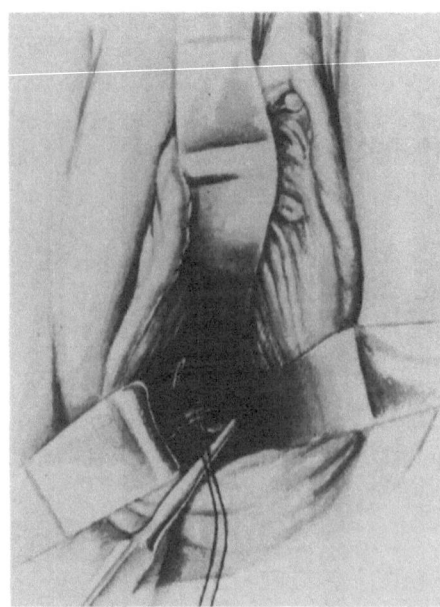

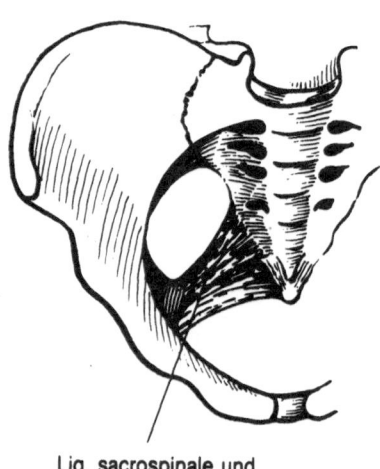

Lig. sacrospinale und
M. coccygeus

Fig. 9a. Sacrospinal fixation of the vagina after Amreich and Richter.

Fig. 9b. Lig. sacrospinal and m., coccygeus (from Käser, Atlas d. gyn. Op.).

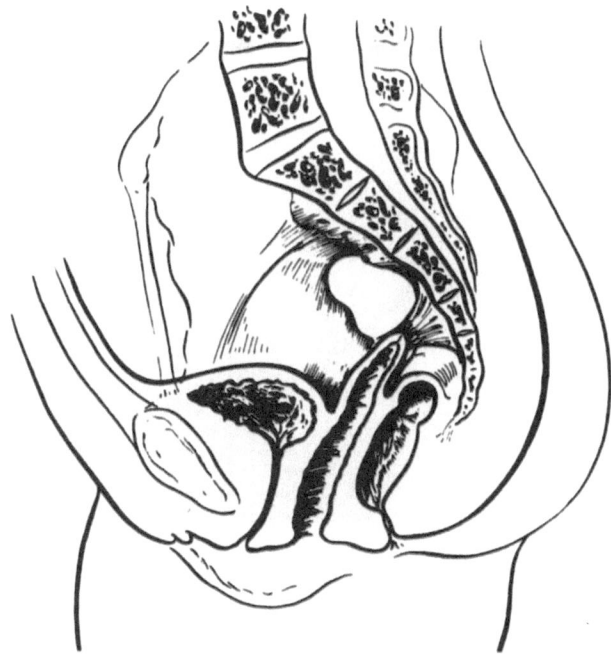

Fig. 10. The end of the vagina has been sutured to the sacrospinal ligament (from Käser, Atlas d. gyn. Op.).

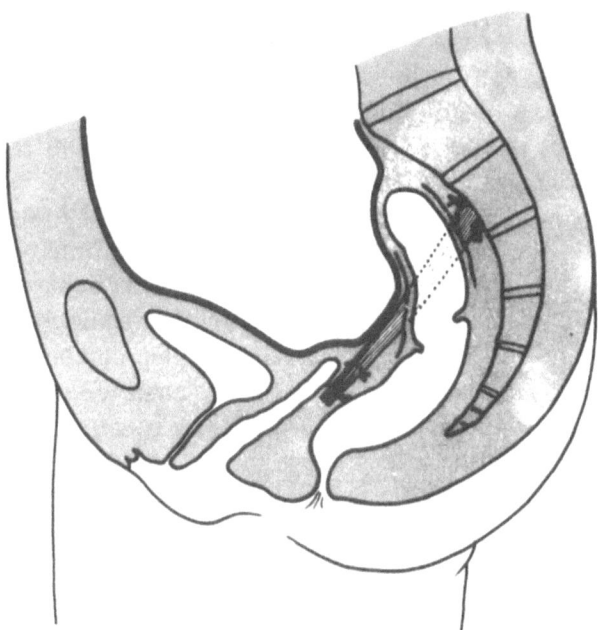

Fig. 11. Principle of the sacropexy by using plastic material (from Käser, Atlas d. gyn. Op.).

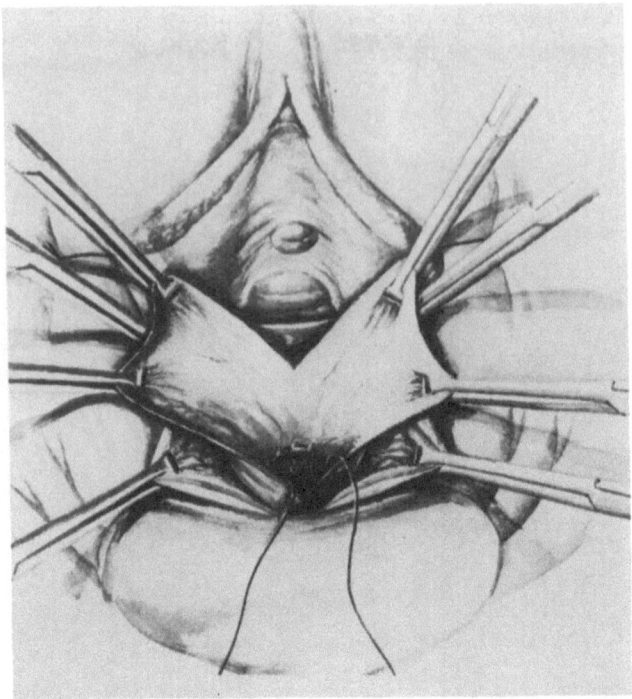

Fig. 12. Closure of the peritoneum after resecting peritoneal sac (from Käser, Atlas d. gyn. Op.).

cystocele. Today the Manchester-Fothergill-operation has limited indications. We use it in women of older age with the presence of a large cystocele where the risk of the surgical procedure should be as limited as possible.

2. *Prolapse of the uterus* is usually treated by vaginal hysterectomy with high fixation of the vaginal vault to the parametrium (uterosacral and cardinal ligament) (Fig. 4, 5). There are rare cases of extreme prolapse of the uterus, where it completely protrudes out of the vagina with oedema and thickening of the surrounding tissue. This is often combined with old age and no desire of intercourse. Under these circumstances more simple techniques have to be considered. We prefer in these situations where the uterus is very mobile, to fix the uterus above the bladder to the abdominal wall, closing the vagina by a high posterior repair including the bulbo-cavernosus. In the German literature this procedure is named hysteropexy after Kocher (Fig. 6).

What we advise not to do anymore in cases of uterine prolapse and anterior wall descent with incontinence is the operation with interposition of the uterus.

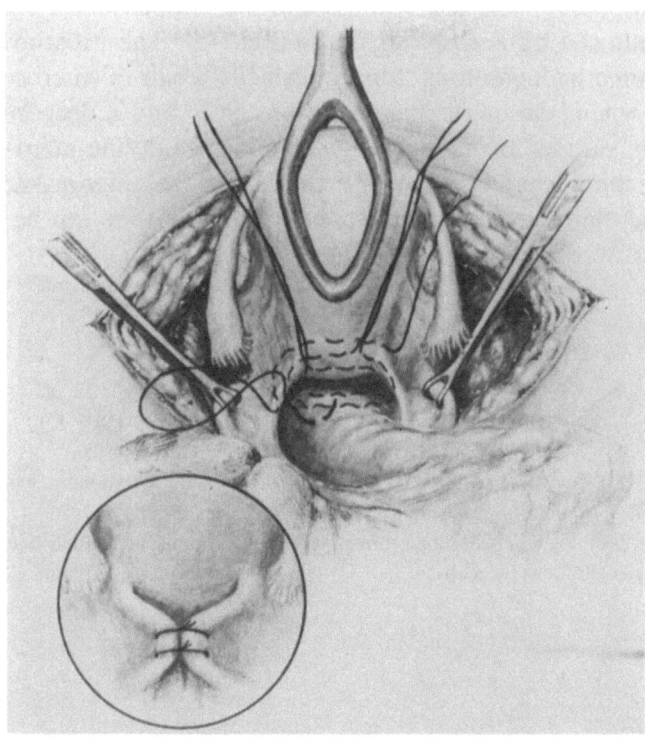

Fig. 13. Principle of the Moschowitz procedure for repair of an enterocele (from Masterson).

Vaginal vault prolapse management after having removed the uterus previously. The choice of the operative procedure depends upon whether the patient desires intercourse and how mobile the prolapsed vagina is. If the patient is of an age where the vaginal function does not have to be preserved, an easy and satisfactory procedure is the anterior and posterior repair in combination with removal of the greatest part of vaginal epithelium (Fig. 7). If the vaginal function should be preserved and if there are still some structures left at the end of the vagina related to the uterosacral and cardinal ligaments, the end of the vagina can be fixed, and an anterior and posterior wall repair can be performed (Fig. 8a, 8b). In cases where no structures are left for fixation of the end of the vagina and if the vagina comes out completely and is very mobile, a sacrospinal fixation after Amreich-Richter can be performed, together with an anterior and posterior repair (Fig. 9a, 9b, 10). If the vagina is not mobile enough the abdominal approach is necessary to achieve an adequate fixation of the vaginal vault to the sacrum by means of a Dacron mesh (Fig. 11).

3. Prolapse of the posterior part of the vagina. One has to distinguish between a rectocele and an enterocele. Usually the vaginal approach is

appropriate for both. In case of an enterocele the peritoneal sac has to be removed followed by a posterior repair (Fig. 12). The Moschowitz procedure performed by laparotomy for prophylactic repair of enterocele is useful in patients where the uterus has to stay in place and a deep cul de sac is present. The sutures in this operation should include the utero-sacral ligaments with the posterior part of the uterus and the anterior surface of the colon. If the uterosacral ligaments are very mobile they can be brought to the center of midline (Fig. 13).

References

1. Beck L. Gynäkologische Urologie. In: Käser O., Friedberg V., Ober K.G., Thomsen K., Zander J. (eds) Gynäkologie und Geburtshilfe, Band III. Thieme (1985).
2. Käser O., Iklé F.A., Hirsch H.A. Atlas der gynäkologischen Operationen, Thieme (1983).
3. Masterson B.J. Manual of Gynecologic Surgery, Springer (1979).
4. Richter K.: Pathologie der Streßinkontinenz und die anatomischen Möglichkeiten ihrer chirurgischen Behandlung. In: Petri E. (ed) Gynäkologische Urologie, Thieme (1983).

IV.4. Essentials of the technical aspects of anterior colporrhaphy and colpoperineal plastic repair: a gynaecologic procedure

J. JANSSENS & F.M. KAUER

Introductory remarks

In the presentation of the essentials of the technical aspects of anterior colporrhaphy and colpoperineal plastic repair we will restrict ourselves to the technical surgical aspects.

In performing an anterior colporrhaphy one should ask oneself if there is a need for combining the anterior colporrhaphy with a colpoperineal plastic repair, amputation of the portio or hysterectomy with or without adnexa. From the gynaecologist it may be expected that he can decide what the optimal extent of the operative procedure should be, also taking into account sexuological aspects.

In carrying out additionally a Stamey-Pereyra procedure, controlled with endoscopy, cooperation of the gynaecologist and the urologist may be important for obtaining better results (the urologist being more familiar with endoscopy).

In performing a colporrhaphy in postmenopausal women, it may be useful to stimulate proliferation of the vaginal epithelium by prescribing Oestriol some weeks before the surgical intervention.

The former conception of the existence of a real sphincter which gets torn in case of sphincter insufficiency has given rise to the technical procedure of a circumscript strengthening of the urethra.

Very well known are the operations according to Kelly (1913), Stoeckel (1921) and Marion (1941). They will give incomplete reinforcement of the closing system. It is now clearly understood that there is no sphincter present and that redressing, strengthening and plication of the bladder wall, introversion of the bladder and reinforcement and narrowing of the urethra is of the utmost importance for a proper functioning. One should try to perform in such a way a continuing plate supporting urethra and bladder and uplifting the bladder neck as much as possible. There is much confusion about the origin of the periurethral and perivesical tissue, different authors having different opinions about it.

The periurethral tissue contains collagen, smooth and striated muscle fibres and some elastic tissue derived from condensations of the endopelvic fascia and fibres derived from the musculus pubococcygeus and bulbocavernosus, all these together responsible for what is called the anterior and posterior pubo-urethral ligaments, with slips to the bladder as well. Partly it creates the so-called external sphincter – not separately recognized – and partly it supports the upper urethra and indirectly the urethrovesical junction, which is important for an optimal transmission of the intra-abdominal pressure in stress situations.

Perivesical tissue is a conglomeration of structures, of which the origin is not discernible, but which is connected with the endopelvic fascia and also with the musculus pubococcygeus, the musculus bulbocavernosus and even with the broad ligament – the connection especially manifested as bladder pillars connected with the cervix.

The surgical procedure

Exposure of the operative field should be arranged by grasping and pulling the portio by means of two tenacula anteriorly just below the last transversal vaginal ridge where the end of the bladder is expected and posteriorly not too high, avoiding the pouch of Douglas. One should make a longitudinal midline 'incision' of the anterior vaginal wall, till a few millimeters away from the urethral meatus.

If the most distal portion of the bladder cannot be identified easily one can find it by introducing a catheter and advancing it until the lower border of the cystocele is marked.

The best way to open the anterior wall is to make at first a small transverse incision at the height of the last transverse ridge of the vagina (Fig. 1). Then one should make a midline incision by means of a pair of scissors, thus creating a cleavage in the mainly avascular space between bladder and vaginal wall. The cleaving should be done by pushing the closed pair of scissors with constant pressure against the undersurface of the vaginal wall up to half a centimeter or a little more and then opening it a little bit (Fig. 2).

The small freed area of the vaginal wall should be grasped as high as possible by means of small clamps and held by an assistant, spreading the wound under tension and giving the surgeon the opportunity to open the anterior vaginal wall for another approximately half a centimeter (and so on till one is only a few millimeters away from the urethral orifice). The anterior wall being opened only in the midline, the vaginal wall should be freed from the bladder laterally (Fig. 3); the cystocele should be separated from the vaginal wall using scissors or a knife, leaving as much perivesical and

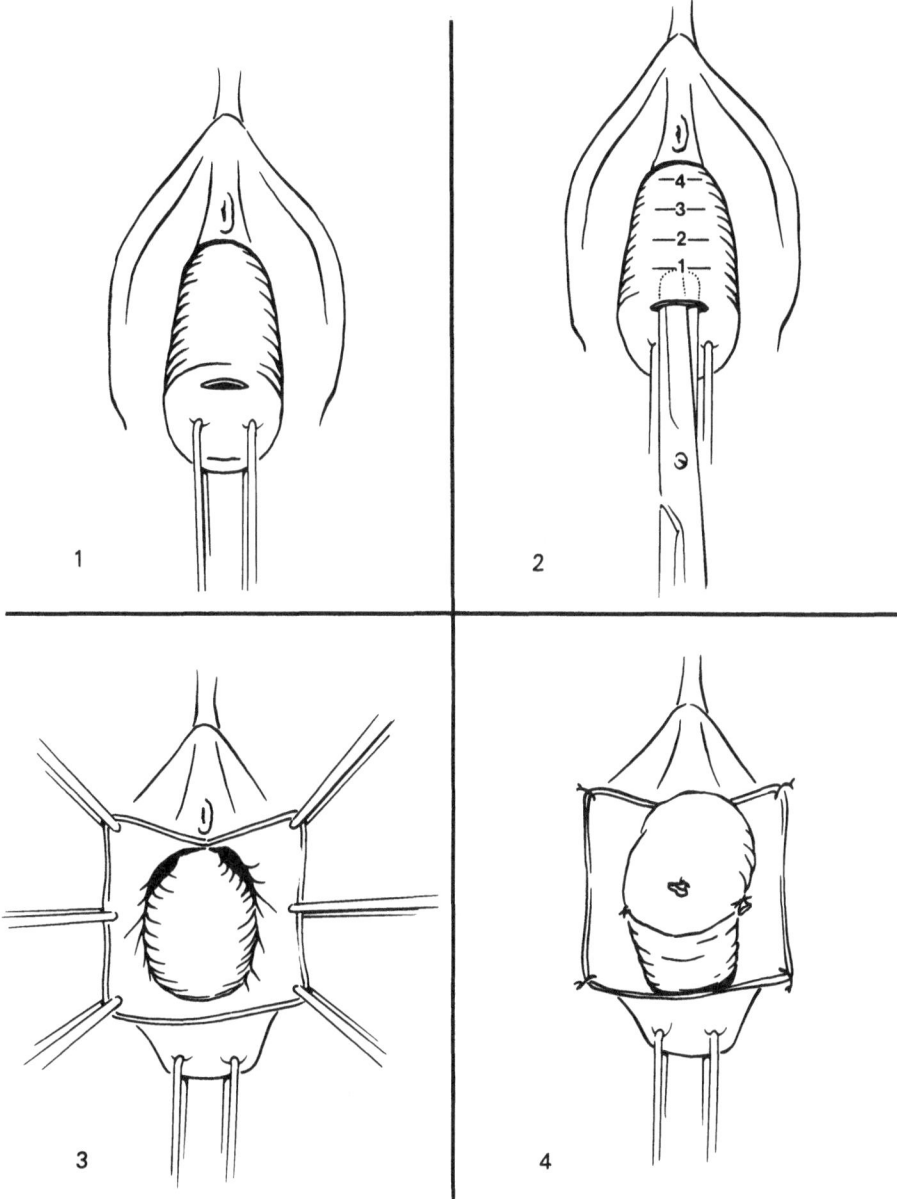

Fig. 1. Exposure of the operative field – Anterior vaginal wall.

Fig. 2. Entering the mainly avascular space between the anterior vaginal wall and cervix or bladder (step by step mobilizing and dividing the vaginal wall).

Fig. 3. Exposure of the cystocele and urethra. The supporting fibro-muscular strands (visible under traction) exposed and cut, leaving perivesical and peri-urethral tissue on bladder and urethra as much as possible.

Fig. 4. The cystocele is freed from the cervix (Partly sharply – ligature – partly bluntly with a Gauze-protected finger).

peri-urethral tissue on the cystocele and urethra as possible, so that it can be used for plication and strengthening of the cystocele and urethra.

The use of scissors or a knife, instead of pushing the cystocele and urethra away from the vaginal wall by means of a finger protected with gauze, should be encouraged because sharp dissection is less traumatic and leaves more perivesical and periurethral tissue on bladder and urethra.

Bleeding vessels should be ligated carefully, avoiding haematomas afterwards. When the cystocele is freed on one side, one should pick up the cystocele with an atraumatic pair of tweezers and place the partly freed cystocele opposite to the side that has not been freed. In this way one will easily be able to find the structures to be dissected for mobilizing the cystocele and urethra on the other side. The supporting fibromuscular strands which bind the bladder and urethra to the vaginal wall will thus be exposed by traction. The cystocele should then be disconnected from the cervix partly sharply by dissecting bladder pillars (eventually ligating bleeding vessels in it) and partly bluntly with a gauze-protected finger (Fig. 4).

Thereafter the freed and mobilized cystocele and urethra should be plicated, strengthened and redressed with the help of mattress sutures arranged in such a way that they overlap each other like rooftiles. The last one should not be placed as a rooftile, tightening the rest of the bladder pillars thus preventing downward displacement of the cystocele (Fig. 5). The sutures should pick up as laterally as possible a substantial part of the periurethral and perivesical tissue, initially left untied in order to give the opportunity to overlook the region optimally. The sutures strengthening, narrowing and redressing the urethra and especially the bladder neck should be placed carefully, using atraumatic needles. If useful a second run of sutures should be placed lateral to the first role. The tissue picked up by the second row may have direct contact with the fascia of the musculus pubococcygeus.

Ingelmann Sundberg has advocated the use of the pubococcygeal muscle for extra support, using anterior portions of it laid free, cut slightly behind the midpoint and united in the midline as a muscular support for the bladder neck.

It is very important not to shorten the length of the urethra. For this reason, tobacco pouch sutures should not be used as they indirectly shorten the urethra through traction.

After removing redundant vaginal wall, being careful in the neighbourhood of the urethral orifice (Fig. 6a, 6b) and removing from there only a small portion, the vagina is closed in the midline with interrupted stitches. The stitches should be inserted at some distance from the cutting line, since they will have to endure postoperative tension produced by oedema and would otherwise tear up.

In this stage of the procedure, one must keep in mind that it should be possible to replace the anterior vaginal wall and uterus. One should there-

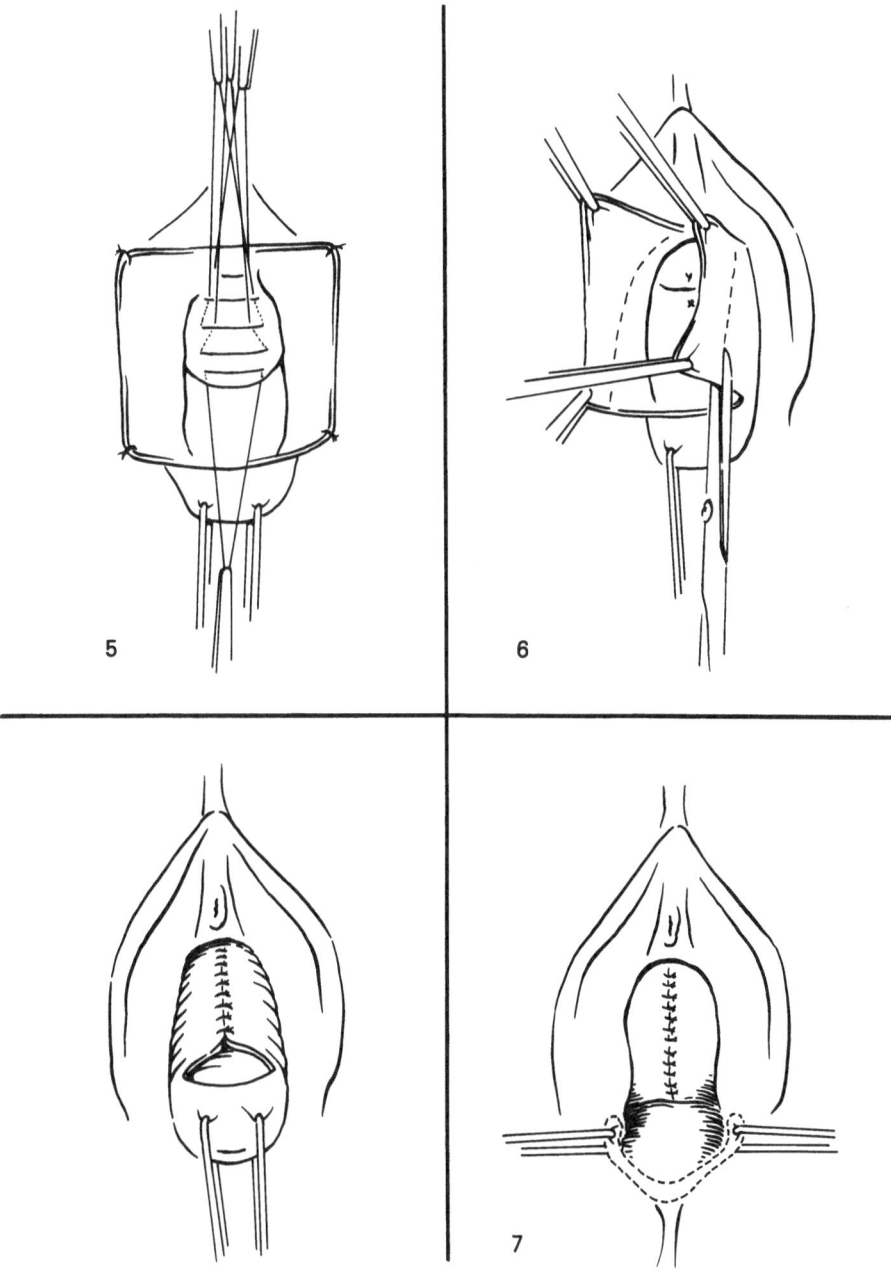

Fig. 5. Reinforcing, narrowing and introverting cystocele mattress sutures, overlapping like roof-tiles, the last one tightening the remainder of bladder pillars.

Fig. 6. Removing redundant vaginal wall and closure of the vagina in the midline.

Fig. 7. Exposure of operative field – colpoperineal region.

200

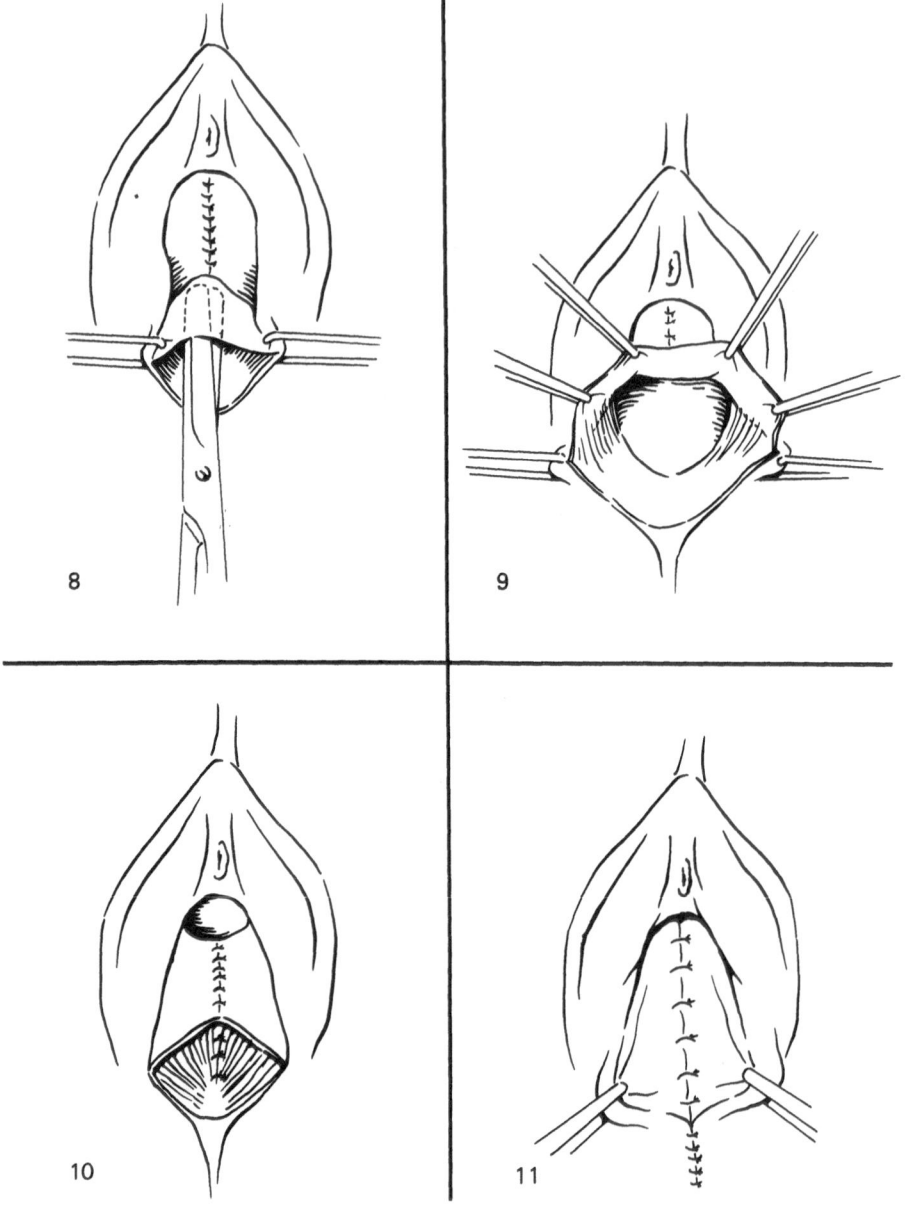

Fig. 8. Entering the mainly avascular space between vagina and rectum.
Fig. 9. The vagina freed from rectum and divided, the rectocele exposed, the levators exposed (incision perineal fasc. and blunt dissection).
Fig. 10. Picking up the levator by insertion of sutures (inverting rectocele and reinforcing the sustaining perineal structures).
Fig. 11. Completion of anterior colporrhaphy and colpoperineal plastic repair.

fore prevent exerting a strong pull on these structures and the uterus.

As already mentioned, a colpoperineal plastic repair should be added almost routinely because it is beneficial for several reasons. We will describe the procedure itself only summarily. The posterior commissura should be incised or, even better, excised completely by means of a knife, in order to have the opportunity to mobilize the posterior vaginal wall (Fig. 7). The edges of the posterior wall should be clamped in order to be able to invert it more and more, using gauze and finger placed on the inner surface of the posterior wall and separating the thus stretched vaginal wall from the rectocele, partly sharply with closed scissors to be opened by pushing it against the inner surface of the vagina in the mainly avascular cleavage plane (Fig. 8) and partly bluntly using a gauze-protected finger.

One should take care not to injure the rectum in the midline; lateral cleavage should always be done first, step by step, followed by the cleavage in the midline. Bloodvessels should carefully be ligated to avoid haematomas afterwards.

The posterior vaginal wall should be mobilized till the end of the rectocele is reached. Then one should expose the levator muscles partly by dissecting the fascia sharply and partly bluntly with the finger (Fig. 9). When in doubt one should check the situation by rectal examination. Thereafter the levator bundles should be picked up deeply with a suture on both sides of the rectum, to be tied afterwards. It depends on the degree of relaxation and the preferred width of the introitus vaginae how many 'levator sutures' should be used and how high the most proximal suture should be laid.

By pulling the threads on the left and right sides and adapting the musculus levator in the midline, one can test the width and correct number and position of these structures. Excess vaginal wall should then be removed in such a way that there remains enough vaginal wall material to prepare ample room and an adequate new commissura posterior. The vagina is then closed in the midline (Fig. 10); in order to prevent stricturation just before tieing the levator sutures, again the width of the introitus vaginae should be checked and if necessary corrected.

Then commissura posterior and perineal structures and skin are sutured (Fig. 11). We prefer using a tampon for 24-48 h and a suprapubic catheter for approximately 5-7 days when the patient in general can evacuate her bladder almost completely.

IV.5. Criterial review of the surgical techniques in the management of vaginal prolapse and urinary incontinence

J.M.J. DONY

Stress urinary incontinence (SUI) can be due to different anatomic aberrations such as loss of the posterior urethrovesical angle, loss of the appropriate urethral axis and stability, urethral funneling and telescoping. Usually more than one of these aberrations play a part in the development of genuine SUI. The surgical procedure which results in repair of all the anatomical aberrations which contribute to stress urinary continence will be the most successful. Only a thorough preoperative investigation will disclose the underlying pathology and result in a proper diagnosis and an adequate therapy.

Vaginal prolapse also can be due to different anatomic aberrations. Relaxation and lengthening of the cardinal and sacrouterine ligaments results in uterine and upper vaginal prolapse (inversion) while damage of the urogenital diaphragm and pelvic floor results in lower vaginal prolapse (eversion) as does the isolated weakening of the vaginal wall with herniation of the bladder base. As is the case in SUI, mostly a combination of different aberrations exists.

Although SUI and genital prolapse share as a rule the same aetiology, being the obstetrical damage to the supports of uterus, vagina and urethra, it is more an exception than a rule that the genital prolapse is the cause of SUI. This misunderstanding has contributed to the philosophy 'Do a vaginal operation first and if it fails go above' and resulted in many postoperative failures, but worse has invalidated patients for life.

An example of such a dramatic event is the woman in her fortieth who has suffered of moderate genuine SUI without genital prolapse and to whom has been told that the chance of success would be enhanced by combining an anterior repair with vaginal hysterectomy. Following the operation, urinary incontinence has been established, however, she considered herself a sexual cripple missing the uterine sensations. These are probably due to uterine lifting and contractions, which in her case were of paramount interest for the experience of profound orgasm.

This patient may be comforted by the fact that another patient who had a comparable preoperative condition got an overzealous anterior repair resulting in intractable sensory urge and after several operative procedures finally ended on with a Bricker bladder. Fortunately these examples are more exception than the women who after a too tight sling operation are condemned to long lasting voiding in bizar positions, or self catheterisation. The mentioned examples are caused by inappropriate preoperative diagnostic investigations, faulty assumptions, bad choice of operative procedure or inadequate execution of the operation.

The choices of operation for the treatment of genuine SUI, without genital prolapse after a thorough investigation, is mostly based on more than one consideration. Considerations taken into account are: the chance of postoperative failure, the duration of the hospital stay and reconvalescence, and recovery of the possibility of spontaneous voiding.

However, the combination of genuine SUI and genital prolapse deserves further consideration beside those already mentioned. Repair of genital prolapse carries true risk of postoperative sexual impairment. Even more important is the risk that if the primary operation fails, especially after anterior colporrhaphy, there is a chance that it becomes nearly impossible to cure the recurrence of SUI. Severe cicatrisation in the urethrovesical region and abnormal shortening of the anterior vaginal wall with loss of mobility is the result of the primary surgical intervention. It is therefore of the utmost importance to establish before operation what kind of genital prolapse is present. While diagnosing of lower vaginal wall prolapse presents mostly no problem, prolapse of the uterus and upper vagina is sometimes more difficult to establish. During the day uterovaginal prolapse becomes more prominent due to continuous traction on the supports of the uterus and upper vagina.

Therefore it is well possible that examination in the morning will not reveal any significant descent of the uterus while at the end of a strenuous day the cervix can be seen in the vaginal outlet without straining. It is advisable if the patient presents herself in the morning for examination to be aware of this fact. If during straining there is no significant descent of the uterus one may place a tenaculum on the uterine cervix. Gentle traction will establish the degree of prolapse which will probably exists at the end of a strenuous day. Furthermore the possibility of traction with the tenaculum on the cervix makes it possible to position the cervix at the normal level. Straining of a patient under this condition will manifest the contribution and severeness of lower vaginal prolapse and the needs for repair of the anterior and posterior vaginal wall and pelvic floor.

The operative choice for repair of genital prolapse and cure of genuine SUI was in the past based on the consideration that the combination of vaginal and abdominal surgery implies more per- and postoperative morbidity. However, perioperative prophylactic antibiotic therapy and the use of suction drains have lowered this risk so far that a combined abdomino-vaginal operation is often the better choice. Nowadays there is no valid reason to desist of a pelvic floor repair after a Burch colposuspension. There exists a fear for a combined abdomino-vaginal operative procedure which holds the risk of improper preoperative examination and judgement. Such an example is the growing tendency to correct the combinations of SUI and a moderate cystocele irrespective of the aetiology of the cystocele with the Burch colposuspension. However this results in traction on the posterior vaginal wall which is evidenced by the ridge at some distance of the vaginal inlet in the posterior wall after the operation. Preoperative examination may reveal that during straining there is already some bulging of the posterior vault. This may indicate a deep pouch of Douglas or begin of an enterocele. It is then advisable to follow Burch and correct the anomaly which predisposes to an enterocele sooner or later. It seems likely that the rate of enterocele development as late complication of the Burch colposuspension will increase in the coming years. The growing tendency to correct even large cystoceles by placing the sutures as lateral as possible in the anterior vaginal wall contribute to this risk.

Taking into account the changing appreciation of uterine preservation by women based on identification of the uterus with feminity and undispensability for sexual satisfaction and the wish to be urinary stress continent even during the most strenuous sports, the choice of the most satisfactory type of operation will become more difficult.

It has become clear that only the vesicourethral neck pull-up type of operation will cure moderate and severe SUI with an acceptable cure rate especially when there is urethral rotation. Therefore it is injudicious to rely on bladder neck plication and overzealous anterior repair. In spite of the seriousness of the genital prolapse it is better to perform a vesicourethral neck pull-up procedure in combination with operative repair of the genital prolapse than to rely on vaginally established push-up of the bladder neck. The author is convinced that the best operative results may be achieved in patients with moderate or severe genital prolapse and SUI when the gynaecologist and urologist combine their efforts together, with the adage 'let to the gynaecologist the repair of the vaginal supports and to the urologist the repair of the bladder neck and urethral supports'.

CHAPTER FIVE

Vesico-vaginal fistulae

V.1. Female incontinence due to urethro- and vesico-vaginal fistulae

A.A. HASPELS

Introduction

Women who have a vesico-vaginal fistula (VVF) are sometimes told that this condition cannot be treated and that they will have to learn to live with it. This statement is mostly incorrect except in inoperable cancer patients. In most instances the occurrence of a fistula could have been prevented and most VVF's are amenable to treatment.

VVF and recto-vaginal fistulae are fortunately seen rarely in the Western countries. If they do occur then they are nearly always a result of gynaeco-

Table 1.

	Haspels Indonesia 1956–1961 Nigeria 1961–1964	Bastiaanse/Quispel Amsterdam 1938–1948	Haspels Utrecht 1969–1983
Total number of fistulae	145	34	104
Obstetrical causes			
Ischaemic necrosis	140	1	1*
Trauma from forceps	3	13	3*
Trauma from caesarean section	1	–	4
Gynaecological causes			
Prolapse repair	–	17	31
Radical hysterectomy	–	1	5
Abdominal hysterectomy	–	1	39
Vaginal hysterectomy	–	1	15
McIndoe plasty	–	–	2
Endoresection urological	–	–	2
Schistosomiasis	1	–	–
Vaginal cyst extirpation	–	–	1
Foreign body	–	–	1

* From North Africa.

logical operative surgery. 40 years ago obstetric causes were still important as the maternal mortality in Caesarean section was high (5.4%) and therefore difficult forceps deliveries were frequently performed.

In honour of Prof. Moonen it may be mentioned that no other urologist in The Netherlands has closed more VVF's by the vaginal route than Prof. Moonen. Modestly I may add that the same is true for myself as a gynaecologist. We gathered experience in tropical countries operating more than 300 VVF patients after complicated obstetrics. A detailed report can be given of 104 patients operated on in Holland from 1969–1983.

Table 2. Duration of fistula.	
Duration	No
Up to 1 year	64
2 - 5	24
6 - 10	8
11 - 15	6
Over 15	2
Total	104

Table 3. Age at time of operation.	
Age	No
18 - 20	4
21 - 30	8
31 - 40	27
41 - 50	32
51 - 60	21
61 - 70	9
70 and over	3
Total	104

Duration of fistula

The first attempt to repair a fistula has the best chance of success, since repeated attempts at repair produce more scarring and further impair the blood supply of the tissue. 61 patients had been unsuccessfully operated before by gynaecologists or urologists or both before they were referred to our department. 38 had one previous unsuccessful repair, 23 had two to four trials of repair before referred. Parallel with this is the duration of the fistulae (Table 2), as well as the age at the time of the VVF repair (Table 3).

Route of operations

Repair by the vaginal route was successfully carried out in 99 patients and by the abdominal route in 5 patients.
    Advantages of vaginal approach:
1. Smaller wound.
2. Vaginal wall and bladder are easy to separate and dissect.
3. Closure of fistulae without tension.

4. Good haemostasis can be achieved.
5. Small wound in bladder results in little intra-vesical bleeding. Urine is usually clear the same day.
6. Therefore intra-vesical clots are rare. Consequently there is less chance of blockage of catheter.
7. If fistula is near bladder-sphincter area a pubococcygeus-sphincter repair can be performed during the same operative procedure.
8. Postoperative pain occurs much less. Patient feels therefore much more comfortable.
9. Urethral fistula cannot be reached via the transabdominal route.

There are a few instances where the transabdominal approach is preferable:

1. In cases where the ureter is included in the VVF.
2. In patients with vesico-cervical-vaginal fistulae after Caesarean section.

In the latter one can make a choice between the transvesical approach and the transabdominal one between bladder and uterus, after careful dissection the fistula can be located and closed.

Anatomic extension of the lesion

The anatomic extension of the lesions are listed: There were 65 cases of VVF, 35 cases of urethra and bladder neck, 3 cases of vesico-cervical fistulae, 1 combined VVF-RVF fistula after trauma. All 35 patients with fistulae of the urethra and bladder neck required a sphincter plasty. The preferred method being the pubococcygeus plasty that can be performed directly after closing the fistula.

Results

An important factor in the surgical management of VVF is the fact that over 50 per cent of those in whom closure was feasible had had one or more attempts at closure with resultant searring prior to admission. Our initial success was 92 patients; 11 patients required a second operation and one patient had three repairs for a final success rate of 100 per cent.

Comment

This study indicates that while obstetric complications are now an infrequent cause, the number of referred patients after gynaecological-urological surgery has increased due to increase of the number of hysterectomies (to a certain extent unnecessary!) What precautions should the surgeon take to avoid this complication? One must recognize that with large fibroids, particularly in the cervical region with endometriosis or previous surgery, there may be bladder distortion which if not recognized may result in bladder injury.

One of the main causes of direct injury to the bladder is its forceful, blunt separation from the uterus. The bladder should be removed from the uterus by careful separation with small snips of the dissecting scissors followed by careful separation with the tip of the index finger. This method should be employed whether the operative approach is abdominal or vaginal. It is in particular required if the patient has had a previous operation in the bladder region such as Caesarean section or anterior colporrhaphy. The Richardson technique of intrafascial hysterectomy is also very useful in this respect, as it provides a safeguard for both the bladder and the ureters. It should therefore not only be used in teaching hospitals!

Good haemostasis is essential for the prevention of fistula formation. Chasser Moir [1] pointed out that haematomata in the vaginal vault are an important cause, especially if they become infected and cause necrosis of surrounding tissues. After hysterectomy the vault of the vagina should therefore remain open and only the peritoneum should be closed. After a few weeks the open-cuff will close spontaneously. If a haematoma does form – and this is perhaps more likely to happen since prophylactic anticoagulant therapy has been routine – then blood or even pus can easily drain into the vagina.

Two patients had fistulae due to urological endoresection. Moreover I have seen several patients with total incontinence after this urethrotomia! I would suggest to the urologist to be very careful with this operation.

Physicians should recognize that the majority of VVF can be repaired vaginally with an excellent cure rate and a low morbidity rate as compared to transvesico- or transabdominal approach. We have an excellent cooperation with our urological department and they refer such cases to us for repair.

This is of course especially true for urethro-vaginal fistulae. An indwelling catheter during the repair of prolapse is important. It should be inserted after the separation of the bladder from the vagina and before the bladder is sutured and the vagina is repaired. This prevents the urethra from being caught in the sutures and from becoming partly necrotic.

A fistula should never be repaired within the first three months following its formation or following a previous operation. After repair I prefer urethral drainage [2]. We have dubious experience with suprapubic drainage. With urethral drainage one avoids a pool of urine over the suture line at the trigone. A few patients with the fistula near the trigone will develop bladder spasm which can be relaxed successfully with probanthine.

For patients near or beyond the menopause, oestrogenic therapy before and after surgery enhances healing. Antibiotic usage is not used routinely. Daily urinary examination is done and chemotherapy is given on indication only. In the western world obstetric trauma as an aetiologic factor has declined in the past quarter century, so will hopefully such fistula following gynaecologic-urologic surgery.

References

1. Chassar Moir J. Journ. Obstet. Gynaec. Br. Emp. 80 (1973): 598.
2. Haspels A.A. Ned. T. Geneesk. 120 (1976): 129.

V.2. The omental repair of complex vesico-vaginal fistulae

R. TURNER-WARWICK

Introduction

It is almost always possible to close a vesico-vaginal fistula; meticulous technique is naturally essential but success with the more complicated problems is dependent upon the ability of the surgeon to select the procedure that is best suited to the particular clinical situation and furthermore to vary it appropriately during the course of the operation, according to the findings, on the basis of a wide personal experience.

Simple traumatic vesico-vaginal fistulae can often be resolved reliably by simple closure in layers either from a vaginal or from an abdominal approach. However, even complex recurrent fistulae and those associated with tissue loss and irradiated healing are repairable by the addition of a vascular omental-interposition graft: thus *any* recurrent fistula after a relatively limited vaginal-approach layer-closure procedure should cause a surgeon to reflect upon the choice of procedure.

The choice of approach

An exaggerated lithotomy position is commonly used for a vaginal repair; the disadvantage of this is that it does not offer the ready facility of extension to a synchronous abdominal exploration, consequently it is generally inappropriate unless the surgeon is quite certain that a simple vaginal repair will be sufficient – which must be rare.

There are many advantages in positioning the patient for a synchronous abdomino-perineal procedure, irrespective of whether a primary approach from the perineum or from the abdomen is planned. With the patient on the operating table in a flat, slightly head-down position, with the legs widely abducted and with only moderate hipflexion, good exposure for vaginal surgery can be achieved, particularly with an appropriate retractor. The patient is draped, with sterile skin and vaginal preparation so that both the abdomen and the perineum are included in the one operating field.

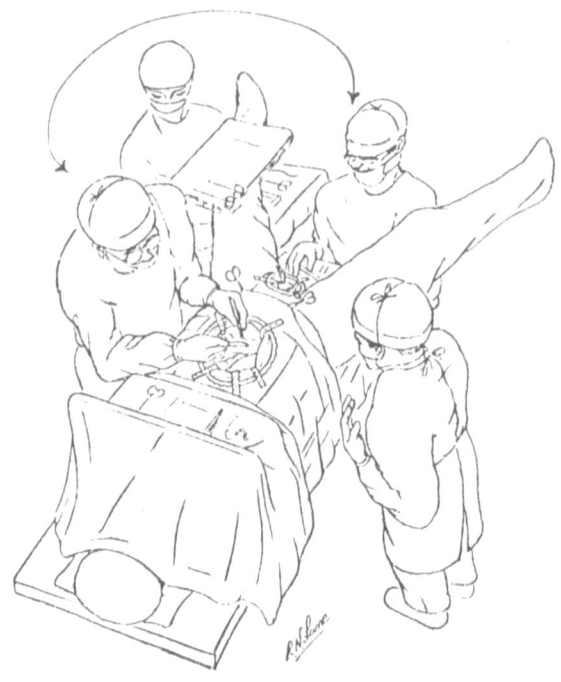

During a vaginal procedure the surgeon is seated with the scrub nurse and instrument tabel immediately to the right (or left, if left handed). If an appropriate retractor is used, one assistant is more than enough. If the vaginal-approach repair proves difficult or inappropriate, the surgeon simply walks round to the abdominal approach position and the scrub nurse repositions the instrument table between the legs (Fig. 1). It is rarely necessary to have a two surgeon synchronous approach. The same patient positioning and preparation is used for a primary abdominal approach; the advantage of including the perineum in the operating field is that an orientating finger in the vagina greatly facilitates the separation of the bladder and vagina around the fistula. A synchronous vaginal approach is also required for the creation of a wide abdomino-perineal tunnel to receive and to fix-distally an adequate bulk of omental pedicle graft when an interpositional support of a vesical or a vesico-urethral closure proves necessary.

The vaginal approach

Because the vaginal approach to a vesico-vaginal fistula is relatively limited, wide retraction and exposure is important. The Turner-Warwick perineal ring retractor with appropriate deep blades and stay-suture trachon guide-knobs generally provides a better exposure for fistula repair than the time-honoured weighted Auvard retractor.

The Turner-Warwick angulated needle holder which allows the needle to be visualised continuously without moving the hand grip facilitates suturing in deep cavities.

The curved Turner-Warwick fibrelight sucker combines two important facilities. The connections of the suction tube and the light cable provide the handle, there is an air bleed hole to adjust the suction immediately in front of the finger ring and another distal air-bleed helps to clear the blood film from the distal fibre-light face.

The abdominal approach

The abdominal approach can be used for the repair of any vesico-vaginal fistula, high or low; many surgeons find it technically easier than the vaginal approach, it is more reliable for repair of a difficult fistula and it is essential for the repair of complex fistulae that are dependent upon an interpositional omental graft. A midline abdominal-wall incision should always be used for an abdominal approach to a vesical fistula repair because it is often necessary to extend this up to the xiphisternum to provide access for mobilisation of the right gastroepiploic pedicle vessels of the omentum when mobilisation of this is necessary to enable a short-omentum to reach the pelvis. However, for the scar-conscious, a preliminary lower-abdominal-wall midline incision can be achieved through a horizontal skin incision so that it is only necessary to combine this with an upper abdominal midline skin incision when an extended mobilisation of the omental pedicle proves necessary.

The universal Turner-Warwick abdomino-perineal ring retractor provides maximal retraction and pelvic floor exposure without the intervention of an assistant. The ring is retained in position by four fully curved abdominal-wall retractor blades of appropriate size; additional deep blades between these retract the abdominal contents efficiently, a sliding clip onto the inner margin of the ring locks them down to prevent them from lifting. A particular advantage of a ring retractor is that appropriate directional tension on elevating traction-stay sutures can be achieved by hooking the tip of the haemostat clips under its margin (Fig. 2A).

Trans-peritoneal supra-vesical fistula exposure (Fig. 2B)

The transperitoneal posterior vesical approach is always preferable for the abdominal repair of vesico-vaginal fistulae; the time-honoured anterior trans-vesical approach provides a relatively poor exposure. The initial

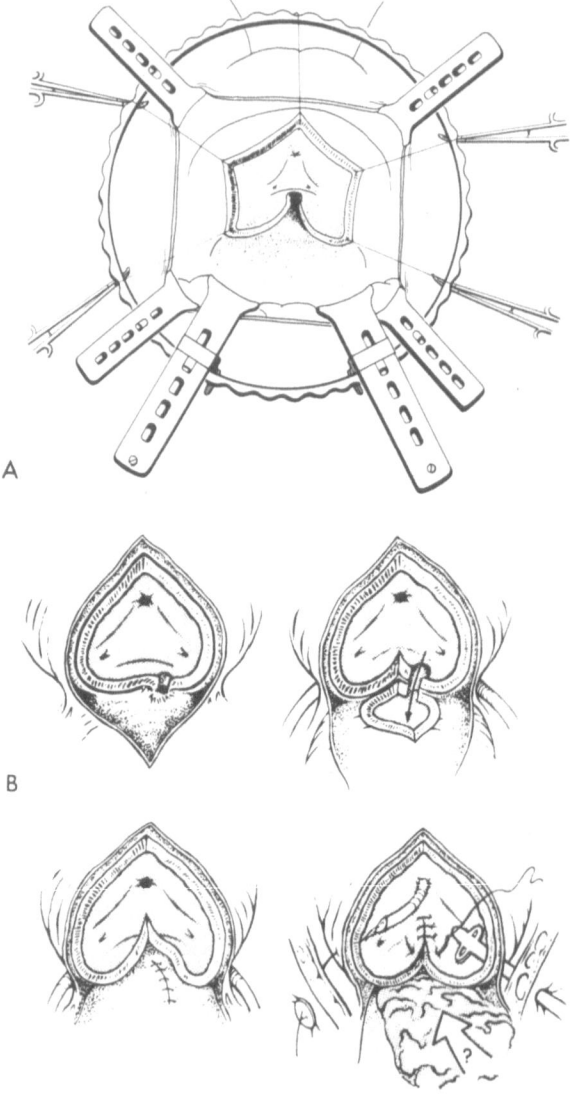

Fig. 2.

intra-peritoneal incision is made in the vesico-vaginal peritoneal fold and the posterior wall of the bladder is opened in the midline just above the fistula. The separation of the vagina from the bladder around the fistula is facilitated by an orientating finger in the vaginal vault. The vaginal vault and the bladder are closed with 3×0 PGA sutures.

A wide exposure of the fistula area is thus provided and a direct extra-vesical exposure of the terminal ureter is easily obtained if its reimplantation into the bladder is indicated. Efficient retraction is maintained by the elevating stay-sutures.

The trans-peritoneal supra-vesical approach to a fistula is also basic to the creation of the abdomino-perineal tunnel when this is required for an interposition omental pedicle graft to support the closure of a complex fistula.

When the posterior wall of the bladder is found to be indurated and fibrotic as it often proves to be in irradiated fistulae, it is important that the fistula-exposing incision in the posterior wall of the bladder should be midline but curved laterally as far as possible to achieve a tension-free sutureline closure of the fistula by rotating the eccentric bladder flap: under such circumstances, a vertical incision in a scarred posterior bladder wall sometimes proves difficult or impossible to close.

The closure of complex fistulae by omental interposition grafts

If the healing potential of the tissue margins of a fistula is compromised by scarring due to infection, to previous attempts at repair, or to irradiation, the success rate of simple layer closure falls abruptly so that some form of additional viable tissue-interposition graft is required; the advisability of this is generally predictable at operation so that a significant incidence of recurrent fistulae after simple layer closure techniques is inacceptable.

Sizeable flaps of parapelvic peritoneum sometimes provide sufficient extra support for a layer-closure but they are obviously inappropriate when they are also affected by the local pathology, especially irradiation. Pedicle grafts of skeletal muscle such as gracilis can be used for simple tissue interposition but are ill adapted to resist infection and inflammation and contribute little to the healing reachon of the local tissues. The omentum is, however, uniquely adapted for the resolution of local inflammatory processes, not only on account of its blood supply, but also its abundant lymphatic drainage which re-absorbs inflammatory cell debris and macro-molecular protein exudates that would otherwise result in purulent accumulations. Thus, quite apart from its value in closing complex fistulae due to irradiation, the omentum has a well established place in complex urinary tract reconstruction in general (Turner-Warwick, 1967, 1976).

The reliability of omental interposition graft repair (Fig. 3)

The reliability of an omental pedicle graft repair depends upon achieving a large interpositional bulk with a wide lateral overlap of the closure suture lines of the bladder and the vagina – it is not just an 'omental plug'. The basic essential of the procedure is therefore to achieve a 3–4 finger-wide abdomino-perineal interposition tunnel and to mobilise a sufficient bulk of the omental apron to fill it.

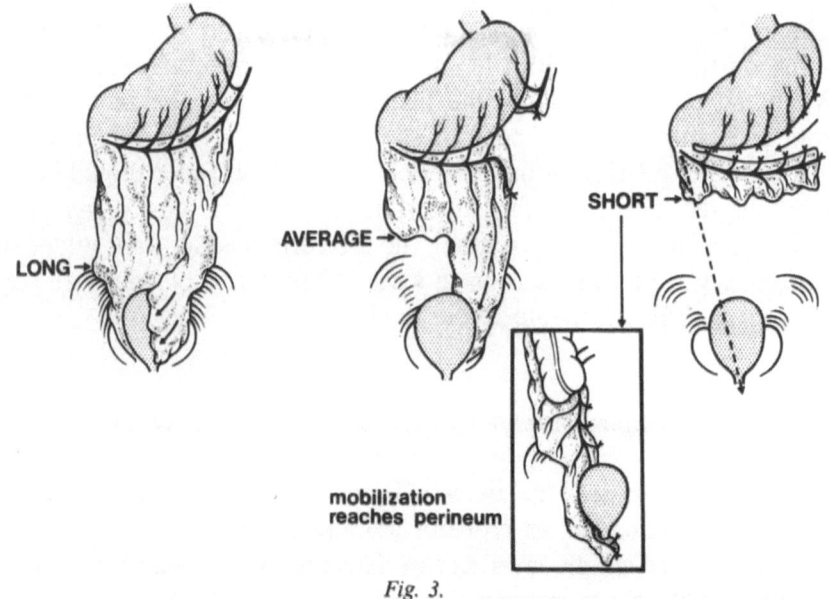

LONG

AVERAGE →

SHORT →

mobilization
reaches perineum

Fig. 3.

It is also essential to appreciate that the magic of the omental pedicle graft is fundamentally dependent upon an arterial blood supply that is efficiently pulsatingly, and upon its unimpaired venous and lymphatic drainage: any impairment of any of these diminish its potential.

Because it is necessary to elongate the vascular pedicle of the omentum in more than 50% of cases to enable it to reach the pelvis, it is fundamentally important to know some basic anatomical features of its vascular supply.

1. The blood supply of the omental apron is derived from vertically running vessels arising from the gastro-epiploic arch with relatively poor arcade communications between them – thus, when dividing the omental apron in the midline to provide a graft support for the reconstruction of an upper urinary tract on one side, the two halves can often be separated without the division of a blood vessel that is sufficiently large to require ligation. It follows that elongation of the omental apron by a horizontal incision below the gastroepiploic arch that it involves division of its vertical vessels, to some extent impairs the blood supply of the extremely of the graft.

2. The main origin of the gastroepiploic vascular area is always from the right side; in fact the junction between the right and the left gastroepiploic vessels that usually forms in a complete gastroepiploic arch is deficient in about 10% of cases at a point to the left of the greater curvature.

It follows that the mobilisation of a short-apron must be based on the right gastroepiploic vessels, not the left; this is fortunate for mechanical reasons because the origin of the right gastroepiploic vessels from the gastroduodenal vessels is much lower in the abdomen than the origin of the left gastroepiploic vessels from the splenic vessels so that when the full length of the gastroepiploic arch is mobilised from the greater curvature of the stomach by the individual ligation division of its 30–40 short gastric branches, its divided left extremely is long enough to reach the pelvis, irrespective of the omental apron itself – thus the omentum can be used in children when the apron is often underdeveloped.

Failure of omental pedicle graft repairs

The reliability of an omental pedicle graft fistula repair can and should be very high so that it is generally possible to attribute a failure to one or more of three shortcomings.
1. Failure to develop an abdomino-perineal interposition tunnel of sufficient dimensions.
2. Failure to mobilise an adequate bulk of omentum.
3. Impairment of the blood supply of the omentum by inappropriate mobilisation of its vascular pedicle.

Mobilisation of the omentum

The lower margin of the omentum apron is long enough to reach the pelvic floor and the perineum without vascular mobilisation in about 30% of cases: however, the omentum should always be separated from its natural adhesion to the transverse colon and mesocolic vessels to avoid the possibility that postoperative gaseous distention of the bowl might dislocate the interposition graft (Fig. 4A).

In about 30% of cases sufficient elongation of a moderate length apron can be achieved by dividing the left gastroepiploic pedicle vessels and those of the direct left lateral branches to the left omentum (Fig. 4B).

Formal full length mobilisation of the right gastroepiploic pedicle is required to enable the omentum to reach the pelvis in about 30% of patients. The fundamental principles of this mobilisation are:

1. Appropriate access through an upward extension of a midline incision.

2. Individual ligation of the 20–40 short gastric branches with absorbable suture material without damaging the main gastro-epiploic vessels.

   a) ligation of a bunch of branches shortens the pedicle and adds the risk that one may escape and bleed.

   b) non-absorbable sutures should never be used on an omental pedicle-graft – anyone could come to lie exposed within the fistulous area and cause stone formation.

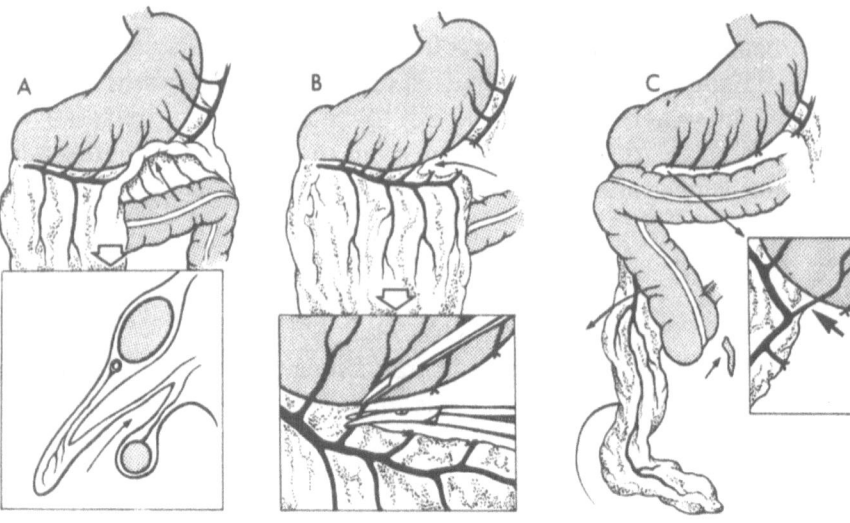

Fig. 4.

c) the technique of division must be meticulous to avoid damage to the parent gastroepiploic vessels. Thus the proximal end should be ligated in continuity before division, not by haemostat ligation because loss of this results in an interstitial haematoma and great care is then necessary to retrieve the bleeding end for secure religation if damage to the main pedicle vessels is to be avoided. Haemostat ligation can be used for the gastric end which is easy to retrieve in case of a slip-off.

d) Once started mobilisation of the gastroepiploic arch should be completed to its gastroduodenal origin otherwise there is a risk that traction on the pedicle might tear the last undivided branch.

3. The run of the slender pedicle of omental vessels down to the pelvic repositioning of the omentum should be protected by relocating it behind the mobilised ascending colon (Fig. 4C).

4. A prophylactic appendicectomy is generally advisable to avoid the risk of secondary damage to the pedicle as a result of a fortituous acute appendicectomy immediately adjacent to it.

5. Gastric suction for a mild ileus is often required for three of four days after an extended mobilisation of the gastroepiploic pedicle. A gastrostomy tube is a humane alternative to a naso-gastric tube and, because the stomach is exposed, this is a quite simple procedure; however, a gastrostomy is prone to leak after removal of the catheter, unless an appropriate technique is used so it is not advocated to urologists who do not have an appropriate training in gastrointestinal surgery.

6. It is fundamentally important to remember that there is only one omentum and that it is a disaster to the patient if the blood supply of this is

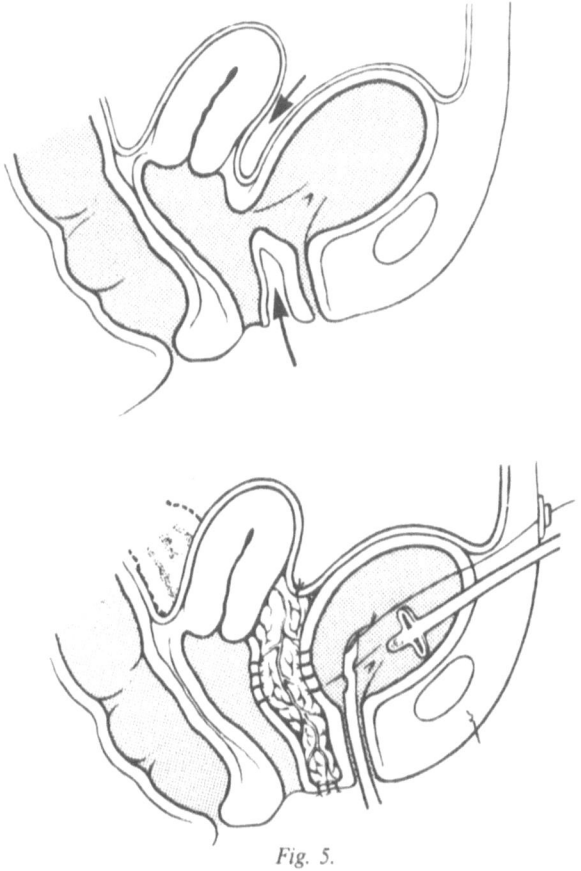

Fig. 5.

damaged by inappropriate mobilisation of its vascular pedicle roof-strip anastomosis.

Omental interposition repair of vesico-vaginal fistulae (Fig. 5)

A wide abdomino-perineal tunnel, that will accept four fingers in the adult, is created in the tissue plane between the vagina and the bladder. The bladder and vagina are closed with interrupted PGA sutures, the knots of which lie within the respective lumina as far as possible so that their summated bulk is detached and voided thus reducing the tissue reaction to a minimum. A maximum bulk of omental graft is interposed and its distal margin included in the introital skin sutures.

Provided there is an adequate bulk of well vascularised omental graft, with a good lateral overlap of the suture line, the recurrence of a urine fistula is exceedingly rare; even if the suture line of a heavily irradiated

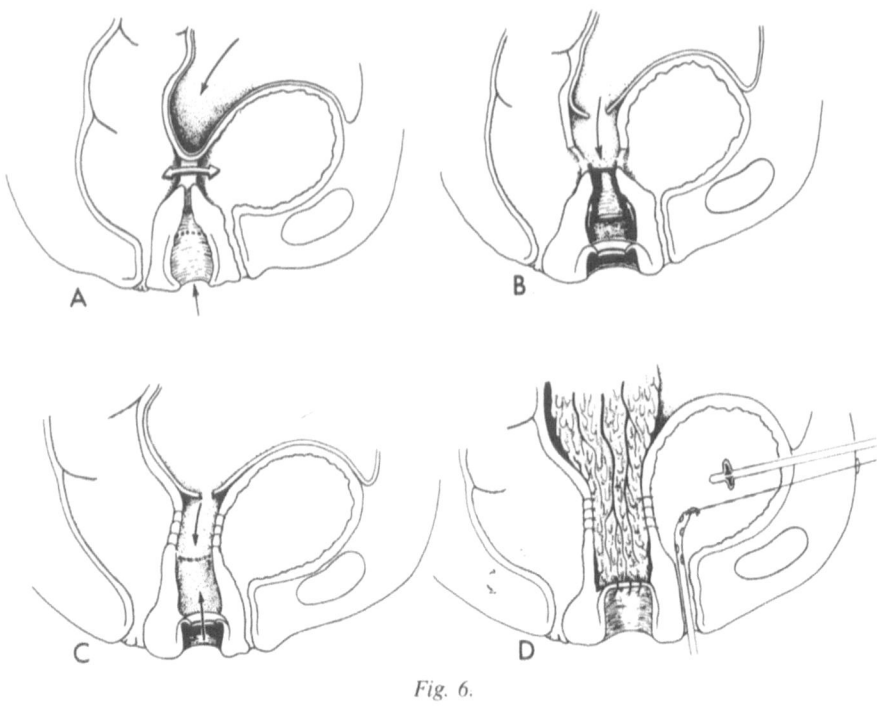

Fig. 6.

bladder breaks down the omentum exposed to the lumen of the bladder rapidly uretheliases.

Omental interposition repair of vesico-urethral-vaginal fistulae

Complicated fistulae extending from the bladder base into the urethra can also be closed with omental support but urinary continence is of course, dependent upon the reconstruction of either an efficient bladder neck sphincter or an efficient urethral sphincter; this in turn depends not only upon meticulous urethral reconstruction but also upon the survival of its intrinsic sphincter function (Turner-Warwick, 1977).

Omental interposition repair of vesico-vaginal rectal fistulae (Fig. 6)

The omentum can be used to repair extensive post-irradiation vesico-vaginal fistulae extending into the rectum, such complex fistulae most commonly are the result of treatment of carcinoma of the cervix by combination of a radical hysterectomy and irradiation. In these cases the vault of the residual vagina is usually stenosed and surrounded by dense irradiation fibrosis; the simplest way of resolving this situation is to circumcise the lower vagina, removing its scarred vault and interposing the bulk of the omentum between the fistula-closure suture lines of the bladder and the rectum. In such cases it is particularly important that the width of the abdomino-perineal tunnel should extend across the full width of the pelvic cavity and the creation of this often involves extensive resection of the irradiation fibrosis of a 'frozen' pelvis laterally.

Omento-caeco-vaginoplasty

In younger patients it is sometimes appropriate to reconstruct the stenosed vault of the vagina with a synchronous caecovagino-plasty supported by an omental wrap (Turner-Warwick et al., 1967). In such cases the suture line between the inverted ascending colon and the lower margin of the vagina usually heals quite well because they are relatively unaffected by the irradiation.

A caecovaginoplasty is sometimes especially valuable in the surgical management of a 'frozen' irradiation pelvis when, for instance, even after full mobilisation of its pedicle, there is an insufficient bulk of omentum available to fill the 'dead space' in the pelvis after the resection of a stenotic rectum and restoration of bowel continuity by a colo-anal anastomosis: in such cases the well vascularised wall of the transposed caecum and its mucosal lining subserves a space-occupying cavity-lining function.

Incarcerated 'obstruction' of the lower ureter associated with irradiation fibrosis

The functional drainage of the lower segment of the ureter is commonly impaired in association with extensive irradiation fibrosis; this is not always the result of a stricture – it sometimes results from fibrotic encasement of a somewhat dilated ureter which compromises the peristaltic activity of the residual muscle of the irradiated ureter. In such cases it is sometimes possible to restore functional drainage by 'hemi-lysis' – carefully resecting the dense fibrosis overlying its medial surface replacing this with the supple omental graft. Owing to the increased risk of necrosis it is generally inappropriate to attempt to mobilise such an irradiated ureter from its fibrotic bed – in the manner of the management of benign retro-peritoneal fibrosis – by lisis, transposition and omental wrap (Turner-Warwick, 1967).

The technique of hemi-omental-support after the hemi-lysis of an irradiated ureter emphasises the urodynamic value of the omentum which, because it never 'sets solid' and so ensures the subsequent freedom of urodynamic movement of any urinary tract repair that is wrapped in it – ureter, bladder or urethral sphincter mechanisms, by preventing immobilisation as a result of recurrent secondary fibrosis (Turner-Warwick, 1976).

A *fenestrated* ureteric stent is generally advisable to cover the early postoperative course after hemi-lysis of an irradiated ureter.

Irradiation fistulae and residual tumour

There is always a possibility that there are residual tumour cells in the fibrosis associated with an irradiation fistula, even when a preliminary biopsy proved negative and even if the treatment was concluded ten or twenty years previously. The presence of microscopic tumour in dense irradiated fibrosis is not necessarily a contraindication to the omental closure of a fistula; however, this situation requires thoughtful qualification and considered clinical judgment.

It is clearly inappropriate to attempt to close a fistula when the bulk of the induration associated with it is active recurrent macroscopic tumour. However, when a representative biopsy simply shows a few residual cells in extensive irradiation fibrosis, this may indicate that the local tumour situation is relatively quiescent and, under these circumstances, because the prognosis is consequently poor, it is all the more important to resolve the incapacitating incontinence as swiftly and as efficiently as possible. Closure of the fistula with omental support is not only a considerably simpler surgical procedure than a uretero-ileal surface conduit but it offers patients a good chance of normal urinary voiding and control for their remaining months.

Postoperative urinary drainage

Suprapubic urinary catheter drainage should be used as a routine postoperative procedure after any vesical fistula repair: it is efficient, reliable, and less uncomfortable than a urethral catheter. Furthermore, at the conclusion of the drainage period it is easy to verify the restoration of voiding efficiency by clamping the suprapubic drainage and checking the post voiding residual volumes before removing it; this compares favourably with the emotionally charged situation which arises when a urethral catheter has to be re-inserted repeatedly – the 'yoyo catheter'.

An additional urethral catheter may be advisable, however this must be retained by a sling-suture with a button on the abdominal wall: a balloon-retained urethral catheter is most inadvisable because inadvertent traction upon it can be disastrously disruptive.

Suction urinary drainage systems are unnecessary. Unfortunately, however, the calibre of the connecting tube of many standard drainage bag systems is so large that they have a tendency to retain air bubbles, and fluid levels in a hanging loop at the bedside can create a positive hydrostatic resistance to the flow of urine. If the internal diameter of a connecting tubing is not much larger than the lumen of the catheter it is draining it remains bubble free and creates a natural syphonic suction; however unobstructed urinary drainage is all that a fistula repair requires – hence the added safety of using both suprapubic and urethral catheter drainage.

The timing of a fistula repair

It is impossible to generalise usefully about the timing of a fistula repair, this is determined by clinical estimation of the healing potention of the local tissues of a particular case in relation to the proposed procedure.

If a repair is to be entirely dependent upon a layered closure it is obviously very important that the local tissue be in the best possible condition. It is often possible to resolve the problem of a simple traumatic or postoperative fistula by early exploration, within a few days, before a compromising degree of tissue healing reaction has developed. However, once this is established, it is usually better to wait several months until the local inflammatory response has stabilised as much as possible.

The main disadvantage of delaying a closure is the discomfort that it causes the unfortunate patient – she is likely to be intractably wet until the fistula is closed; nevertheless if this course of action is necessary it must be carried through with determination because disaster can result from impatience and premature intervention. Reasonably efficient interim collection of urine can sometimes be achieved by a Foley catheter drainage of the *vagina* if the introitus is narrow enough to retain a large balloon.

Although it is obviously important to ensure that any acute inflammatory element or haematoma is resolved, the timing of a fistula repair is relatively less critical when the success of the procedure is largely dependent upon an interposed omental pedicle graft; just as this procedure has enabled us to repair fistulae resulting from permanent severe tissue damage, or loss due to infection, trauma or irradiation, that were way beyond the potential of a layer closure procedure, so it can also make us somewhat less time-dependent on the local tissue healing of a relatively simple fistula repair.

Thus the timing of a repair must be considered carefully in relation to each individual fistula. It is generally unjustifiable to use a relatively major abdomino-perineal procedure involving a full length median incision for the repair of a simple fistula when, by waiting a few months, this can be simply repaired by a vaginal approach layer-closure procedure. However, there are

224

occasions when it may be quite clear that the ultimate repair is going to require the omental position anyway, so that, provided any coincident infection has been reduced to a minimum and there is no haematoma-mass, it may be unnecessary to wait for maximal resolution of the local tissue reaction.

References

1. Turner-Warwick R., Wynne E.J.C. and Handley Ashken M. The use of the omental pedicle graft in urinary tract reconstruction. Brit. J. Surg. 54 (1967): 849.
2. Turner-Warwick R. The use of pedicle grafts in the repair of urinary tract fistulae. Brit. J. Urol. 44 (1972): 644–656.
3. Turner-Warwick R. The use of the omentum in urinary tract reconstruction. J. Urol. 116 (1976): 341.
4. Turner-Warwick R. The repair of urinary vaginal fistulae. In 3rd edition of Operative Surgery, Rob, C. and Smith, R., 1977): 206–218.
5. Turner-Warwick R. Urinary fistula in the female. In: Harrison Ed. et al. (eds) Campbells Urology. Saunders, chapter 85 (1979).
6. Turner-Warwick R. Surgical access. In: Chisholm Ed., Heineman G.D. (eds) Urology. Heineman, London, (1980) 401–422.

V.3. Technical considerations in the vaginal approach of vesico-vaginal fistulae

G.H. BRILLENBURG WURTH

Twenty years ago, vesico-vaginal fistulae were regarded as doom... 'You should not cause a vaginal fistula because you could not repair it'. One mighty person, Boudijk Bastiaanse from Amsterdam, controlled the art of repairing fistulae through the vagina; during that time he was regarded as the Guru of the vesico-vaginal fistulae in our country.

In those years, gynaecologists used to have splendid ability in vaginal surgery but fistula-closing was reserved for academic Big Shots. Urologists – on the other hand – skilful in operating via the abdomen had no experience in vaginal surgery.

Since those early years circumstances have changed somewhat. A generation of Dutch surgeons and gynaecologists came back from African countries and brought with them a wealth of experience in fistula surgery. Today, you do not have problems as to where you can have your fistula repaired. Furthermore, fistulae seem to have become rare in this country.

The choice between the vaginal – or the abdominal route should not merely depend on specific ability of the surgeon. Strict indications for both procedures have to be respected. In general: big ulcerating fistulae, radiation complications, and fistulae with connection to the ureter should be operated in all cases abdominally.

Smaller fistulae including those at the top – mostly caused during abdominal hysterectomy, and peripheric leasions in the bladder neck – sometimes caused by vacuum extractors during delivery, can be operated via the vagina.

Some words about the patient's position on the table. The 'stone-cut position' is not that easy for the surgeon. He experiences the same problems as a mechanic in the garage who is always doing his work from the wrong position.

We decided to solve the problem by turning the patient on her front with spread upper legs. Working in this position saves the cervical spine of the urologist. Using ureteral catheters may be helpful for security but is not absolutely necessary. The application of a suprapubic indwelling catheter is a prime and absolute condition for the vaginal operation.

A mediolateral episiotomy or Suchardt incision is sometimes helpful in the deep or narrow vagina. A perfect haemostasis is necessary.

Through the vaginal fistula-opening a 5 cc balloon no. 8 Foley catheter is brought into the bladder; the operation area can be brought into the reach of your instruments by slight traction on the catheter. With much care and prudence the dissection of the vaginal epithelium from the bladder all around the fistula is completed. 'How far should the dissection be done??' 'Extremely far!!', Wim Moonen used to teach me. 'The really important thing is to free the bladder flaps fully and allow them to come together without any tension'.

The epithelialised fistula is excised from the bladder wall; the hole in the bladder is closed with a first layer of number 3–0 vicryl. A second layer of number 2–0 vicryl interrupted mattress sutures is placed so as to bury the first row. The vaginal mucosa is closed with everted interrupted sutures of number 2–0 vicryl. Care should be taken that the vaginal scar is placed slightly distal from the bladder closing. If possible, an extra layer of peritoneum can be placed between bladder and vagina. In ideal patients the pubo-coccigetus muscles can be interposed. A large tampon is placed post-operatively in the vagina. Drains are not used, care is taken for accurate haemostasis. Intravenous infusions are not necessary. We seldom use pro-phylactic antibiotics. With the suprapubic catheter the patient is mobile directly after the operation. After 4 or 5 days she can be discharged from the hospital. The catheter will be removed after 10 days. Sexual intercourse can be resumed 4 weeks after the operation.

The time-interval between the first operation and the repair of the fistula varies to between 8 and 12 weeks, depending on the degree of inflammation. The success of the treatment could be dependent on the amount of time between the two operations. If in the pre-operative period an indwelling catheter is desired, a suprapubic system is preferable. The fistula is mostly located at the bottom of the bladder, just proximal of the trigone. No in-dwelling catheter prevents the loss of urine through the vagina. The patient is wet in all circumstances. However, this problem has one advantage: 'urine-leakage cleans the fistula and the operation area'.

Some complications after fistula-closing

Occlusion of the catheter means disaster. Take care that very obese ladies do not fall a-sleep with their weight on the drainage tube. Because of this stupid reason, we had to reoperate 3 or 4 cases. Bladder spasms are also to be avoided assiduously. Against this problem Probantine or Antrenyl du-plex are good choises. In one case we were confronted with repeated incrus-trations of the scar inside the bladder, caused perhaps by insufficient closing or wrong closing material. A postoperative stress or urge incontinence is sometimes a depressing side-effect after a successful fistula-closing, the cause may be from the previous situation. Closing of the pubo-coccigeus muscles, especially in distal fistulae, could be very useful in preventing stress incontinence. In general however, complications are rare, and the success-rate of this procedure is high, if precise preoperative indication has been stated about the way of operating.

References

1. Brillenburg Wurth G.H. Sluiten van vesico-vaginalé fistels langs vaginale weg. Tijdschr. voor Geneesk. 124, 15 (1980): 23.
2. Cattegno B. et al. Position opératoire et décubitis ventral dans la chirurgie du bas appareil urinaire féminin. La Presse Médical, 31 (10 sept. 1983): 12.
3. Friedberg V., Altwein J.E. and Petri E. Vaginaler oder Abdominaler Verschluss von Blasen-Scheiden-Fisteln. Gynäkologischen Urologie, Thieme Verlag, Stuttgart-New York, (1983) 73–85.
4. Hohenfellner R. and Wulff H.N. Urologische Komplikationen. Inter- und postoperative Komplikationen in der Gynäkologie, Thieme Verlag, Stuttgart, (1979) 179–181.
5. Hurd Fr.J.K. Vaginal repair of vesico-vaginal fistula. Reconstructive urologic surgery, The Williams and Wilkins Company, Baltimore, (1977) 232–238.
6. Mack W.S. Repair of vesico-vaginal fistula. XVe Congrès de la Société International d'Urologie, Tokio (12–18 July, 1970).
7. Oderwald W.H.J. Experiences with injuries of the urinary pathways caused by gynaecological surgery. Current and future trends in urology: a book in honour of Prof. P.J. Donker at his retirement from office 1979.
8. Roberson J.R. Vesico-vaginal fistula: gynaecologists responsibility. Obstet. and Gynaec. 42 (1973): 611.
9. Turner-Warwick R. The use of pedicle grafts in the repair of urinary tract fistulae. Brit. J. Urol. 44 (1972): 644.

CHAPTER SIX

Male incontinence

VI.1. The sphincter mechanisms of the male and the prevention of postprostatectomy incontinence

R. TURNER-WARWICK

Introduction

The whole length of the posterior urethra of the male is sphincter-active and the feasibility of operations upon it such as the resolution of prostatic obstruction and the repair of pelvic fracture strictures depends upon two facts:

1. The *occlusive competence of the bladder neck mechanism* (formerly known as the internal sphincter), which extends from the internal meatus down to the level of the verumontanum, is *structurally and functionally distinct from the distal urethral mechanism* (formerly known as the external sphincter), which extends from the membranous urethra up to level of the verumontanum on the inside of the prostate.

The commonest cause of intermittent urine leakage after prostatectomy is in fact the result of persistent instability of the detrusor, with or without an element of sphincter impairment.

2. The functionally distinct mechanisms of the *bladder neck* and of the distal urethral mechanism are both independently competent and individually capable of maintaining continence in the absence of the other (Turner-Warwick, 1968, 1970).

Continence after prostatectomy

After prostatectomy the bladder neck mechanism is almost invariably functionally incompetent, not only because it is ablated by routine prostatectomy procedures, both endoscopic and open, but also because the preceeding progressive upward enlargement of the lateral and middle 'lobes' have commonly expanded it widely and over-stretched it. Even in the course of a definitive reconstructive prostatectomy it is in fact very difficult to reconstruct a functionally occlusive and competent bladder neck mechanism without it becoming obstructive (Turner-Warwick, 1984).

Consequently urinary continence after prostatectomy is entirely dependent upon the functional competence of the distal sphincter mechanism and this is a prime consideration of every prostatectomy procedure.

A normal distal sphincter mechanism that is uninjured and functioning normally under volitional control can contain intravesical pressure rises due to postural changes, coughing, straining and also those resulting from detrusor contractions up to a level of about 120 cm H_2O.

With proper understanding of the anatomy and appropriate technique it is generally possible to avoid injury to the distal sphincter mechanism during surgical procedures for the relief of non-malignant prostatic obstruction; however distal sphincter incompetence can also result from abnormalities of it that existed preoperatively. Thus postprostatectomy incontinence should be regarded as potentially preventable or predictable.

It is a remarkable fact that, in symposia held across the world, much time is spent discussing relatively unsuccessful methods of the after treatment of postprostatectomy incontinence and little or none on the principles and techniques of avoiding the surgical damage to the distal sphincter mechanisms that is commonly responsible for, or contributes to, unpredicted urine leakage.

Predictable postprostatectomy incontinence

The possibility of urinary leakage after prostatectomy is sometimes predictable.

Unstable high-pressure detrusor dysfunction

Leakage may occur in spite of an entirely normally functioning distal mechanism when abnormally high intravesical pressures are created by involuntary contractions of an over-powerful unstable detrusor mechanism during bladder filling. However although it forewarns of the possibility, the preoperative demonstration of high-pressure (over 100–120 cm H_2O) is not a contra-indication to the relief of prostatic obstruction, partly because there is a better-than-even chance that the unstable detrusor behaviour will revert to stability following the relief of the obstruction (Turner-Warwick, 1970, 1979) and partly because the contraction may well increase still further in response to persistent outlet obstruction.

Pre-existing distal sphincter impairment

Techniques for the preservation of the sphincter mechanism distal to the verumontanum are unavailing if its mechanism has already been impaired by a pre-existing condition. The identification of this situation often requires a high index of suspicion because the patient's continence will have been maintained by the bladder neck mechanism and subsequently by the prostatic enlargement. Furthermore, when partial distal sphincter incompetence is suspected, it is often impossible to predetermine with certainty whether there is sufficient residual function to maintain continence. In general therefore when there is doubt about the efficiency of the distal sphincter mechanism, the indications for prostatectomy should be retention of urine rather than symptoms that can be lived with.

Pelvic fracture urethral injuries. Pelvic fracture injuries of the sub-prostatic urethra almost invariably impair or destroy the competence of the distal sphincter mechanism even if they do not create a stricture (Turner-Warwick, 1973). Such patients are usually unaware of their sphincter damage and may not volunteer a history of injury. However, radiological evidence of an old fracture should be noted and the distal sphincter mechanism carefully reviewed endoscopically for evidence of scarring or rigidity. The 'stop-test' on videovoiding cystourethrography (Turner-Warwick, 1979) may be helpful with the caution that, although the peri-urethral pelvic floor musculature is incapable of sustained urethral occlusion, it can interrupt the voiding stream and briefly simulate a functional distal urethral mechanism.

Following the spatulated anastomotic repair of an occlusive sub-prostatic stricture the distal mechanism is overtly absent and continence entirely dependent upon the bladder neck mechanism (Turner-Warwick, 1973, 1982). The treatment of subsequent prostatic enlargement by a transurethral resection will inevitably result in functional ablation of any surviving element of the bladder neck mechanism and result in incontinence. In such cases a transcapsular dissection enucleation with definitive bladder neck reconstruction offers the best chance of subsequent sphincter-competence (Turner-Warwick, 1984).

Internal urethrotomy of bulbo-membranous strictures. The current enthusiasm for extensive endoscopic urethrotomy may create postprostatectomy incontinence problems in the long term (Turner-Warwick, 1979, 1981). We have seen examples of the treatment of posterior bulbar strictures resulting from urethritis by endoscopic urethrotomy that extends posteriorly through the full thickness of the entire length of the distal mechanism, rendering it so incompetent that during a subsequent definitive repair of the residual distal stricture the verumontanum could be viewed without the aid of a speculum.

Trans-sphincter bulbo-membranous urethroplasty. Urethritis rarely results in significant damage to the distal urethra, however in the course of a definitive repair of the stricture the membranous urethra may be found to be sufficiently narrow to require recalibration and a trans-sphincter extension of a substitute graft to avoid proximal restenosis. Special instruments are required to achieve this within a calibre of 34–36F to avoid compromising its sphincteric function; however incompetence of a distal sphincter mechanism is likely to result when a posterior flap is inlaid up to the verumontanum by relaxing incisions sufficient to enable standard instruments to be used (Turner-Warwick, 1982).

Urethral valves. Previous treatment of urethral valves always raises the suspicion of distal sphincter incompetence because the only techniques for this involve the use of button electrodes or loop-resection which are apt to electro-coagulate the intramural thickness of the distal sphincter mechanism.

Prostatic carcinoma

Invasion of the distal urethra by prostatic tumour can create a compromising degree of distal sphincter rigidity or stricture, however, mild degrees of this can often be controlled by a titrated dose of local irradiation which does not significantly increase the local sphincter damage (Turner-Warwick, 1984).

Neuropathy

The coincidence of prostatic obstruction and neuropathy requires detailed urodynamic evaluation and every case must be considered individually. A significant bladder outlet obstruction rarely contributes a useful element of urinary control in neuropathic bladder dysfunction; more often it compromises emptying by an under-active detrusor dysfunction or by an over-active detrusor when unstable neuropathic detrusor contractions are not sustained. When it is necessary to relieve a prostatic obstruction associated with detrusor dysfunction and neuropathy it is particularly important to ensure both maximum sphincter preservation and the complete resolution of residual apical tissue obstruction; this may be more easily achieved by an intra-urethral sphincter-preserving enucleation (Turner-Warwick, 1983) than by a transurethral resection but this is a matter of individual surgical judgement.

The avoidance of damage to the distal sphincter mechanism during prostatectomy

Although preservation of functional competence of the distal urethral sphincter mechanism has always been a prime consideration in prostatic surgery its mechanism has often been damaged in the course of generally accepted procedures for enucleation prostatectomy, radical prostatectomy, optical urethrotomy and wide-access urethroplasty. Many of the problems have arisen as a result of a false sense of security derived from the incredibly erroneous supposition that the mechanism of the intrinsic distal urethral mechanism is supported by an effective sphincter mechanism 'external' to the membranous urethra.

The myth of the 'urogenital diaphragm' and the concept of the 'external sphincter'

Descriptions of the macro-anatomy of the distal sphincter mechanism, both in traditional and current anatomical and surgical texts, are generally grossly inaccurate and surgically misleading, indeed it is quite remarkable that they have survived unchallenged for so long.

There is in fact a dearth of accurate anatomical description. Almost all the illustrations are diagrammatic and subject to both erroneous traditional concept and to artistic licence (Fig. 1).

The commonly described and illustrated concept of two fascial layers of 'urogenital diaphragm' enclosing an encircling bulk of peri-urethral striated muscle – through which the membranous urethra is supposed to pass and to the undersurface of which the spongy tissue of the bulb is supposed to be applied is frankly mythological.

Ambiguous nomenclature has also contributed to the erroneous concept of the distal urethral sphincter mechanism (Turner-Warwick et al., 1973).

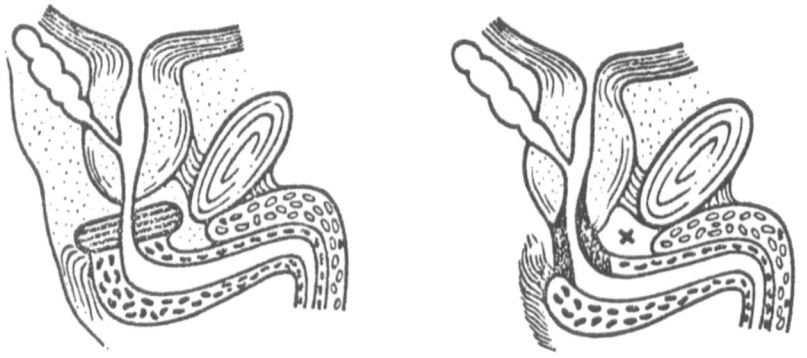

Fig. 1. The distal sphincter mechanism – fiction and fact.

The term 'external sphincter' was originally intended to denote that it was external (i.e. distal) to the 'internal sphincter' – the bladder neck mechanism. Unfortunately this has often been misconceived as denoting a mythical circumferential sphincter muscle 'external' to (i.e. surrounding) the membranous urethra – the 'compressor urethrae'.

To add to the terminological confusion Tanagho has also used the term 'external sphincter' to denote the external (i.e. outer) striated muscle layer of the intramural urethral mechanism to distinguish it from the inner layer of the smooth muscle and the term 'rhabdo-sphincter' is no great improvement as it is impossible to distinguish the electromyographic activity of the continence-competent 'slow twitch' striated muscle fibres of the intrinsic urethral mechanism from the continent-incompetent 'fast-twitch' striated muscle fibers of the posteriorly located pubo-urethral element of the pelvic floor musculature.

Once a word is in generally misconceived mis-use it is virtually impossible to retrieve and redefine it – thus there is good reason to abandon the term 'external sphincter' in favour of the distal urethral sphincter mechanism (DUSM).

During the development of anastomotic bulbo-prostatic stricture repairs, Turner-Warwick (1973) observed that far from being surrounded by muscle, the antero-lateral surface of the membranous urethra relates to a surgically significant sub-pubo prostatic space (Turner-Warwick, 1982, 1984) (Fig. 2). This, coupled with the introduction of objective urodynamic evaluation has led to a fundamental revision of sphincter anatomy and function and to the adoption of appropriate sphincter-preserving procedures during prostatic and stricture surgery (Turner-Warwick, 1968, 1970, 1981, 1983; Turner-Warwick et al., 1973).

The distal urethral mechanism

The distal urethral mechanism is composed of an inner layer of smooth muscle and an external layer of striated muscle – together they form the 3–4 mm thickness of the wall of the membranous urethra and they extend upwards through the apex of the prostate up to the level of the verumontanum. As the lateral lobes of 'prostatic enlargement' form from microscopic sub-urothelial glands in the mid-prostatic urethra (McNeal, 1972), the verumontanum is carried upwards so that the distal extent of the 'lateral lobe hypertrophy' lies outside the proximal part of the distal sphincter mechanism although the real extent of this is not apparent endoscopically (Fig. 3).

Thus in the surgical resolution of obstructive prostatic hypertrophy it is helpful to consider the distal mechanism in three equal parts, the distal

236

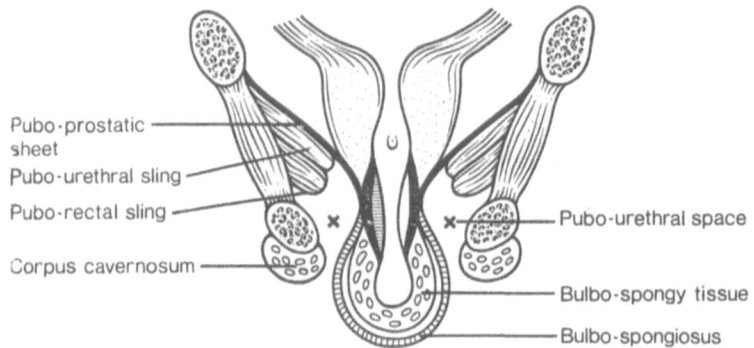

Pubo·prostatic sheet

Pubo·urethral sling

Pubo·rectal sling

Corpus cavernosum

Pubo-urethral space

Bulbo·spongy tissue

Bulbo·spongiosus

Fig. 2. The distal 'external' sphincter muscles (coronal section).

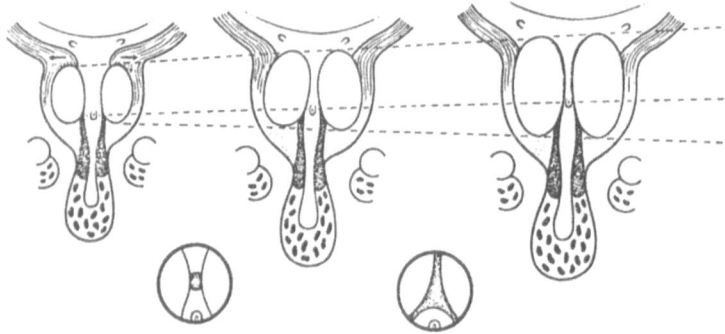

Fig. 3. Prostatic enlargement and its relation to the distal sphincter mechanism.

third being the membranous urethra, the middle third lying within the apical 'prostatic capsule' and the proximal third extending upwards on the inner surface of the 'lateral lobe'.

Under the circumstances of prostatic enlargement the proximal third of the distal urethral mechanism is the least efficient as it is spread thinly over the lateral lobe. However, so far as the surgical relief of the lobar obstruction is concerned, whether by transurethral resection or by enucleation, technical endeavours to preserve the proximal third are undoubtedly the best way of ensuring that the function of the important middle third, and the all-important distal third, survive.

Damage to the distal urethral sphincter mechanism during classic open enucleation procedures

a) *Finger-breaking the distal urethra* (Fig. 4). The time-honoured technique of breaking across the distal urethra by finger-pressure in the course of a

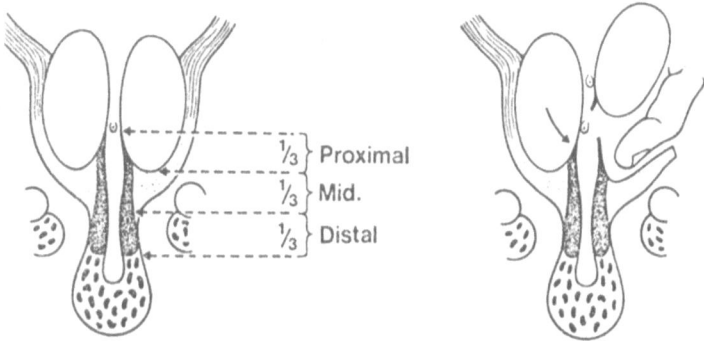

Fig. 4. Three areas of the distal sphincter mechanism.

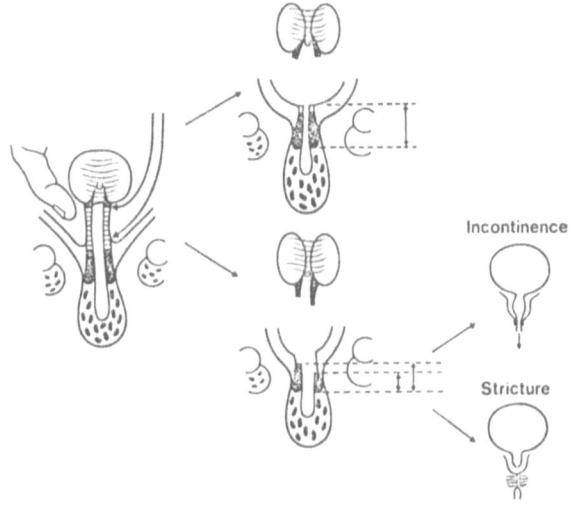

Fig. 5. Division of the distal sphincter mechanism by sub-apical finger-breaking and scissor transection.

transvesical prostatectomy or a sub-capsular retropubic prostatic enuclea-tion risks extensive damage to its intramural sphincter mechanism. When the prostate is grossly enlarged, the risks of finger-breaking the urethra is diminished because the proximal third of the urethra becomes progressively stretched to paper-thinness so that it automatically tends to break in the region of its proximal extent on the inside of the lateral lobes. However, when the prostate is not much enlarged, there is no particular differential weakness of the distal mechanism so that its whole length may be avulsed after a distal breakage in the course of attempts to enucleate a 'small fibrous prostate'.

b) *Sharp transection of the distal urethra during sub-capsular retropubic enucleation* (Fig. 5). Awareness of the problems associated with finger-breaking of the urethra led to the development of the Millin technique of dividing the distal urethra with scissors after it had been isolated in the course of a sub-capsular retropubic enucleation; however, although this avoids the possibility of complete avulsion of the distal third of the sphincter, the middle third is inevitably dislocated to some extent by the interposition of the finger between the apex of the lower lobe and the capsule. Furthermore, this sphincter-active segment of the urethra is cut-on-the-stretch at a point determined by the curvature of the scissors, so that the verumontanum and the proximal third of the urethral sphincter which lies on the inside of the lower lobes is removed with the specimen together with a proportion of the urodynamically important middle third of the sphincter mechanism, the actual extent of which depends upon the angle of the curve of the scissors used.

Preservation of the distal urethral sphincter by intra-urethral pre-enucleation division (Fig. 6)

By far the safest way of preserving the distal urethral sphincter mechanism during retropubic enucleation of the prostate is to extend the transcapsular incision into the lumen of the urethra and to transect the urethra on the inside of the lateral lobes at the level of the verumontanum before proceeding to any enucleation (Turner-Warwick, 1968; Turner-Warwick et al., 1973); while the proximal third of the urethral sphincter mechanism thus preserved may not itself have much residual function, its preservation, undislocated, ensures that the middle third remains undamaged. The verumontanum and the ejaculatory ducts are left in situ and intact after an intra-urethral enucleation of the lateral lobes.

Preservation of the distal sphincter mechanism during a radical prostatectomy (Fig. 7)

The standard procedure of a radical prostatectomy involves transection of the urethra below the apex of the prostatic capsule; the proximal and middle thirds of the distal sphincter mechanism are therefore removed with the specimen. The distal third of the intramural sphincter remains in situ within the stump of the residual membranous urethra. The fictitious concept of an 'external' sphincter, lying within the 'uro-genital diaphragm' and surrounding the membranous urethra has, over the years, encouraged many urologists to treat this precious distal third of the intramural sphincter mechanism in a most cavalier manner during total prostatectomy, effectively dividing it into segments in the course of restoring continuity of the urinary

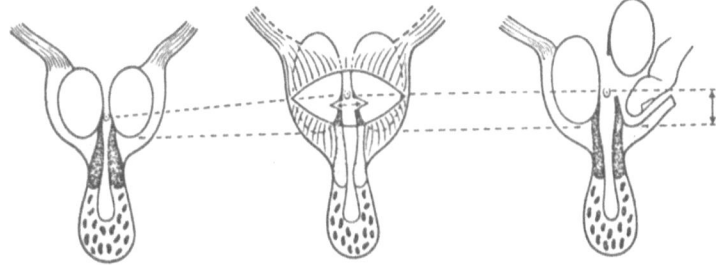

Fig. 6. Pre-enucleation intra-urethral division of the distal sphincter mechanism.

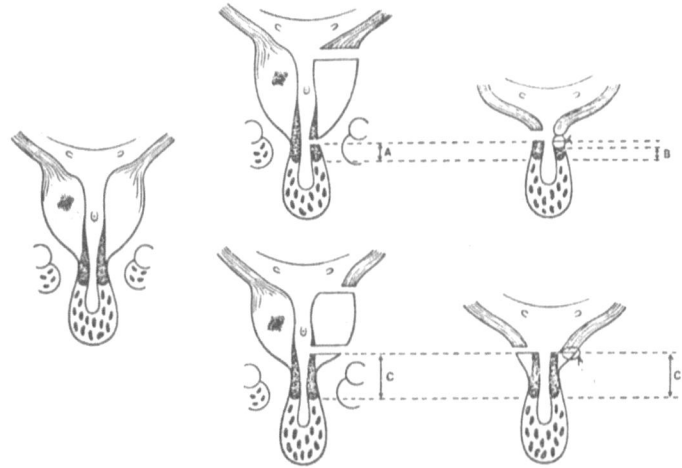

Fig. 7. Radical prostatectomy and the distal sphincter mechanism.

tract by approximating the bladder base to it with 'five or six well placed anastomotic sutures' – it is not surprising that patients treated in this way not infrequently suffer from varying degrees of 'impaired urinary control'.

If a surgeons concept of 'cancer surgery' requires him to remove the proximal two-thirds of the distal mechanism by transecting the urethra below the apex of the prostatic tissue, then the function of the residual distal third of the sphincter mechanism is best preserved by inserting the anastomotic sutures in the fascial layer around it, not into it. However, since the surgical treatment of cancer and prostatic cancer in particular must surely be a compromise, the functional advantages of transecting the prostate a few millimeters above the distal extent of the capsule must be considered because this not only preserves an additional length of the middle third of the distal mechanism, but the margin of the capsule surrounding it provides good anchorage for the anastomotic sutures without inserting them through the functional mechanism itself (Elmer Belt's procedure).

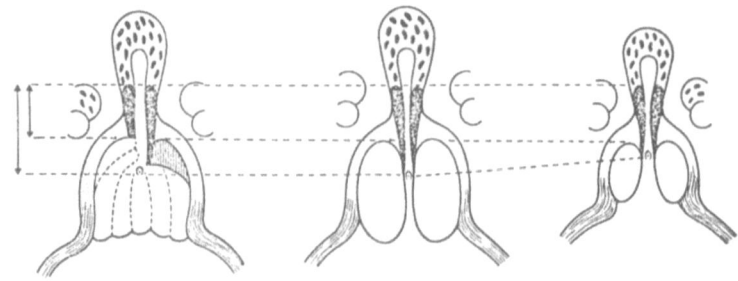

Fig. 8. Transurethral resection; the apical 'lobar' tissue and the distal sphincter mechanism.

Preservation of distal urethral sphincter mechanism during transurethral resection

Most texts on transurethral resection show diagrams illustrating the distal extent of the lateral lobes to be situated at the verumontanum; as previously mentioned, this is because their true distal extent is hidden from endoscopic view by the proximal extent of the urethral sphincter mechanism lying within (Turner-Warwick, 1968; Turner-Warwick et al., 1973; Turner-Warwick, 1979).

This relationship creates a surgical dilemma which is most easily solved by those who have not quite understood the problem. Few resectionists believe that they leave a significant amount of hypertrophic tissue at the apex of the lateral lobes and few accept that they resect a significant amount of the sphincter mechanism; yet even with rectal finger-displacement of the lobes, it is almost impossible to resect the apical lobe tissue completely without sacrificing that part of the sphincter mechanism that is overlying it (Fig. 8).

In practice, a great majority of resectionists leave the unseen apical tissue and this accounts for the fact that the post-operative voiding flow-rates after transurethral resections tend to be marginally less good than those in a comparable series of patients after treatment by enucleation prostatectomy (Turner-Warwick, 1979; Shah et al., 1979). Of the two faults, the sins of omission are far better than the sins of comission, especially in the training-stages of an endoscopic resectionist (which lasts for many years).

The 30° beaked-sheath resectoscope is much the most widely used for transurethral resection – its beaked sheath has certain positive advantages, especially for large-volume resections and for the ease of sector-localisation of bleeding points during haemostasis. However the beak obscures the verumontanum during antero-lateral resection and anterior incision of the bladder neck, and this compromises the accurate location of the distal limit of the resection in this sector – furthermore it distorts the functional occlusion of the distal urethral mechanism so that it is impossible to visualise this circumferentially. These deficiencies are resolved by changing to a 0° beak-less resectoscope for the final precision-resection of the apical lobar tissue and maximum preservation of the distal sphincter mechanism – the two problems which give rise to the majority of complications after transure-thral resection.

Conclusion

It is to be hoped that an accurate knowledge of the anatomy of the sphincter mechanism and the replacement of some of the time-honoured but sphinc-ter-risking prostatectomy techniques (open, endoscopic and radical) by more appropriate sphincter-preserving variations, together with a better understanding of urodynamic function and dysfunction, will significantly reduce the incidence of post-prostatectomy incontinence.

References

1. McNeal J.E. The prostate and prostatic urethra – a morphological synthesis. J. Urol. 107 (1972): 1008.
2. Shah P.J.R., Abrams P.H., Feneley R.C.L. and Green N.A. The influence of prostatic ana-tomy and the differing results of prostatectomy according to the surgical approach. Brit. J. Urol. 51 (1979): 549–551.
3. Turner-Warwick R.T. The repair of urethral strictures in the region of the membranous urethra. J. Urol., 100 (1968): 303–314.
4. Turner-Warwick R. Clinical problems associated with urodynamic abnormalities. First Internat. Urodynamics Symposium, Aachen. In: Lutzyer-W. & Melchior H. (eds) Urody-namics. Berlin. Springer Verlag. (1970) 237–263.
5. Turner-Warwick R., Whiteside C.G., Arnold E.P., Bates E.P., Worth P.H.L., Milroy E.J.G., Webster J.R. and Weir J. A urodynamic view of prostatic obstruction and the results of prostatectomy. Brit. J. Urol. 45 (1973): 631–645.
6. Turner-Warwick R.T. The management of traumatic urethral strictures and injuries. Brit. J. Surg. 60 (1973): 775–781.
7. Turner-Warwick R. Clinical Urodynamics. Urol. Clin. N. America, Ed. Turner-Warwick R. & Whiteside C.G. Vol. 6 (1979).
8. Turner-Warwick R. The sphincter mechanism – the avoidance of post-prostatectomy incon-tinence. Die Post-Operative Harninkontinenz des Mannes. Frankfurt International Sympo-sium, Weber W. & Jonas D. Georg Thieme Verlag. (1979) 17–33.
9. Turner-Warwick R. Lower urinary tract reconstruction. Chapter in Reconstructive Surgery. Ed. Gilroy Bevan, Blackwell, 1981.
10. Turner-Warwick R. Urethral stricture surgery. In: Glenn J. and Boyce G. (eds) Urologic Surgery. Harper & Row, ch. 68 (1982).
11. Turner-Warwick R. The relationship of prostatic enlargement to the distal sphincter mech-anism, the bladder neck mechanism – dyssenergic bladder neck obstruction. Chapter in Benign Prostatic Hypertrophy. Ed. Hinman F. & Chishilm G., Springer Verlag, 1983.
12. Turner-Warwick R. Bladder outflow obstruction. In: Mundy A., Stephenson T.P. and Wein A. (eds) Urodynamics, Churchill Livingstone (1984).

242

VI.2. Postprostatectomy incontinence

E.A. TANAGHO

As Mr. Turner-Warwick previously stated, postprostatectomy incontinence should no longer exist because prostatectomy, done properly and with careful adherence to basic principles, should not lead to incontinence. However, we still encounter these cases, although, fortunately, the incidence is not high. Every now and then, we will see this problem and ask ourselves: 'What is the best remedy?' Is it reconstructive surgery? Integration of the membranous urethra into the genitourinary diaphragm, with compression of it by the resilient tissue of the crura? Bladder neck reconstruction? AMS prosthesis? Electrical stimulation? Kaufman compression or another type of compression procedure on the bulbous urethra? We have a multitude of choices.

If we review the anatomy of this area, we can understand why postprostatectomy incontinence occurs. In the male, the musculature of the sphincteric mechanism is abundant. The main smooth sphincter is embedded in the prostate gland itself. The prostatic glandular stroma and its muscular element constitute the main internal sphincter or smooth sphincteric element. Added to this is a generous segment of membranous urethra composed of two elements – the smooth muscular element and a skeletal element.

Fig. 1 shows a sagittal section of the adult male pelvis, which has not been dissected, just fixed and sliced in the midline. You can see the pubic bone, bladder, internal meatus, prostate gland, and genito-urinary diaphragm area or membranous urethra. Notice its length and muscularity at the beginning of the bulbous spongy tissue and the beginning of the bulbous urethra and the urethra in the penis. You can readily see that, if you discard this entire segment, from the apex of the prostate up to the bladder neck, you leave a one-inch segment of heavily muscularized tube. This is the basic mechanism of control after radical prostatectomy.

If we do simple prostatectomy, enucleation, or transurethral resection, in which the original tissue is preserved, there should be no reason for any incontinence. You take a parasagittal section just to avoid the prostate gland itself, but there is plenty of muscle in the entire length of the urethra from

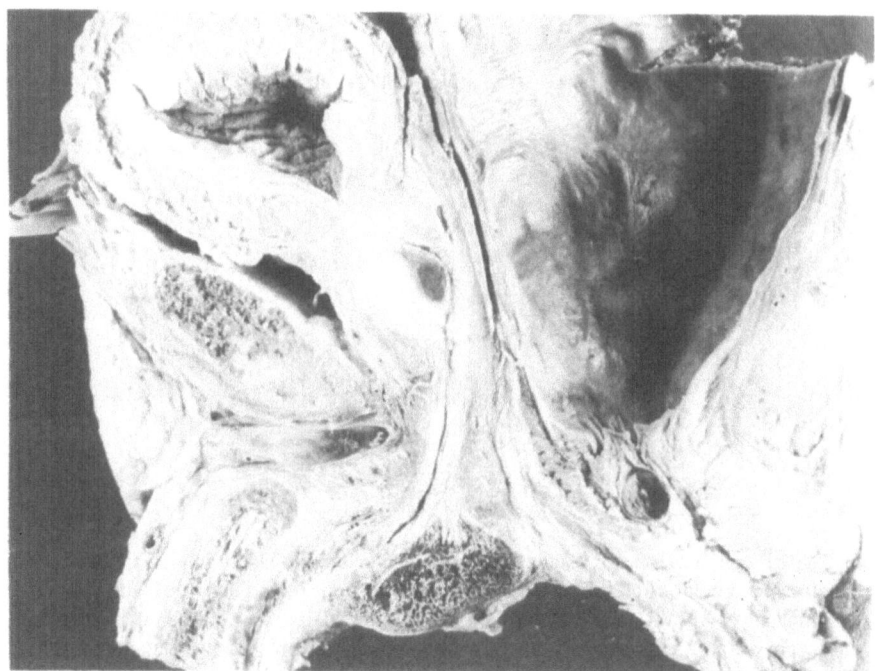

Fig. 1. Sagittal section of a fixed adult male pelvis, cut exactly in the midline to show the anatomic relationship of the pubic bone to the bladder, bladder neck, and prostatic segment as well as the membranous urethra where it enters the spongy tissue of the penis. Also note the prominent anal sphincter as well as the rectum. Most significant is the length of the urethral segment traversing the pelvic floor before entering the spongy tissue of the penis. The distance between the apex of the prostate and the bulbous part of the urethra constitutes the membranous urethra, which is roughly of equal length as the prostatic urethra. (Reprinted with permission from: Tanagho, E.A.: Anatomy of the lower urinary tract. In Campbell's Textbook of Urology (Walsh P.C., Gittes R.E., Perlmutter A.D. and Stamey T.A., eds.) 5th Ed. Philadelphia: W.B. Saunders, 1985.

the bladder neck down to the genito-urinary diaphragm. Do a neat, proper prostatectomy and you leave a prostatic cavity – clean and smooth, with an abundance of smooth-muscle tissue left in the prostate gland itself (Fig. 2). The most valuable segment is left intact: the ejaculatory duct, the apex of the prostate below the verumontanum, and the entire length of the membranous urethra below that. If you do a small glandular resection, you still leave behind an abundance of tissue that should be more than adequate to maintain continence.

Indeed, viewing the anatomy, it seems extremely difficult to make anyone incontinent. In cross-section (Fig. 3), you can see the depth: the membranous urethra, right below the apex of the prostate; and the smooth muscular coat inside it, surrounded by a heavy muscular coat. Magnified a bit more, one can see the two elements very clearly: the smooth-muscle element, the

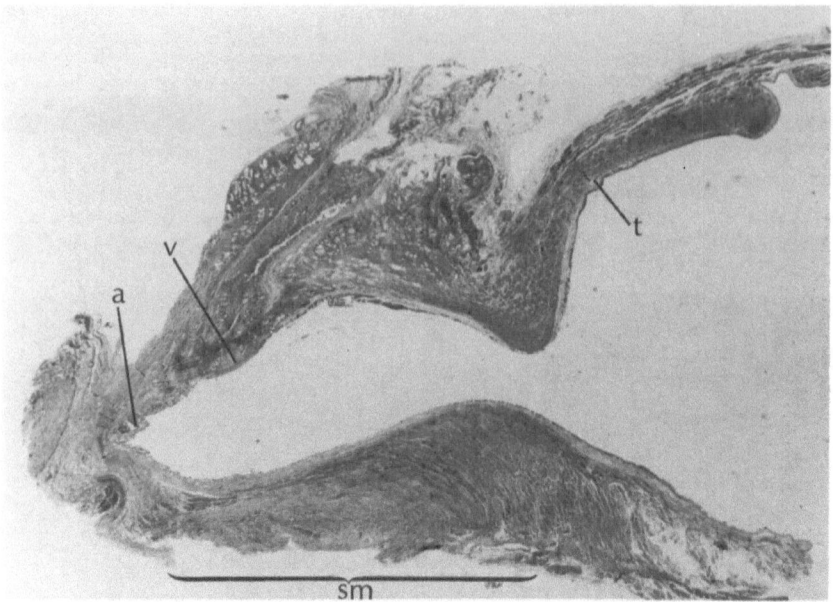

Fig. 2. Sagittal section of a postprostatectomy specimen across the bladder neck, prostatic fossa, and proximal membranous urethra. Note hypertrophied trigone (t) and anterior bladder wall, the smooth prostatic cavity with an abundance of smooth musculature (sm) in the prostatic capsule and in the apex (a) of the prostate. The verumontanum (v) and prostatic utricle and part of the ejaculatory duct are seen posteriorly.

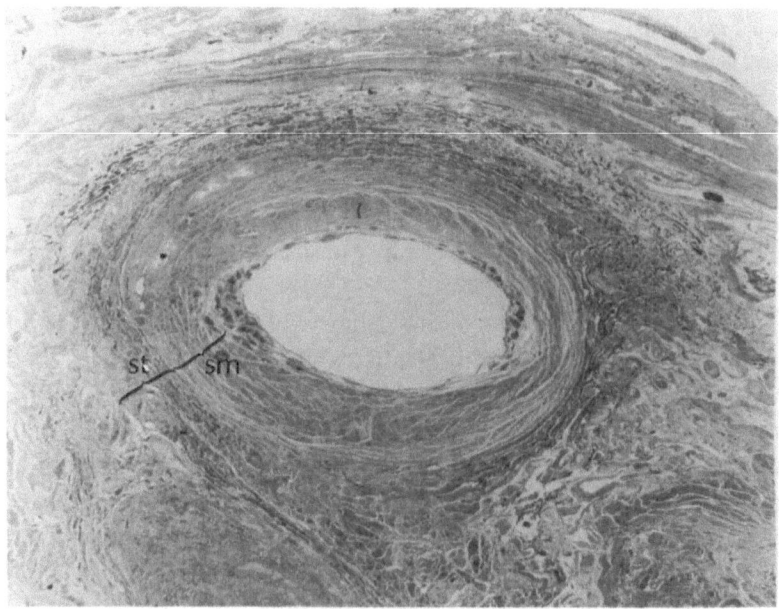

Fig. 3. Histologic cross-section of the membranous urethra of an adult male shows the distribution of the smooth intrinsic musculature (sm) in the urethral wall, with circular fiber orientation; it is surrounded by an equally thick intrinsic coat of striated muscle fibers (st), which converge posteriorly to insert in the perineal body. Note that the external sphincter constitutes an integral part of the musculature of the urethral wall at the level of the membranous urethra.

intrinsic element of the sphincteric mechanism; and the striated muscle around it. Both are intrinsic elements of the sphincter proper; they are not the genitourinary diaphragm, levator ani, or the transversus perinei. This abundant sphincteric musculature is completely below the prostate. For resection to approach the external sphincter – the cause of postprostatectomy incontinence – it would have to be very deep. Clearly, if a patient has been rendered incontinent, this element has been damaged completely.

With appreciation of this anatomy, one wonders why this complication occurs.

VI.3. The mechanisms of continence and incontinence after prostatectomy

C. FRIMODT-MØLLER, H. COLSTRUP & H.-H. MEYHOFF

Introduction

The mechanisms of urinary continence and incontinence in postprostatectomy patients have for many years been an important point of interest. Traditional anatomical concepts of the sphincter function have been rejected gradually as neurophysiological and urodynamic investigations were introduced. Surgery on the bladder neck and the prostate has provided even more knowledge to the anatomy of the continence mechanism. In order to facilitate the understanding of the continence mechanisms following surgery a short review of the anatomical structure of the bladder and urethra is necessary.

The anatomy of the bladder and urethra

The following concept is mainly derived from the studies by Gosling [1]. The *detrusor* muscle consists of numerous intermingling bundles arranged in a complex meshwork of smooth muscle, which makes possible an overall reduction of the bladder volume during contraction. The detrusor muscle is mainly parasympathetically innervated through pelvic nerves from the 2nd, 3rd and 4th segments of the sacral spinal cord, the transmitting substance being acetylcholine.

The *trigone* (Fig. 1) consists of a deep muscle layer indistinguishable from the detrusor muscle, and a superficial muscle layer extending from the ureteric orifices and down to the verumontanum. In contrast to the detrusor this thin layer is composed of relatively small muscle bundles with only minor parasympathetic innervation.

The *bladder neck* smooth muscle is independent of the detrusor muscle. It circumscribes the bladder neck with circular muscle bundles that also extend into the preprostatic portion of the urethra and intermingle with the smooth muscles of the prostatic capsule, and with the smooth muscles of the ejaculatory ducts. Thus, this smooth muscle has the localization and

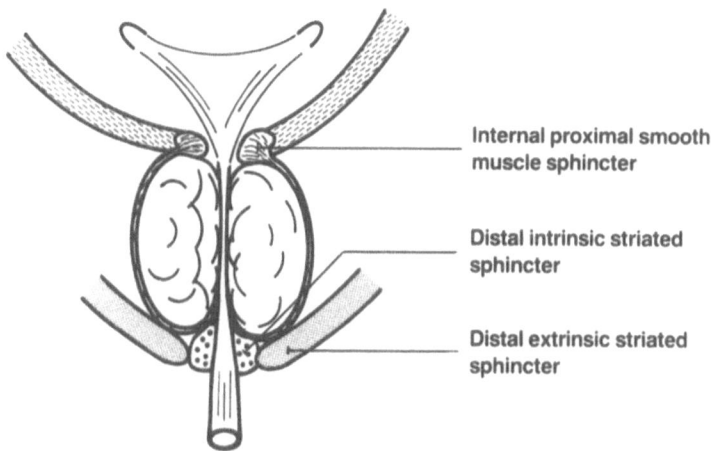

Internal proximal smooth
muscle sphincter

Distal intrinsic striated
sphincter

Distal extrinsic striated
sphincter

Fig. 1. A schematic diagram of the lower urinary tract in a patient with benign prostatic hypertrophy.

orientation of muscle fibres to act as a sphincter. It is termed the *internal proximal* or pre-prostatic urethral sphincter. This sphincter muscle is mainly supplied by sympathetic adrenergic nerves.

The striated muscle of the *membranous urethra* distal to the verumontanum consists of circular muscle fibres that proximally intermingle with the distal part of the prostate. This muscle is not only separate from the periurethral striated muscle included in the pelvic floor, but also in contrast to the pelvic floor it consists of small striated fibres of the 'slow-twitch' type capable of maintaining a sustained contraction for a long period. This muscle, totally different in function from the periurethral sphincter muscle, is termed the *distal intrinsic striated urethral sphincter.* The motor innervation of this sphincter is derived from the pelvic parasympathetic nerves. The periurethral or *distal, extrinsic striated sphincter* of the pelvic floor (previously regarded solely as the external sphincter) contains a mixture of slow- and fast-twitch muscle fibres. In contrast to the distal intrinsic sphincter this sphincter muscle is able to perform rapid contractions over shorter time periods. The motor innervation is through the pudendal nerves.

The physiology of the male proximal urethra

Urethral activity consists of two functions, (*1*) to maintain continence, and (*2*) to act as a urinary conduct. Many factors contribute to the maintenance of continence: active smooth and striated muscular contraction, vascular tissue, periurethral connective tissue, inner urethral softness and – in patients with benign prostatic hypertrophy (BPH) – the bulk of the prostatic tissue.

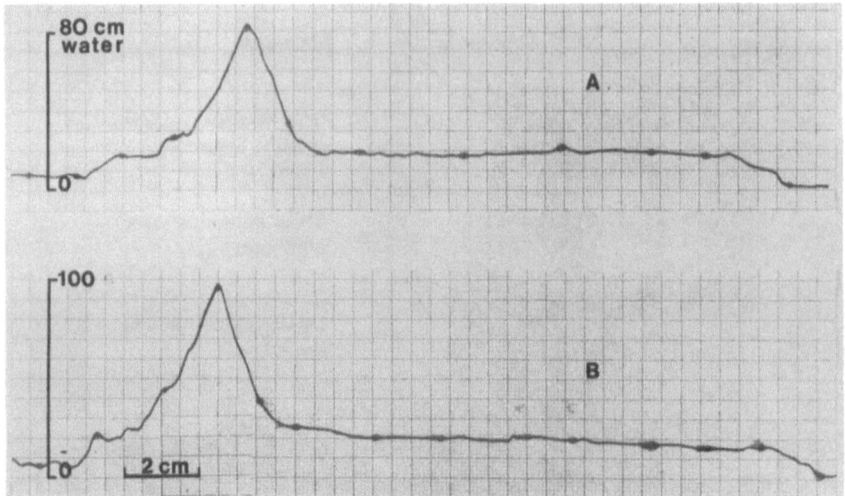

Fig. 2. Urethral profilometry in a normal male. Pump infusion rate 2 ml/sec, catheter withdrawal rate 5 mm/sec. Upper tracing (A) at rest, lower tracing (B) when squeezing.

There are two sphincter systems responsible for continence in the male:

1. The proximal internal smooth muscle sphincter located at the bladder neck and extending down to the verumontanum.

2. The distal urethral sphincter system consisting of

a) the distal intrinsic striated sphincter distal to the verumontanum and consisting of slow-twitch muscle-fibres.

b) the periurethral striated sphincter integrated in the pelvic floor and located at the membranous urethra. The muscle-fibres are mainly of the fast-twitch type.

The normal male continence is mainly achieved by the distal urethral sphincteric system, where the slow-twitch fibres maintain a long-acting contraction of the urethra, a so-called 'passive' continence. The function of the fast-twitch fibres of the peri-urethral sphincter is to perform quick contractions thereby increasing urethral pressure during coughing, straining etc. The role of the proximal internal sphincter at the bladder neck is still not clarified. Of major importance is the contraction of the bladder neck during ejaculation in order to prevent retrograde ejaculation. The influence on continence of this sphincter is, however, still not known.

Urodynamic and neurophysiological studies have increased our knowledge of the continence mechanisms. Urethral profilometry [2] provides a method to determine the urethral closure pressure of the distal urethral sphincter system, an example is shown in Fig. 2. Electromyographic registration of the sphincter system is another method of visualizing sphincter activity [3], but it is difficult to obtain specific recordings from the different

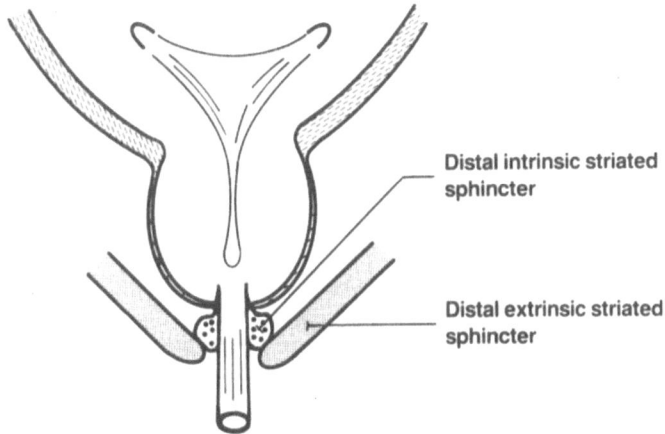

Fig. 3. A schematic diagram of the lower urinary tract following prostatic surgery.

sphincter muscles within the distal sphincter system. A combination of micturition-cysto-urethrography, urethral- and anal-EMG recordings [4] enables the clinician to localize sphincter pathology in the outlet tract.

Blocking of the neural pathways may help to evaluate the importance of the different sphincter systems. Blocking of alpha-adrenergic receptors will decrease bladder neck and urethral smooth muscle activity which is easily visualized on urethral pressure profiles [5, 6] where the presphincteric 'prostatic area' is diminished, while little change is seen in the maximum urethral pressure. The average decrease in total urethral pressure due to alpha adrenergic blocking has been estimated to 40% [7].

Blocking of the smooth and striated muscles in the pelvic floor by means of spinal anaesthesia demonstrated total loss of pressure tone in the sphincteric area as well as a 40% decrease of 'prostatic area'. If striated muscles are anaesthetized by bilateral pudendal blocks, the voluntary sphincter contraction is eliminated, but it does not result in urinary incontinence [8].

Detrusor instability and infravesical obstruction

It is today an established phenomenon that detrusor instability often occurs with infravesical obstruction (Fig. 4). The incidence of detrusor instability has been demonstrated in 40–80% of patients with BPH [9–11], the large range probably indicating different methods of performing the cystometric investigations [12]. The pathophysiology of this phenomenon is still not quite clear, although Chalfin & Bradley [13] have provided convincing proof as to the aetiology. They based their study on the work of Barrington, who stated that nerve pathways relaying through the spinal cord exist between

250

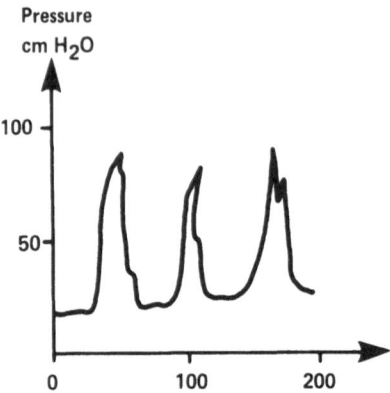

Fig. 4. Cystometrogram from patient with BPH and detrusor instability. Investigation performed with transurethral medium-fill water cystometry.

the proximal urethra and the detrusor muscle. In 11 patients with detrusor instability and BPH they blocked the sensory stimuli from the prostate by injection lidocaine into the prostate. In 10 of the 11 patients the cystometric instability vanished. From this study they conclude that sensory stimuli, but not the enlarged prostate, induce detrusor instability. However, the question still remains whether the resection of sensory afferents of the relief of infra-vesical obstruction is responsible for the decrease in postoperative instability.

The function of the proximal urethra following prostatectomy

Following removal of the prostatic adenoma – whether by suprapubic or transurethral surgery – the anatomy has changed as seen in Fig. 3. The bladder neck and proximal internal sphincter have been removed along with the enlarged prostatic adenoma. The intrinsic and extrinsic sphincter systems on the other hand are untouched.

Previous studies have suggested that continence after prostatectomy also was due to the smooth muscle and elastic tissue in the prostatic capsule. This theory has been turned down by Koyanagi and Tsuji [8], who from their dissection of the posterior urethra could not find any elastic tissue or smooth muscle in the distal end of the prostatic capsule. Many resectionists have experienced numerous lesions of the prostatic capsule in dealing with patients with prostatitis, prostatic calculi or prostatic carcinoma and yet have not experienced postoperative incontinence.

Thus it is evident that postprostatectomy continence is dependent on the distal sphincter system, primarily the intrinsic striated sphincter [8, 14, 15]. With its slow-twitch fibres it maintains the 'passive' continence.

Postprostatectomy incontinence

Incidence

Only very few prospective studies are available indicating exact figures and reasons of postprostatectomy problems (Table 1) [10, 11], however, their size of materials and length of follow-up are unfortunately limited. Retrospective studies [16–19] present impressive numbers of patients, but these studies lack urodynamic investigations at follow-up and they seldom specify the type of incontinence (Table 2).

It is apparent from the studies in table 2 that complaints of incontinence regardless of operative method occurred in approximately 5% at 3–6 months' follow-up, but dropped to levels of 1–4% at 1 year follow-up [16, 17]. On the other hand, in the long-term follow-up studies [18, 19] an incidence of 6–13% of patients with urge incontinence is note-worthy, whereas 3% complained of stress incontinence.

Table 1. Detrusor instability before and after prostatectomy.

References	No. of patients	Preop. instability %	Postop. instability %	Follow-up time
Abrams et al. 1979 [10]	100 92	53 71	36 54	4 months
Meyhoff et al. 1984 [11]	75	80	50	6 months

Table 2. Incidence of postprostatectomy incontinence.

References	No. of patients	Technique*	Follow-up time	Incidence of incontinence
Poulsen et al., 1980 [16]	346	TVP	6 months 12 months	5% stress/urge 3,6% –
Mortensen et al., 1980 [17]	356 242	TURP TVP	3 months 12 months	5% 1% stress
Røder et al., 1981 [18]	143	RPP	30 months (6–72)	3% stress 6% urge
Ball & Smith, 1982 [19]	54	RPP16 TURP 38	60 months (40–71)	13% urge

* TVP = transvesical prostatectomy (Freyer)
  RPP = retropubic prostatectomy (Millin)
  TURP = transurethral prostatectomy

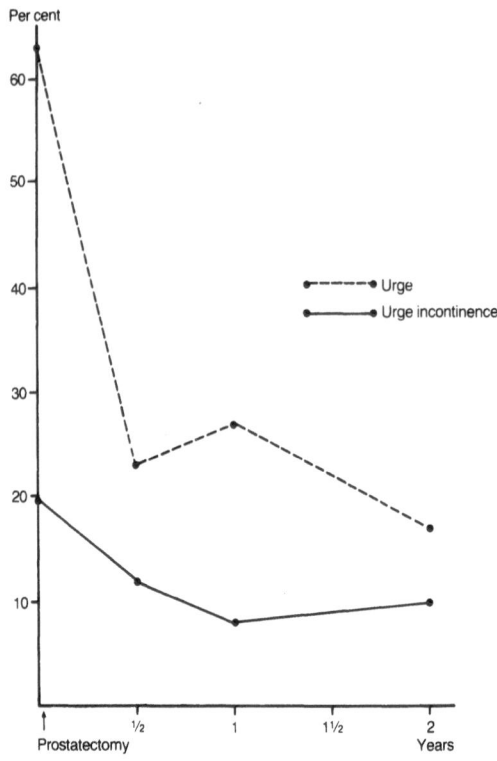

Fig. 5. Incidence of postprostatectomy urge and urge-incontinence in 60 patients. Urge = all patients with the symptom according to the International Continence Society. Urge-incontinence: one or more incontinence episodes within a 14 day-period.

Concurrent diseases such as dementia, diabetes and prostatic malignancy have been demonstrated in many of the incontinent patients.

From Table 2 it is evident that patients with BPH 50–80% also demonstrate detrusor instability on preoperative cystometry. Although these patients are relieved of their infravesical obstruction they still present with a high frequency of detrusor instability, 30–50%. Preoperative symptoms of urge dropped from 49 to 20% postoperatively and urge incontinence from 27 to 10% [10]. In Fig. 5 the incidence of postprostatectomy urge and urge incontinence at different time-intervals is shown [22, 23]. While the incidence of urge incontinence apparently is stable at the 1-year control, a continuous decrease in the number of urge-patients is seen. From these studies it is apparent that postprostatectomy incontinence of the stress type occurs in approximately 1–3% after one year, while urge incontinence is much more common, 6–13%, after two years.

Symptoms. Incontinence is a frequent symptom in the early period following prostatic surgery. Immediate stress incontinence is within a few days

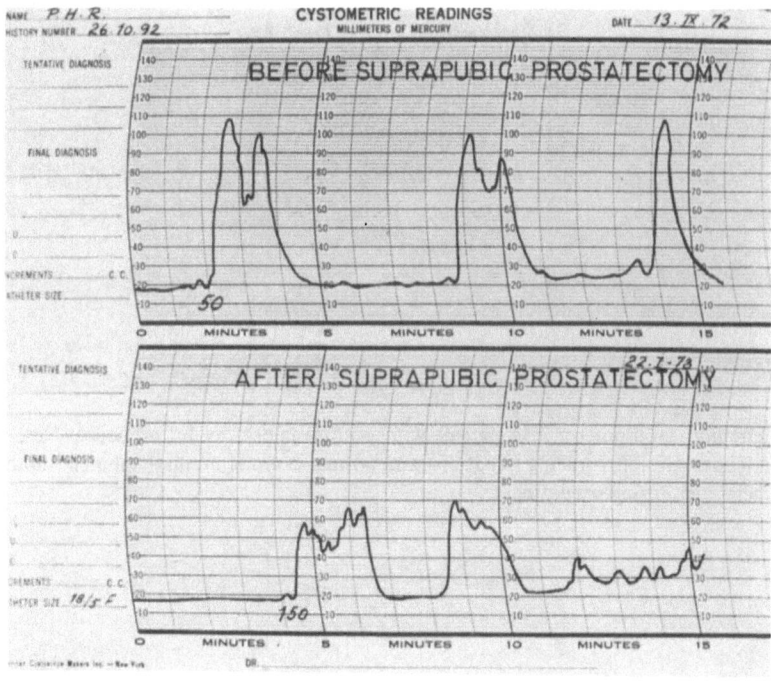

Fig. 6. Medium-fill water cystometry in 80-year old male before and after prostatic surgery. Note uninhibited detrusor contractions 20 cm H_2O at pre- as well as postoperative investigations.

succeeded by urgency and to some extent by urge incontinence. While stress and urge incontinence diminish to values below 10% within the first year the most frequent symptom, urgency, occurs at 20–25%. This is in accordance with a remarkable large number of unstable bladders found at cystometry [10, 11, 23].

In a study of patients with postprostatectomy problems [20] incontinence occurred in 55% of the 60 patients, especially urge incontinence. Among the other symptoms there was one group with slow stream, hesitancy and straining, and another group consisting of frequency, nocturia and urgency.

It is often possible from the complaints by the patient to predict the cause of incontinence. The stress-incontinent patient may be able to sleep without wetting his bed, but must always wear diapers or even a penile clamp during day-time. He is able to perform reasonable small micturitions with changing flow rates. Overflow-incontinence is characterized by continuous wetting, no inhibitory control and often a feeling of retention. Patients complaining of incontinence, dysuria and/or suprapubic pain may have bacteriuria.

Regardless of the type of incontinence these patients are often in despair, because their daily, their social and their marital life is miserable.

254

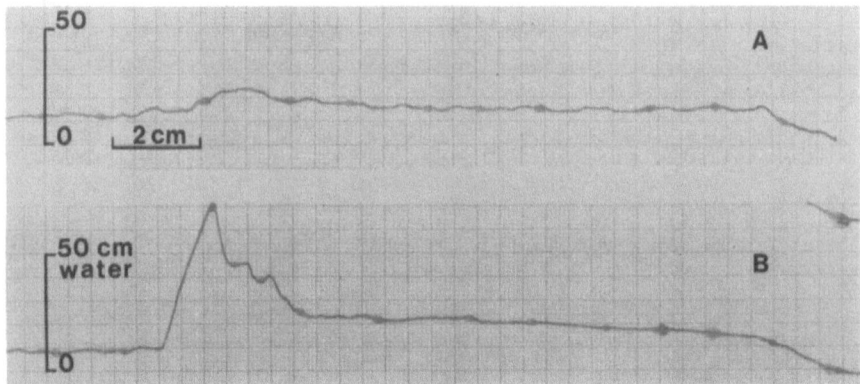

Fig. 7. Urethral profilometry in a patient with postprostatectomy incontinence. Note lack of sphincteric area on upper tracing (A) at rest and normal external urethral sphincter function on lower tracing (B) during squeezing.

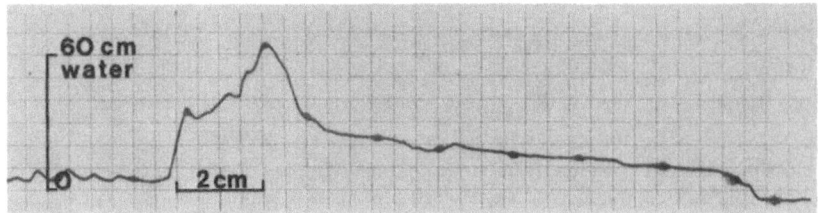

Fig. 8. Urethral profilometry following transurethral prostatectomy. Residual prostate adenoma is clearly seen.

Urodynamic findings. Urodynamic investigations are indispensable to delineate the cause of incontinence. Uroflowmetry demonstrating a reduced flow-rate may indicate obstructed micturition due to urethral stricture or insufficient prostatectomy, but also impaired detrusor function without infravesical obstruction [20, 21]. Cystometry may reveal detrusor instability (Fig. 6), or a decompensated bladder. At the same time the residual volume may be measured. A urethral pressure profile may provide information regarding a lesion of the intrinsic urethral prostatectomy (Fig. 8) or the presence of postoperative urethral stricture. A simultaneous pressure flow study will reveal the quality of detrusor function or any residual infravesical obstruction. Andersen and Nordling [21] were able to demonstrate urodynamic pathology in all of their 34 postprostatectomy-incontinent patients.

Abrams [20] could relate symptoms to urodynamic findings, for instance all of his stress incontinent patients had impaired sphincter pressure on urethral profilometry, at cystometry almost all of his patients with urge demonstrated instability, and at micturition slow stream was associated with obstructed flow and/or underactive detrusor.

Aetiology

A number of aetiological factors are listed at random in Table 3.

Insufficient resection of the prostatic lobes may inevitably lead to urinary retention and incontinence. Mundy [24] found residual prostatic tissue in 37 of 47 postprostatectomy incontinent men and was able to reduce incontinence by a second TURP in 40% of patients.

Lesions of distal intrinsic sphincter system does occur in transurethral as well as supra- or retropubic prostatectomy. Fortunately the incidence is low, regardless of the operative procedure, local fibrosis and pelvic floor excercises contribute to the recommendation of a very conservative attitude towards these patients for 0.5–1 year before final treatment is chosen.

Urethral strictures occur in up to 20–25% of patients following prostatectomy [22] and not infrequently this gives rise to incontinence [20]. Since strictures develop within the first 4–6 months after surgery it is advisable to follow the patients until that time and then relieve them of their stricture.

Detrusor instability has been shown to be present in a considerable number of patients (Table 1) before and after surgery. This explains the relatively large number of patients with urge incontinence that continue with their symptoms for years (Table 2).

Decompensated bladders with high residuals and poor/no detrusor function during voiding constitute a minor group of incontinent patients. Probably a majority of this type of patients were admitted preoperatively with chronic distended bladders and large residual volumes.

Mental disorders including dementia, cerebro-vascular diseases etc. are common in the elderly prostatic population. Now and then the anaesthesia or hospital-stay may prolong the convalescence. The symptoms of incontinence vary, and it is necessary to evaluate this type of patients with urodynamics because of invalid information.

Malignancy of the prostate. Malignant infiltration of the sphincter system

Table 3. Etiology of permanent postprostatectomy incontinence.

Insufficient resection
Lesion of distal intrinsic sphincter system
Urethral stricture
Detrusor instability
Decompensated bladder
Mental disorders
Prostatic malignancy
Pharmacological influence
Infection

is often responsible for incontinence or stricture-formation, but otherwise patients with localized prostatic cancer favour equally with BPH [22].

Infection following prostatectomy occurs in approximately 20% of trans-urethrally operated patients [22, 25]. It is well known that urinary infection may induce symptoms such as frequency, urgency and urge-incontinence, just as cystometry may demonstrate low compliance with reduced function-al capacity. Obviously infection may mimic incontinence symptoms, and it is therefore essential to eradicate any infection before further investigations are initiated.

Pharmacological manipulation. The increased use of tranquillizers, anti-convulsants, antidepressants, antihistaminics, drugs acting on the auto-nomic nervous system, and diuretics may either result in incontinence (usually of the overflow type) or mask established incontinence.

Conclusion

Prostatic surgery belongs to one of the most frequent operations performed in the elderly male, approximately every tenth male will be a candidate for prostatic resection. Although preoperative investigations have improved, surgical techniques have been refined and postoperative control of compli-cations been intensified, there is still a number of patients suffering from postprostatectomy incontinence. This fact calls for continuous efforts in avoiding this problem and in finding suitable solutions for the treatment of postprostatectomy incontinence.

References

1. Gosling J. The structure of the bladder and urethra in relation to function. Urol. Clin. North Am. 6 (1979): 31–38.
2. Abrams P.H. Perfusion urethral profilometry. Urol. Clin. North Am. 6 (1979): 103–110.
3. Nordling J., Meyhoff H.H. Dissociation of urethral and anal sphincter activity in neurogenic bladder dysfunction. J. Urol. 122 (1979): 352–356.
4. McGuire E. Electromyographic evaluation of sphincter function and dysfunction. Urol. Clin. North Am. 6 (1979): 121–124.
5. Abrams P.H., Shah P.J.R., Stone R. and Choa R.G. Bladder outflow obstruction treated with phenoxybenzamine. Br. J. Urol. 54 (1982): 527–530.
6. Tanagho E.A. Membrane and microtransducer catheters: Their effectiveness for profilome-try of the lower urinary tract. Urol. Clin. North Am. 6 (1979): 110–119.
7. Furuya S., Kumamoto Y., Yokoyama E. et al. Alpha-adrenergic activity and urethral pres-sure in prostatic zones in benign prostatic hypertrophy. J. Urol. 128 (1982): 836–839.
8. Koyanagi T. and Tsuji I. The mechanism of urinary continence after prostatectomy. Urol. int. 32 (1977): 353–367.
9. Andersen J.T. Detrusor hyperreflexia in benign infravesical obstruction. A cystometric stu-dy. J. Urol. 115 (1976): 532–534.

10. Abrams P.H., Farrar D.J., Turner-Warwick R.T., Whiteside C.G. and Feneley R.C.L. The results of prostatectomy: a symptomatic and urodynamic analysis of 152 patients. J. Urol. 121 (1979): 640–642.

11. Meyhoff H.H., Nordling J. and Hald T. Urodynamic evaluation of transurethral versus transvesical prostatectomy. Scand. J. Urol. Nephrol. 18 (1984): 27–35.

12. Colstrup H., Andersen J.T. and Walter S. Detrusor reflex instability in the male. Infravesical obstruction: Fact or artefact? Neurol. Urodyn. 1 (1982): 183–185.

13. Chalfin S.A. and Bradley W.E. The etiology of detrusor hyperreflexia in patients with infravesical obstruction. J. Urol. 127 (1982): 938–942.

14. Hauri D. Post-prostatectomy incontinence. Urol. Res. 6 (1978): 113–118.

15. Turner-Warwick R. A urodynamic review of bladder outlet obstruction in the male and its clinical implications. Urol. Clin. North Am. 6 (1979): 171–192.

16. Poulsen S.R., Alsbæk H. and Feldt-Rasmussen B.F. Prostatic hypertrophy. Defence of the transvesical operation. Ugeskr. Læg. 142 (1980): 2257–2261.

17. Mortensen T. and Ellekilde G. Transurethral resection of the prostate and transvesical prostatectomy in the treatment of prostatic hypertrophy. Ugeskr. Læg. 142 (1980): 2261–2264.

18. Røder O.C. and Outzen K.E. Retropubic prostatectomy by Millin's method. A follow-up investigation in 177 patients. Ugeskr. Læg. 143 (1981): 2498–2500.

19. Ball A.J. and Smith P.J.B. The long-term effects of prostatectomy: a uroflowmetric analysis. J. Urol. 128 (1982): 538–540.

20. Abrams P.H. Investigation of postprostatectomy problems. Urology 15 (1980): 209–212.

21. Andersen J.T. and Nordling J. Urinary incontinence after transvesical prostatectomy. Urol. int. 33 (1978): 191–198.

22. Meyhoff H.H., Nordling J. and Hald T. Clinical evaluation of transurethral versus transvesical prostatectomy. Scand. J. Urol. Nephrol. In press.

23. Meyhoff H.H. Unpublished data.

24. Mundy A.R. The best form of treatment for postprostatectomy incontinence is a prostatectomy. Proceedings International Continence Society. Leiden, p. 39.

25. Chilton C.P., Morgan R.J., England H.R., Paris A.M.L. and Blandy J.P. A critical evaluation of the results of transurethral resection of the prostate. Br. J. Urol. 50 (1978): 542–546.

VI.4. Incontinence-operation for postprostatectomy incontinence

D. HAURI

For *theoretical* purposes we demanded two prerequisites for our incontinence operation.
1. A stabilization should result of the posterior urethra and the bladder.
2. An elastic, peripheral resistance has to be installed.

The rigid support

These prerequirities are derived from the following perceptions: In the model experiment we assume that the bladder, the urethra and the pelvic floor form a unity. Therefore the bladder, which is under intra-abdominal pressure changes is comparable to a plain-load on a rigid support, namely the pelvic floor. In the model experiment the bladder, which is filled with liquid, is situated as an elastic, hollow body on a support with constant volume, that is also filled with liquid and that has for the time being rigid walls. The urethra passes through this support as a flaccid tube with mean tonus and has free connection between the bladder and the outside world (Fig. 1). As we know from the technology, pressure produced by plain-loads distributes in a characteristic way in which one can measure vertical and horizontal pressure-gradients. If this bladder-body is charged from outside, the interior pressure of the support will increase in like manner. The pressure caused distributes in the support equally in all directions and produces a closing strength orientated towards the urethra. This is recognized by the identical pressure-development measured simultaneously in the bladder and in the urethra. The model, when charged, is continent.

The prerequisite for this condition lies in the rigidity of the support. If the rigid base of the support is replaced by an elastic one (Fig. 2), a totally different pressure transmission results. Pressure now causes a considerable pressure loss in the support. The horizontal pressure gradient which is directed against the urethra is decreased, which is obvious from the comparison of the lowered urethral pressure to the bladder pressure (Fig. 2). Consequently a positive pressure gradient arises between the bladder and the outside world and the model becomes incontinent.

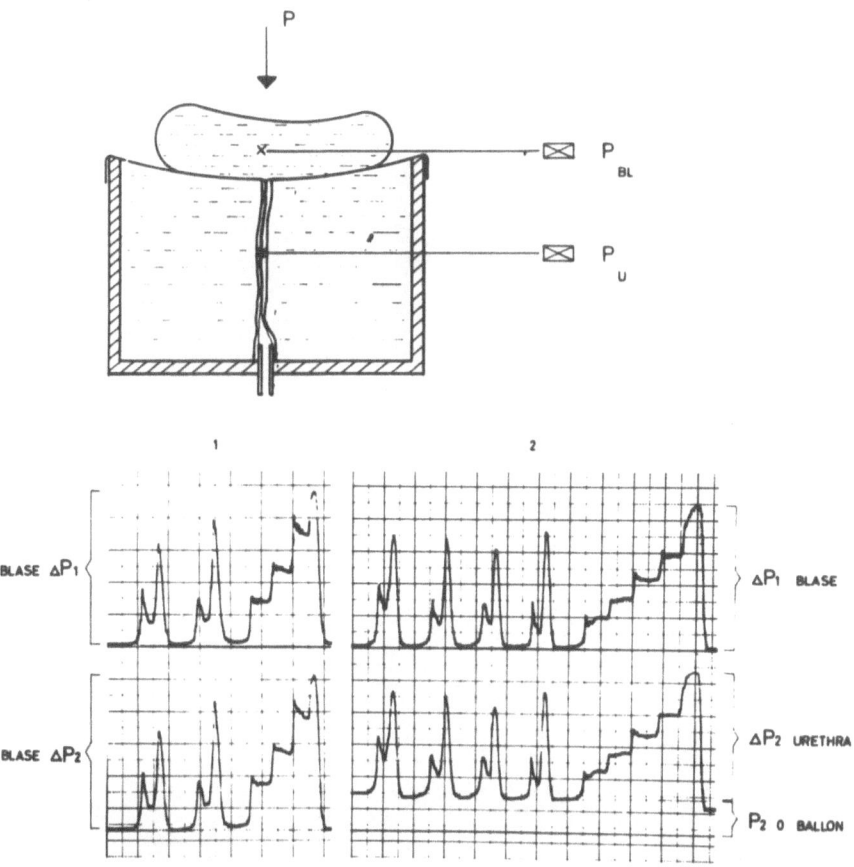

Fig. 1. Bladder-model, where the walls of the support are rigid, according to Graber [1]. See details in the text.

260

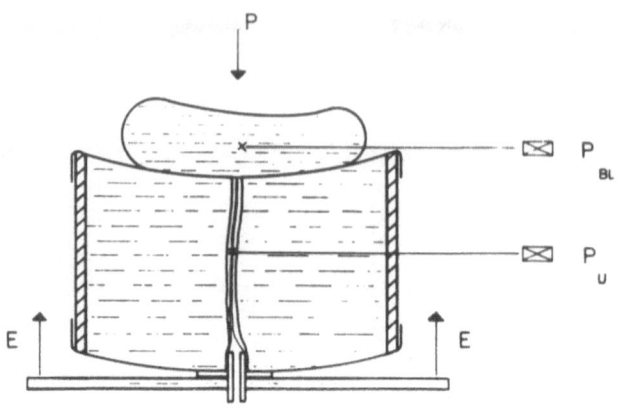

E = ELASTISCHE ZUGE ZUR UNTERSTÜTZUNG DER BODENFLACHE

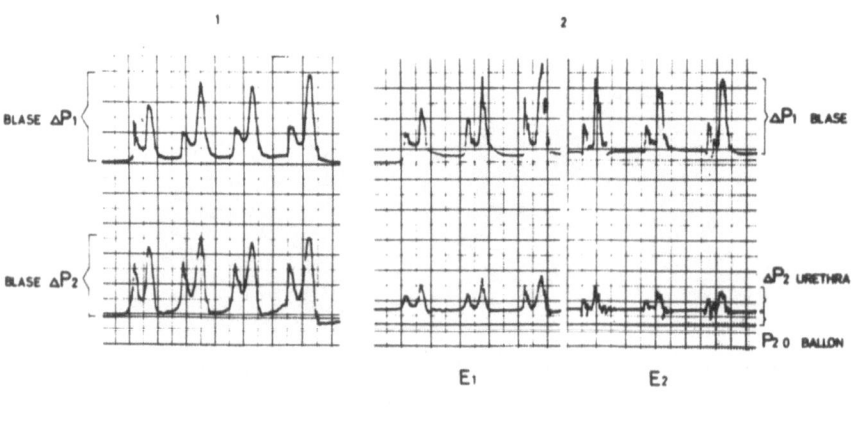

Fig. 2. Bladder-model with elastic floor in the support, according to Graber [1]. See details in the text.

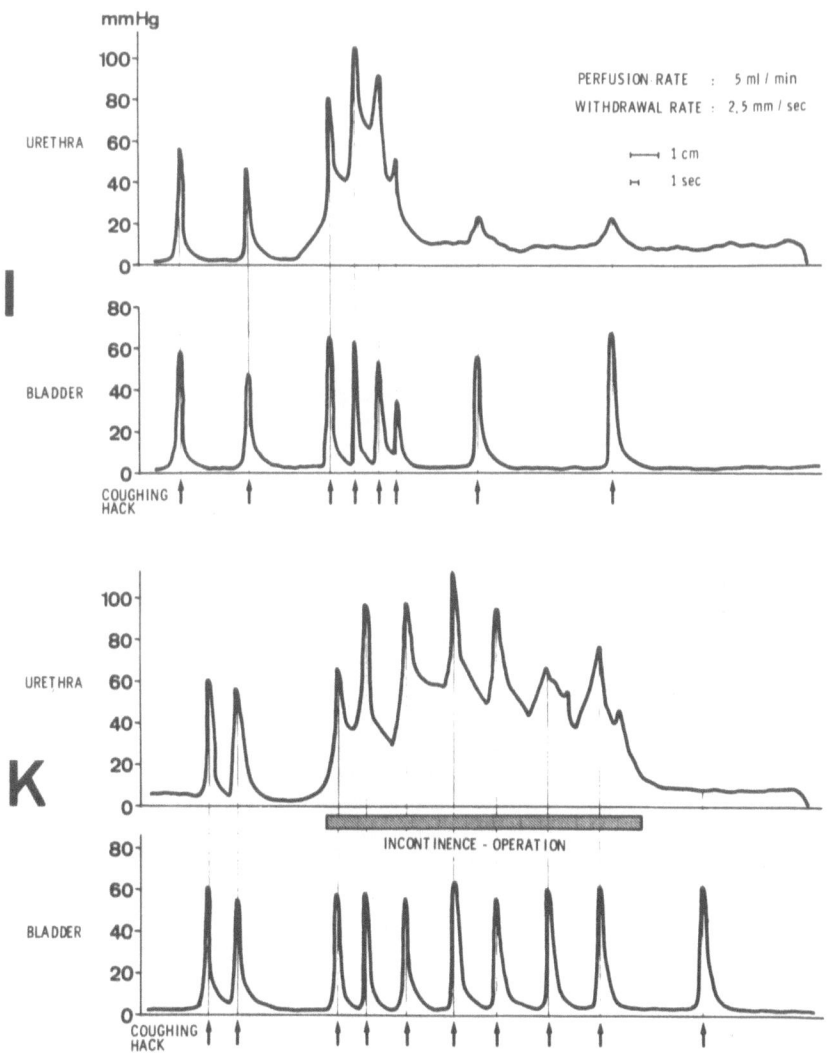

Fig. 3. Urethra-stress-profile: The whole posterior urethra reacts upon coughing-hacks, what means that the urethra is integrated in the pelvic floor.

I = preoparetively incontinence

K = postoperatively continence

This model shows the situation after occured prostatectomy. Here too, the free movable, little fixed bladder and the posterior urethra which is no longer supported by the prostate are directly exposed to the influences of intra-abdominal pressure and to the gravitation. At first we tried to achieve this stabilization of the pelvic floor by advancing in the perineal way. In this way a necrosis of the posterior urethra occurred several times because the corresponding vessels, which are end arteries, were damaged [2]. Since we

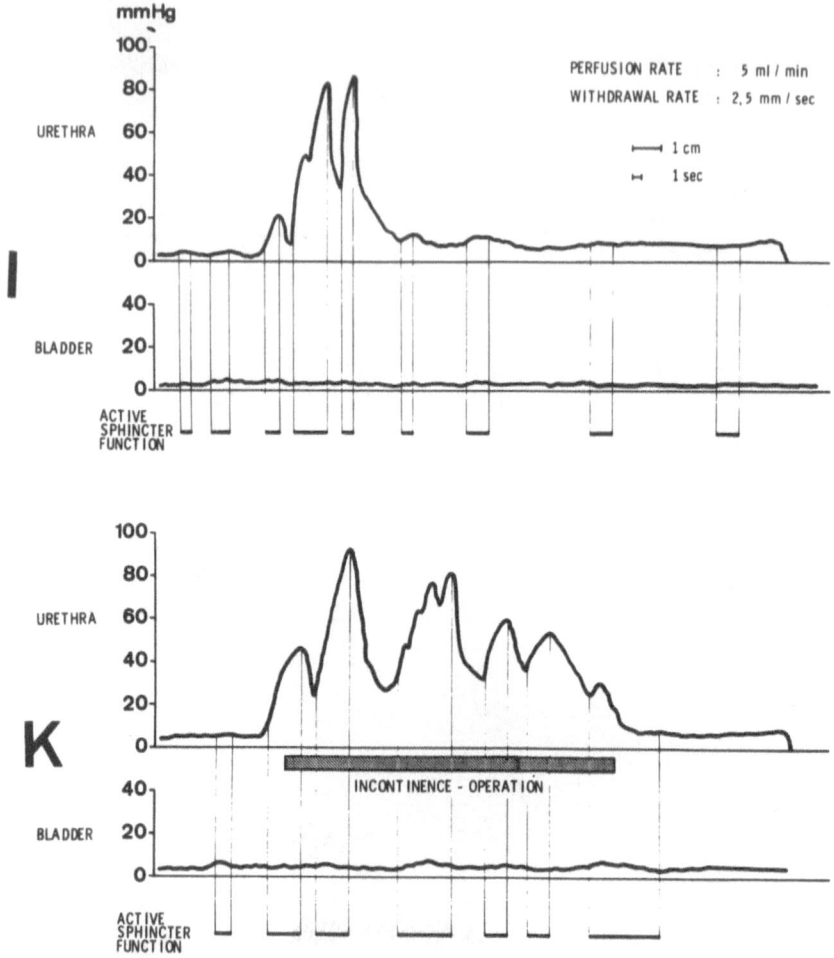

Fig. 4. Urethra-working-profile: The whole integrated urethra reacts upon the voluntary active sphincter-function.
I = preoperatively incontinence
K = postoperatively continence

have performed this surgical step by retropubic access (Fig. 6–8) our results have improved [3]. We can prove by the urethra profile that after our incontinence-operation the urethra is integrated again in a stable support. In the urethra-stress-profile one can perceive that the whole displaced posterior urethra reacts to coughing (Fig. 3). On the other hand, in the working-profile the posterior urethra also co-operates when requested in the sphincteric activity (Fig. 4).

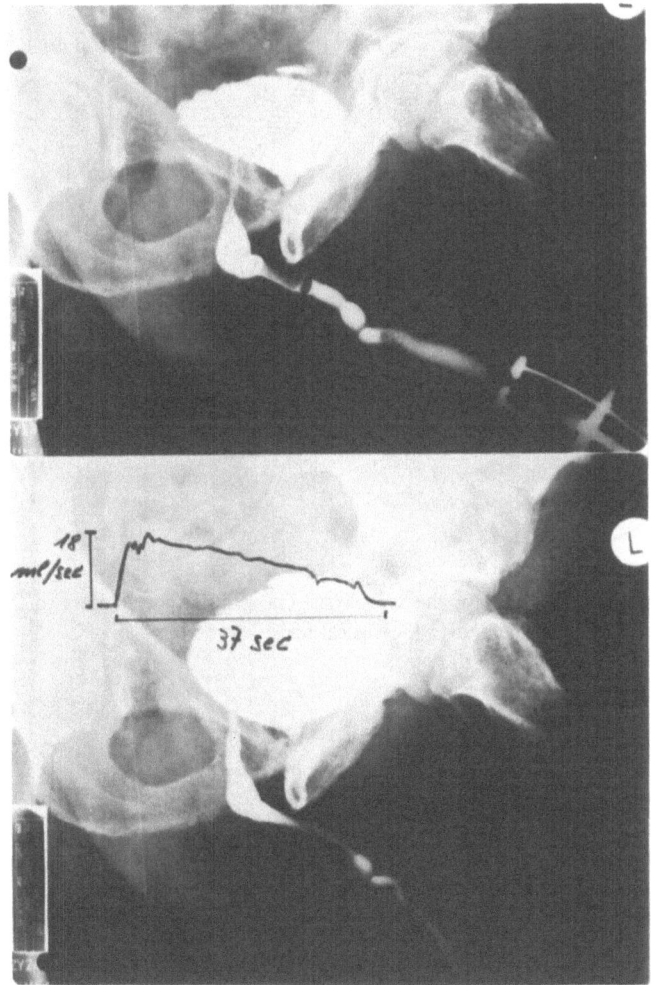

Fig. 5. Urethrographies after a successful incontinence-operation. Above: Retrograde urethrography: The not stenosed urethra, which is displaced between the corpora cavernosa is to perceive.
Below: Urethrography during micturition combined with uroflowmetry: The micturition is possible without disturbances and with approximatively normal flow-values.

The peripheral elastic resistance

With a peripheral elastic resistance we follow the functional imitation of the normal, continence-conserving sphincter system with smooth muscles. The advantage of this is that this doesn't cause an obstruction of the urethra – which is not a remedy for incontinence anyway – but that it is a system which opens during micturition and decreases the peripheral resistance.

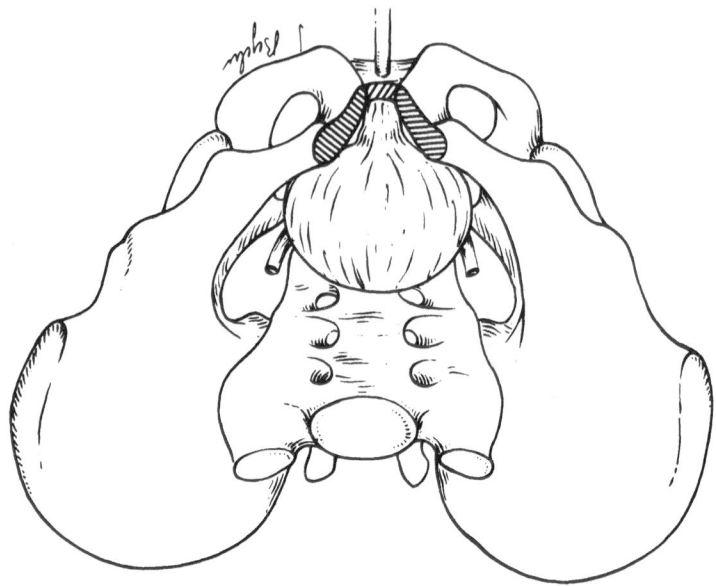

Fig. 6. After chiseling out a part of the symphysis, one gains a good access to the posterior urethra, to the prostatic capsule and to the vesical neck.

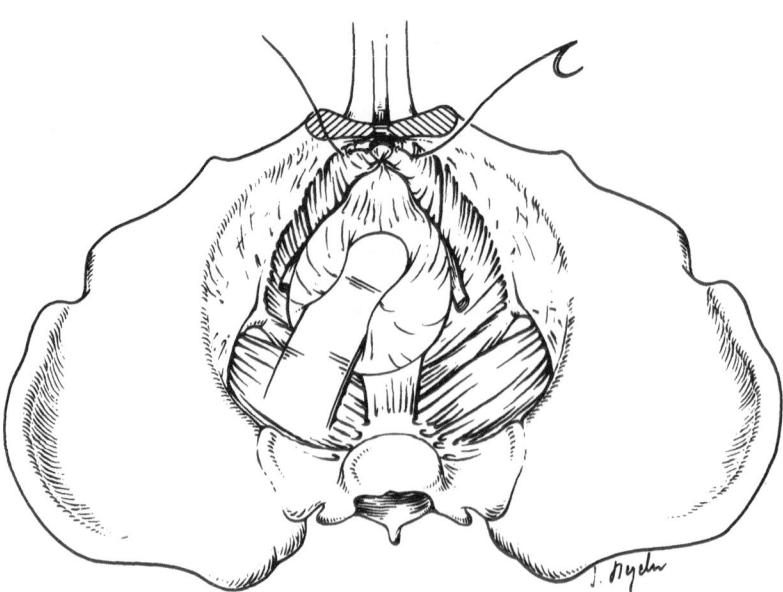

Fig. 7. The muscles of the pelvic floor are unified ventrally to the posterior urethra by means of no resorbable sutures.

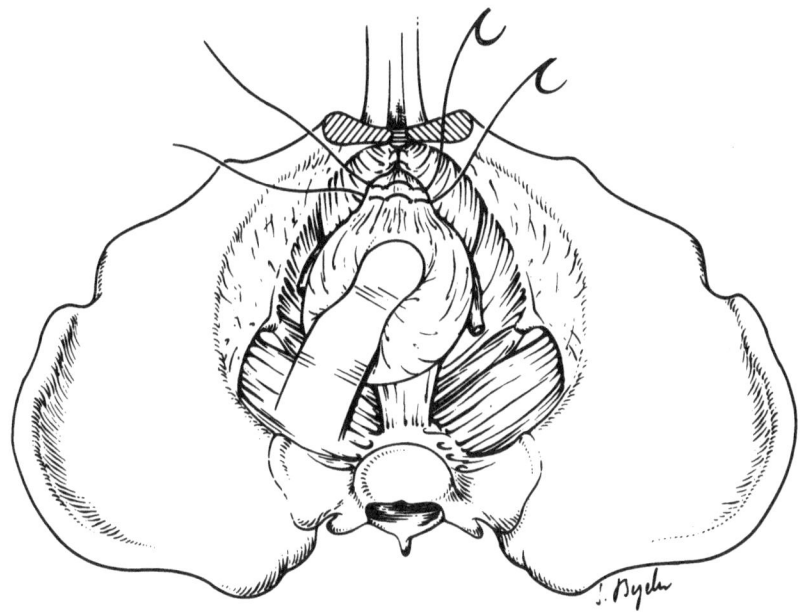

Fig. 8. Simultaneously the prostatic capsule gets reduced.

For this purpose the urethra is embedded between the corpora cavernosa (Fig. 11–13). As shown by the model experiments, it is clear that with diminution of the cross-section of the urethra by 50 % the resistance increases at most by the factor 2 [4]. Consequently it is necessary to embed the urethra at as long a distance as possible into the corpora cavernosa. In our experience, this distance should amount to at least 6 centimeters. The proof that it is really a matter of an elastic resistance can be demonstrated by postoperative urethrographies combined with a uroflowmetry (Fig. 5).

Method

1. The patient is put in supine position. Next the bladder and the symphysis are emptied by an inferior, mediane laparotomy. After having carefully separated the Mm. recti from the symphysis, a part of the symphysis is removed by a gouge. In doing so we are careful not to be tangent to the Foramina obduratoria to avoid static problems postoperatively. We now have an optimal view of the vesical neck, the prostatic capsule and the posterior urethra (Fig. 6). After having prepared the prostatic capsule and the posterior urethra, the muscles of the pelvic floor, which are situated laterally to the urethra, and their fascia are unified ventrally to the urethra with no resorbable sutures (Fig. 7). Simultaneously the prostatic capsule is reduced by the same sutures (Fig. 8). At this point one must be careful not

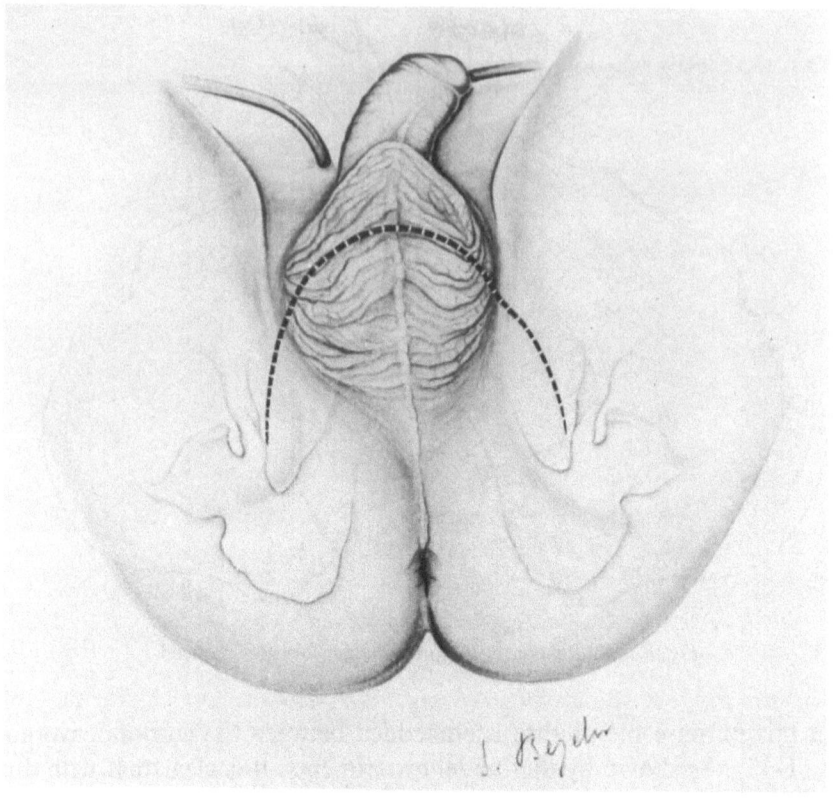

Fig. 9. Perineoscrotal access.

to be tangent to the vesical neck to avoid neurogenic disturbances during micturition. With this step of the operation we attain the stabilization of the pelvic floor. After installing a cystostomy and the drainage of the Cavum Retzii by means of two thick Redon-Drains, the excised part of the symphysis is re-inserted and fixed with resorbable sutures. This part of the symphysis will grow in again within about 3 months and guarantee the stability of the pelvis.

2. The patient is now placed in lithotomy position and the urethra freed through a perineoscrotal incision (Fig. 9, 10). After having cut the M. bulbocavernosus lengthwise, the urethra, which is splinted with a catheter Charr. 12, is separated carefully from the corpora cavernosa at a distance of 6–10 centimeters (Fig. 11). Now the corpora cavernosa are separated from their bifurcation along their septum nearly up to the dorsal-side of the penis (Fig. 12). Subsequently the urethra is displaced between the corpora cavernosa whilst these are unified again over the urethra by no resorbable sutures (Fig. 13). After a slight mediorotation of both Crura of the cavernous bodies with the ischiacavernous muscles situated upon them they are unified addi-

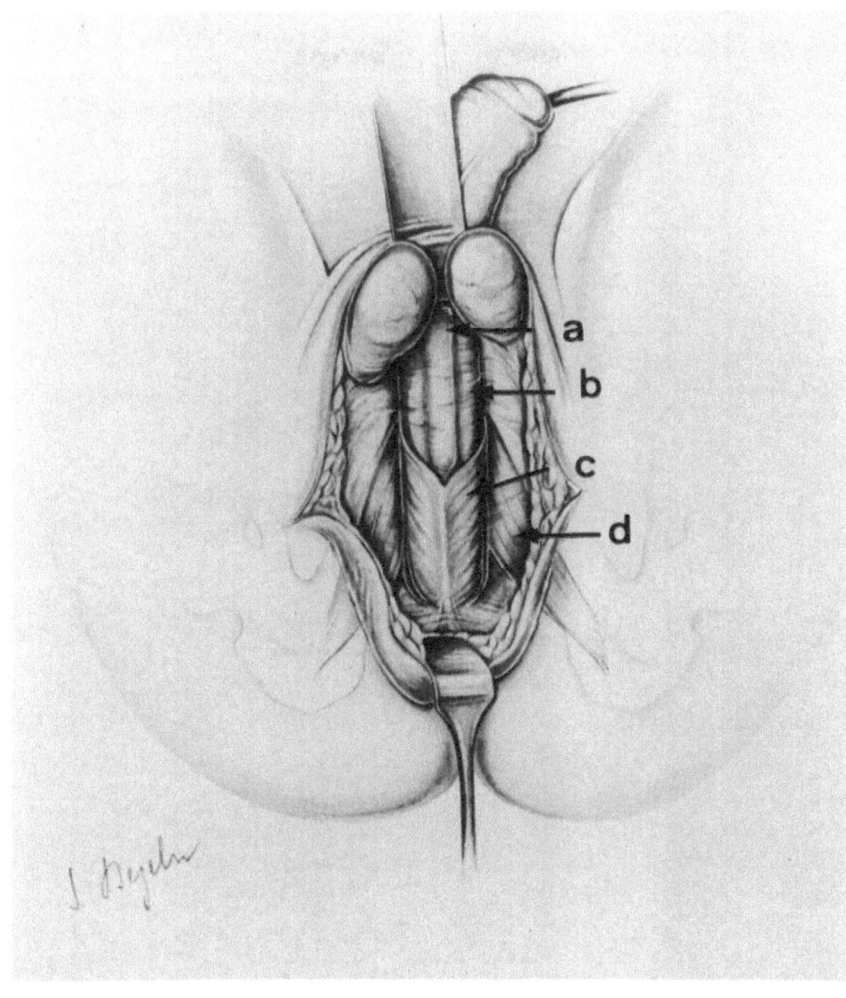

Fig. 10. The prepared posterior and middle urethra: a) urethra, b) left corpus cavernosum, c) M. bulbocavernosus, d) left M. ischiocavernosus.

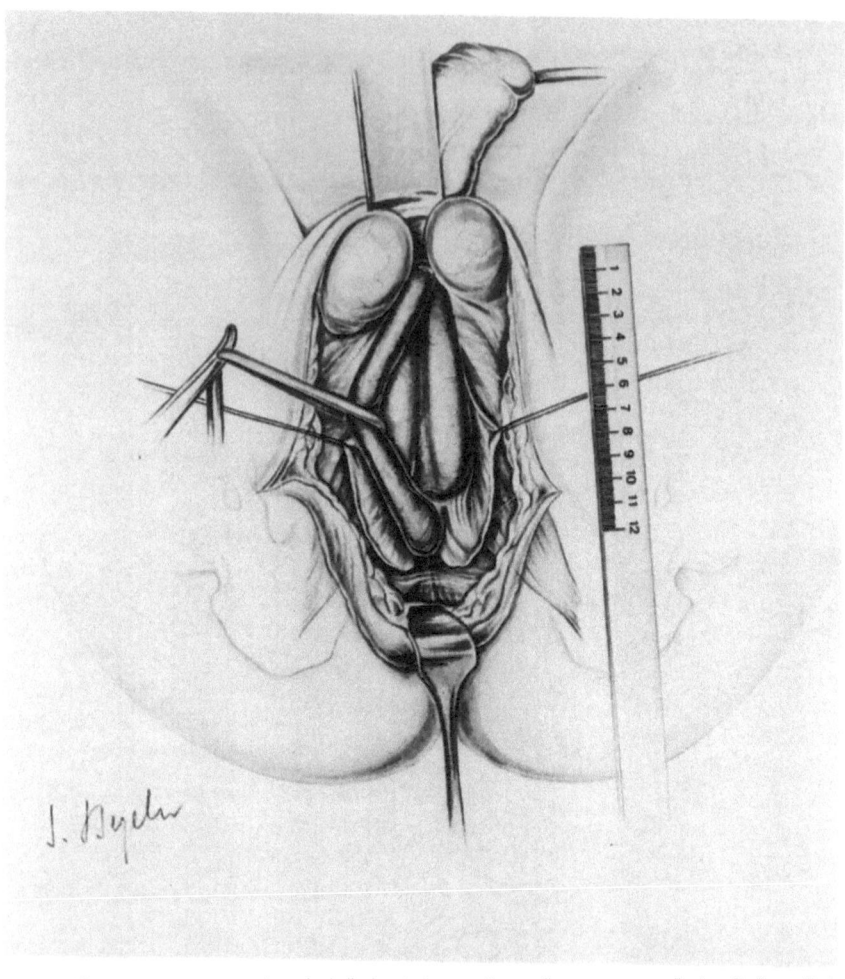

Fig. 11. The M. bulbocavernosus is cleaved lengthwise and it is kept open by attachement-sutures. Now the urethra gets separated of the corpora cavernosa.

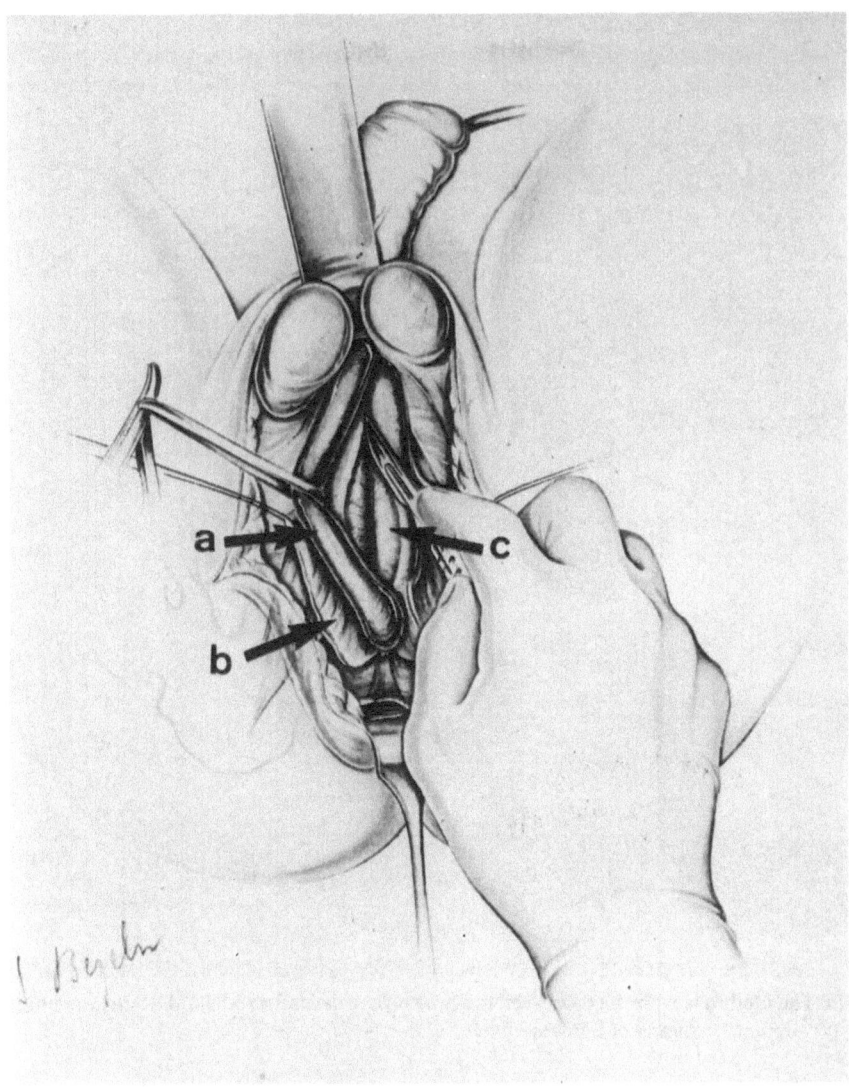

Fig. 12. The corpora cavernosa are separated along their septum on a distance of at least 6 centimeters. a) urethra, which is pulled aside slightly, b) lengthwise cleaved M. bulbocavernosus, c) left corpus cavernosum.

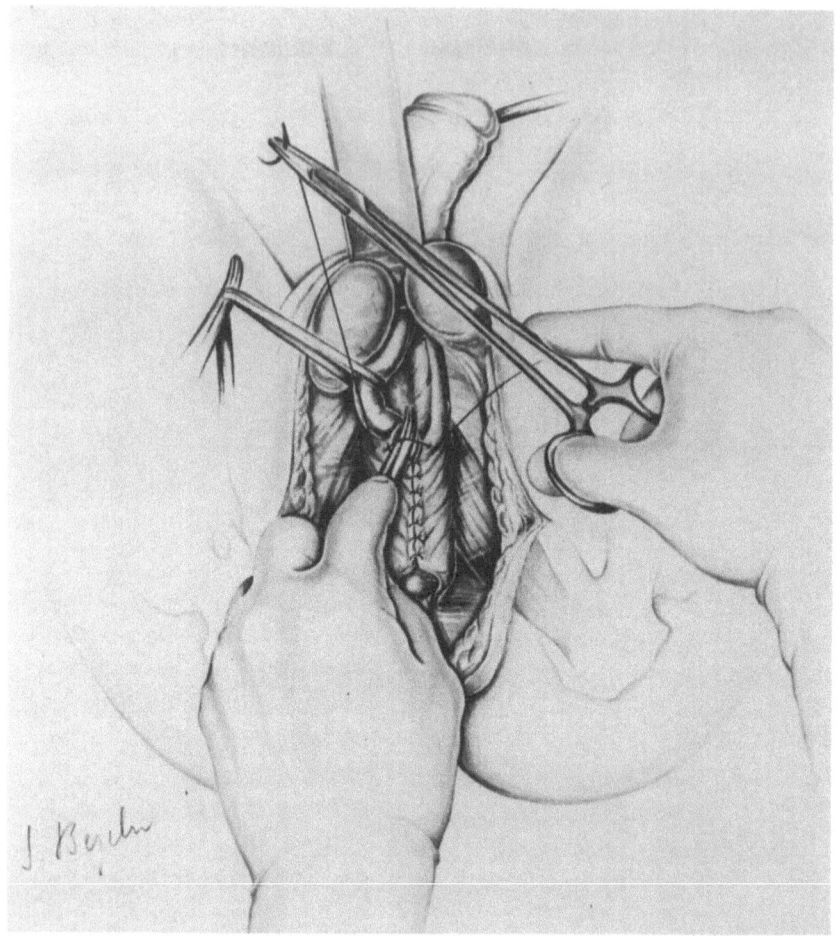

Fig. 13. The urethra is embedded between the two corpora cavernosa whilst the latter are unified over the urethra by means of non-resorbable sutures.

tionally in the medianline (Fig. 14). We thereby achieve the peripheral, elastic resistance. The wound is closed by laying in two thin Redon-Drains. Postoperatively the patient is immobilized for 10 days because the part resection of the symphysis, could occasionally cause pain during walking. However, after 10 days mobilization is possible without pain or disturbance of the healing process. After 10 days we also begin the micturition experiments. For this purpose the cystostomy, which was kept open immediately after the operation, is closed and the patient is ordered to void on feeling a full bladder. For the first time this is often difficult because of the postoperative oedema on the one hand, and on the other hand because the patient has to get used again to normal micturition. We leave the cystosto-

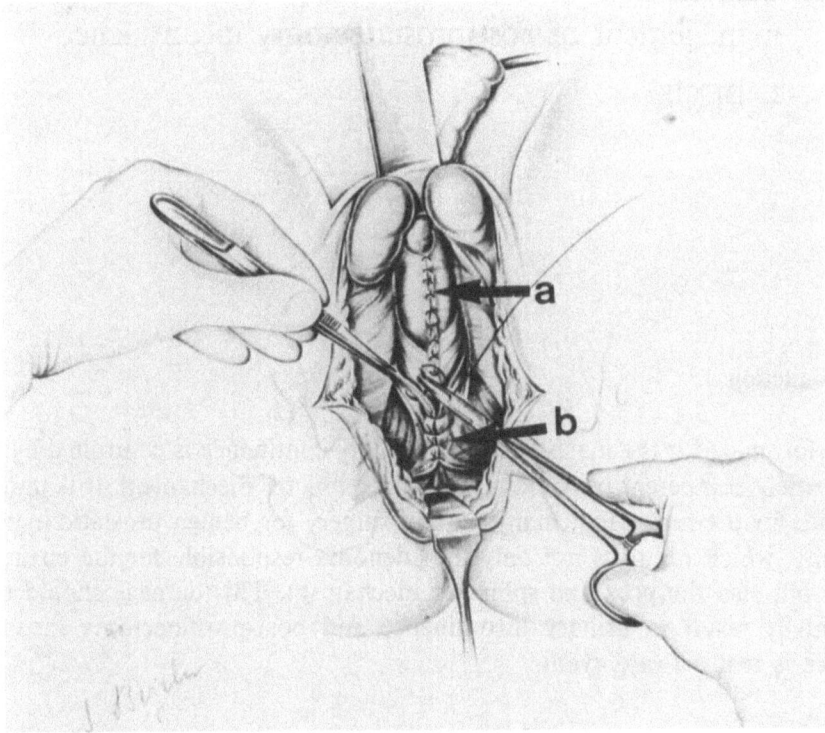

Fig. 14. The Mm. ischiocavernosi are unified in the medianline: a) suture of the unified corpora cavernosa, b) suture of the adapted Mm. ischiocavernosi.

my as a safety valve. Usually normal micturition occurs within the following 2–3 days and the cystostomy is removed.

Results

Over a period of 2–7 years we operated on 19 patients with the described method. Of these, 16 patients were completely continent post-operatively, which shows a healing quota of just over 80%. It is particularly important to note that we showed no complications post-operatively, and that continence once achieved appeared to be lasting.

Since we installed the stabilization of the pelvic floor transpubically we improved our success rate and lowered the complication rate. We had previously encountered occasional problems with partial or complete necrosis of the displaced urethra. Today, however, we have encountered only one fistula of the urethra which required an operative revision, and two slight strictures of the urethra which were cured by an internal urethrotomy. The current complication rate is 15%.

VI.5. Critical analysis of the surgical procedures in the management of post-prostatectomy incontinence

L. DENIS

Introduction

It is fortunate for the males that their urinary continence is controlled by an extremely competent proximal and distal sphincter mechanism. It is unfortunate for the males that many require surgery for benign prostatic hypertrophy, which removes not only the adenoma responsible for the obstruction but also the proximal sphincter mechanism. This damage should not normally result in urinary incontinence and post-prostatectomy incontinence is really a rare event.

Definition

Urodynamic studies in postprostatectomy incontinence demonstrate a considerable fall in the closure pressure of the apex of the prostate and a reduction in the length of the functional segment of the membranous urethra [1]. Most frequently seen is a situation where detrusor hyperreflexia and pelvic floor irritability cause urinary incontinence associated with urgency. Bladder instability can be caused by the previous obstruction, infection, insufficient surgical procedures and postoperative strictures. This condition should be treated by appropriate medical treatment and patience for both patient and surgeon [2]. Prevention of course is still the better treatment and a detailed history, a complete diagnostic work-up, a meticulous surgical technique and antimicrobial prophylaxis may prevent these curable but annoying episodes of urinary incontinence after surgery.

The true postprostatectomy incontinence, which is of the stress or dribbling type, depends then on the absence of all anomalies couplied to a serious loss of closure pressure in the standing position. This diagnostic work-up is performed from two to four weeks after surgery and conservative treatment instituted. Failure to respond to these conservative measures for at least six months to one year is mandatory before consideration is given to surgical correction.

Patient and treatment selection

The initial investigation immediately after the removal of the catheter a few days after surgery will exclude urinary tract infection by urine culture and residual outflow obstruction by a mictiogram. The ever present possibility of prostatitis requires of course appropriate treatment. Reassurance of the patient and a solution for his incontinence by incontinence devices or penile clamps control the immediate problem. Continuous moral support and motivation of the patient will ultimately help to decide on the choice of treatment.

This treatment will include:
1. More patience and training.
2. Drugs to relax the detrusor and/or strengthen the sphincter.
3. Permanent incontinence devices or clamps.
4. Electrical stimulation.
5. Surgical procedures.

Selection of surgical procedures

The multitude of surgical procedures devised to improve postprostatectomy incontinence is proof of the failure to achieve satisfactory results; all procedures rely on the principle that the urethral resistance to detrusor pressure should be increased. A list of the procedures is presented in Table 1. A few techniques have withstood the passage of time and Tanagho is the most outstanding proponent of his technique of anterior flap bladder neck reconstruction [3]. Out of 44 anterior repairs for postprostatectomy incontinence 17 had excellent and 16 good results or 75% of overall good results. The results after previous transurethral resection were better than after open surgery. Transient and functional obstruction are common complications. More information is available in the procedures utilizing passive compression of the urethra. The procedure advocated by Hauri utilizes the presence of the corpora cavernosa to bury the urethra in these structures and fix the posterior urethra to the musculature in the pelvis [4].

He reports a success rate of 70% in 31 cases with a 20% complication rate. The second phase brought the percentage up to 80%. The intercavernous embedding of the entire length of the bulboperineal urethra brought 75% of excellent results with a 30% complication rate in 30 patients in the hands of Lenzi et al. [5].

Politano popularized the teflon paste peri-urethral injections and has reported good results in 73% of 75 cases [6]. Most patients require more than one injection and it is advised to wait from 4 to 6 months before repeating the injection. Migration of the paste has been reported but no

Table 1. Overview of surgical procedures for cure of male incontinence.

1. *Vesico-urethral suspension:*
Kelley	1929
Marshall	1949
Küss	1955

2. *Allongation of the posterior urethra:*
Young-Dees	1919
Barnes	1949
Thompson	1964
Leadbetter	1964

3. *Plication / torsion urethra:*
Young	1907
Lowsley	1935
Beneventi	1966
Petersen	1967

4. *Passive compression urethra:*
Quackels	1955	paraffin
Berny	1961	acrylic, silastic
Girgis	1965	collagen
Schmaelze	1968	autologous bone
Millin	1968	fascia lata
Kaufmann	1973	ischio-cavernosus
	1973	polyprophylene
	1976	silicone gel
Politano	1973	teflon paste
Hauri	1977	corpora cavernosa
Jonas	1984	artifical clamp

5. *Reconstructive urinary sphincters:*
Goebel-Stockel	1917
Deming	1926
Flochs	1953
Tanagho	1962
Mathisen	1970

6. *Artificial urinary sphincters:*
Foley sphincter	1947
Scott inflatable sphincter	1973
Rosen sphincter	1976

serious complications have been encountered. The first artificial sphincter implantation was performed by Scott in 1972 [7]. The device was commercially produced by the American Medical Systems as AS 721. Subsequent experience introduced technological improvements which brought the latest AMS sphincter 800™.

Pressure regulation, deactivation and newer cuff design are expected to reduce the 20% complications described in earlier series with other models. The best results can be anticipated with cuff placement about the vesical neck if the prostate is intact. It is advisable to evaluate carefully the indications after prostatectomy and cuff placement around the urethra may be indicated in some patients [8]. The results were listed as good in 91 % of 229 patients followed for three months decreasing to 81 % of 90 patients followed for 18 months [9].

Discussion and conclusions

It is obvious from the long list of possible surgical techniques to cure male incontinence that simple techniques will just not produce successful results. The only exception to this general rule is the peri-urethral teflon paste injection. The method has been perfected by Politano. Most important is that the injection does not interfere with later surgery which makes this technique an option for urologists with a lack of experience in reconstructive procedures or without access to artificial sphincter implantation.

Still the 73 % success rate runs parallel with the success rate reported by Tanagho and Hauri with their reconstructive procedures. This fact indicates that the surgical techniques fail constantly in 30 % of the cases. This high figure in the best of hands will even be higher when the procedure is performed by unexperienced surgeons. The conclusion is that extensive training is required to perform the procedure and that a variety of factors may be responsible for the final results. The diagnostic workup of these patients should be meticulous and the absence of proper neuro-muscular innervation or a complete degree of sphincter insufficiency will doom any surgical reconstruction from the start. The reported series are all limited and a publication of data analyzed by life table methods would expose the realistic success rates regardless of time of follow-up [10].

The increasing popularity of the artifical sphincter implantation with more than 8 000 implants performed to this date led to the publication of a quarterly colleagues in Urology designed for surgeons implanting these devices. The voluminous literature on the subject testifies to its success and several chapters in this volume will deal with all the aspects of artificial sphincter implantations.

Again the conclusion is that extra training is required to perform this procedure and that a minimum of experience will inevitably reduce the complication rate of the surgery. Mechanical complications are inherent to artificial devices but are subject to improvement by future technology.

In conclusion we may state that the teflon paste injection might be a first choice for the general urologist while the second choice and the first choice for patients with neuro-muscular lesions or complete loss of the sphincter system will benefit from the artificial sphincter implantation especially if the procedure is performed in experienced centers.

276

References

1. Tanagho E.A. Postprostatectomy Incontinence: Urodynamic Evaluation. In: Hinman F. (ed), Benign Hypertrophy, Springer-Verlag, New York (1983). pp. 985–996.
2. Vergès-Flaqué A. Urinary Incontinence following Prostatectomy. Cure by non-operative treatment. J. Urol. 92 (1984): 203–205.
3. Tanagho E.A. Bladder Neck Reconstruction for Total Urinary Incontinence: 10 Years of Experience. J. Urol. 125 (1981): 321–326.
4. Hauri D. Die operative Korrektur der männlichen Inkontinenz. Helv. Chir. Acta 49 (1982): 493–503.
5. Lenzi R., Barbagli G., Stomaci N. and Selli C. Surgical Treatment of Male Urinary Incontinence. J. Urol. 130 (1983): 463–465.
6. Politano V.A. Periurethral teflon injection for urinary incontinence. Urol. Clin. North Am. 5 (1978): 415–422.
7. Scott F.B., Bradley W.E., Timm G.W. Treatment of urinary incontinence by an implantable prostatic sphincter. Urology 1 (1973): 252–259.
8. Furlow W.L. Postprostatectomy Urinary Incontinence. Urol. Clin. North Am. 5 (1978): 347–352.
9. Scott F.B., Light J.K., Fishmann I.F. and West J.E. Implantation of an artificial sphincter for urinary incontinence. Contemp. Surg. 18 (1981): 11–34.
10. Scott F.B. Treatment of urinary incontinence. J. Urol. 125 (1981): 799.

CHAPTER SEVEN

Artificial sphincters in
the management of urinary incontinence

VII.1. The bladder neck artificial sphincter

T. HALD

Introduction

The artificial urinary sphincter developed by American Medical Systems offers a chance of rehabilitating selected patients with severe incontinence.

The prosthesis has undergone several changes since the first model which appeared in 1973 [1]. The present device (AS 800) (Fig. 1) features a combined pump and control unit, a choice of 5 different pressure balloons ranging from 50 to 90 cm H_2O and a line of occlusive cuffs ranging from 4.5 to 11 cm. In the following 10 years experience with six different models (AS 721, 761, 742, 791, 792 and 800) is presented.

Material

From May 1, 1974 to May 1, 1984 83 patients were treated by a total of 114 sphincter implants. The type of prostheses used are listed in Table 1 and the age distribution in Fig. 2. There were 60 men and 23 women. Thirty-three patients had neuropathic bladder dysfunction and 50 non-neuropathic urinary incontinence. The diagnoses are shown in Table 2. A complete urodynamic work-up, including cystometry with sphincter EMG pressure-flow

Table 1. Artificial urinary sphincter.

Type of prosthesis	No of patients
AS 721	15
AS 761	4
AS 742	22
AS 791 ⎫ AS 792 ⎬	58
AS 800	15

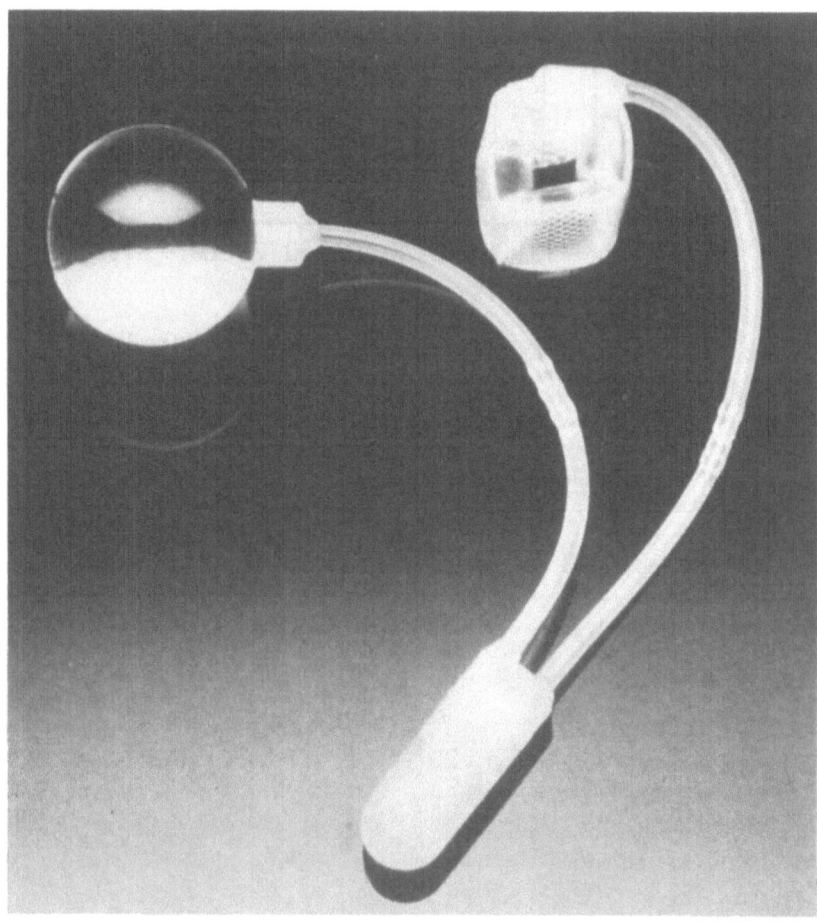

Fig. 1. The AS 800 artificial urinary sphincter.

studies and micturition cysto-urethrography, was made in order to secure the feasability of the procedure. 64 of the implants were performed with the cuff around the bladder neck. The cuff sizes and the balloon pressures used are listed in Table 3 and 4. In the female the bladder neck position of the

Table 2. Artificial urinary sphincter: diagnosis. (Patients n = 83).

Neuropathic bladder		Non-neuropathic bladder	
Myelodysplasia	18	Postprostatectomy stress	35
Seq traumatic lesion	8	Extrophy – Epispadias	9
Seq lumbar disc	4	Recurr. fem. genuine stress	2
Seq nervous system tumour	3	Seq urethral rupture	2
	33	Seq recto-urethral fistula	2
			50

280

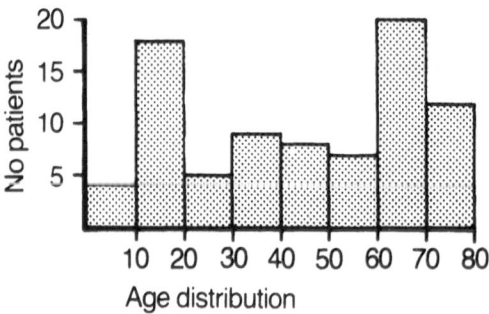

Fig. 2. Distribution per age of the patients (n = 83; male: 60; female: 23).

Table 3. Artificial urinary sphincter: cuff size.

cm	Females (bladder neck)	Males (bladder neck)
4.5	0	
5.0	1	
5.5	0	
6.0	1	
6.5	3	
7.0	7	5
7.5	4	2
8.0	13*	8
9.0	3	8
10.0	1	11
11.0	0	9
12.0	0	1

* 2 were too large.

Table 4. Artificial urinary sphincter: balloon pressures.

| | cm H$_2$O | | | |
	51–60	61–70	71–80	81–90
Females (bladder neck)				
No of implants	1	12	13	2
No of eroded	0	2	2	1
Males (bladder neck)				
No of implants	1	4	9	4
No of eroded	0	0	2	1

Table 5. Patient requirements.

1. Reasonably good physical condition
2. Reasonably good mental condition
3. Upper extremity dexterity
4. Boys > 10; girls > 14–15
5. No UTI
6. No decubitus
7. Fair upper urinary tract
8. No outflow obstruction
9. Demonstrable stress incontinence
10. No or insignificant detrusor overactivity

Table 6. Hospital requirements.

1. Urodynamic expertise
2. Willingness to establish a programme
3. Willigness to follow patients life-long
4. Surgical taining in procedure

cuff is the only practical. In the male the alternative is the membranous or bulbous urethra, the latter being the easiest to perform.

The restricting requirements for patients and hospitals are important prerequisites for securing a satisfactory result. These are shown in Table 5 and 6.

Procedure

The patient is prepared for surgery by two whole body scrubs with chlorhexidine soap on the day prior to operation. The urethra is instilled with a chlorhexidine containing gel. The operation is performed in general or epidural anaesthesia after a 15 minutes scrub of the operative field with betadine soap. The patient is positioned in stirrups which can be raised and flattened during surgery for convenient access to the urethra and the vagina. Carbenicillin 5–10 g is administered intravenously during the operation. Otherwise, no antibiotics were used unless the patient had a recent urinary tract infection. A Foley catheter 16 F was placed in the bladder. A Pfannenstiel incision or a low transverse abdominal incision allows the best approach to the bladder neck region. If previous surgery has been performed in the area, the bladder and urethra are dissected with the scalpel from the posterior aspect of the pubic bone. The endopelvic fascia is incised lateral to the bladder neck. In females the help of an assistant's hand in the vagina lifting up the anterolateral wall is highly recommendable. The plane behind the bladder neck is developed by sharp and blunt dissection. In case of difficulty the bladder should be opened to assure that the bladder or urethra are not entered. A cutter clamp has been developed for blind passage around the bladder neck in severely scarred tissue, but it should be used with extreme caution and only when its grip around the bladder neck can be checked endoscopically. The circumference of the bladder neck is measured. The cuff should fit snug but not tight. The inclusion of too much perivesical tissue within the cuff may cause pressure atrophy of fat and connective tissue and with time result in a cuff that cannot close sufficiently on the bladder neck. The cuff is implanted in the empty state but free of air. The balloon can be placed either alongside the bladder or in the peritoneum. It is filled with 16 ml Hypaque 12,5% after the cuff has been filled from the balloon with a temporary volume of 18 ml. A space is created in one labium majus or one side of the scrotum by spreading gently the tissue by the scissors and the control pump brought in place and fixed by a Babcock clamp applied around one of the tubings across the skin. This will prevent accidental dislocation throughout the rest of the procedure. Before leaving the pump out of sight the tubings running to the cuff, respectively the balloon, are carefully identified in order to make the correct connections. The tubings coming from the cuff and the balloon are drawn through the inguinal canal by the use of tubing passers. Finally, the connections are made in the inguinal region, just outside the external inguinal ring. 3-0 prolene is used for this purpose. The wound is closed in layers using 2-0 prolene in the fascia, 3-0 Dexon® in the subcutaneous tissue and an intracuticular 2-0 prolene. The prosthesis is checked for good function and deactivated by pushing the small button on the side of the basis of the control pump. The catheter is left in place until the activation of the sphincter can be started without too much discomfort to the patient. When the condition of the tissue under the cuff is questionable (previous surgery, lesion of the bladder neck) the prosthesis is kept deactivated for 6–8 weeks.

Results

Wound infection occurred in 4.4% of the implants and necessitated in all cases removal of part or of the entire prosthesis.

Of the earliest models (AS 721 and 761) implanted 1974–76 only one patient out of 17 still has a functional good result. The main problems were mechanical in nature. The subsequent prosthesis (AS 742) was considerably more successful. 45% are working well after 5 years. The newest models (AS 791, 792 and 800) have proved reliable although the cuff is still a mechanically weak link, causing leaks in 20–25% of the patients over a 5 year period.

The most serious complication is erosion of the bladder neck. In the entire material the incidence has been 18 % in the females and 8 % in the males.

The overall subjective result is seen in Table 7 which includes bladder neck as well as urethral implants. Using an incontinence quantitation test [2, 3] in 34 patients claiming to have a satisfactory result of the implantation, it was evident that the patients with a bladder neck prosthesis obtained a better and more reliable continence than those with a bulbous urethral implant.

Three patients developed detrusor hyperreflexia postoperatively. In two, high doses of emepromium controlled the problem, but the last patient had the prosthesis removed.

Discussion

An artificial urinary sphincter placed at the bladder neck offers a chance of achieving continence at the level where continence is normally maintained. Although the surgery is more difficult than a bulbous urethral implant a bladder neck sphincter should be a first choice whenever possible.

In the female the bladder neck implant is the only practical and in the young male it is always the best choice. In the elderly male where a prostatectomy has been performed the difficulties that can be encountered with this approach and the comparative ease of a bulbar implant speaks in favour of the latter.

Most complications are relatively easy to deal with. Leaks and kinks can be handled by small surgical procedures. The mechanical failures related to function of the valves and the resistor in the control unit are few, but it is extremely important to prevent the entrance of blood, lint and small tissue bits into the system during surgery.

Urethral erosion remains a problem. The causes are slow infection, bad tissue perfusion or accidental high pressure in the prosthesis. If infection can

Table 7. Overall subjective result.

	No of patients	
Essential dry, satisfied	62	78 %
Improved but not dry	2	
Awaiting repair	4	
Beyond repair (heart, cancer)	2	
Failure	13 ~	16 %
	83	

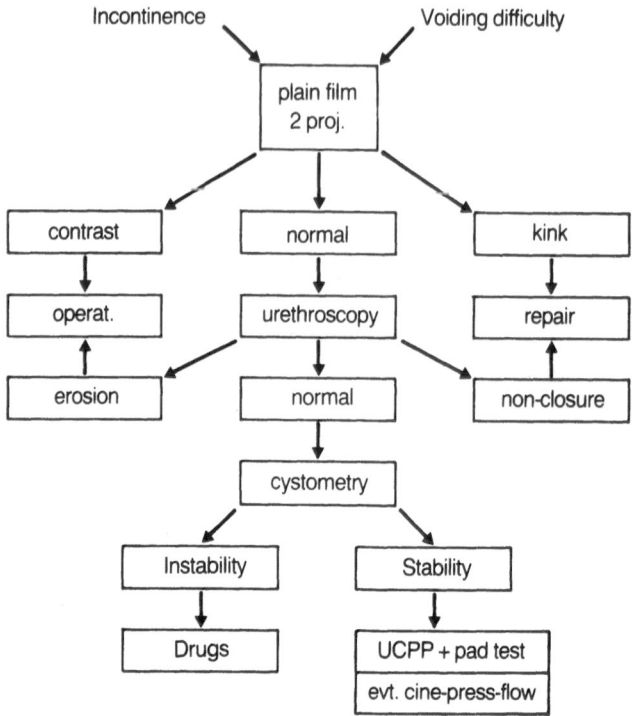

Fig. 3. Fault finding scheme.

be avoided, if balloon pressures are kept low (<70 cm H_2O in females, <80 cm H_2O in males), if kinks of tubing are properly corrected and, if the patients are selected with care (avoidance of irradiated patients and patients with low systemic arterial blood pressure or severe arteriosclerosis) the complication rate is bound to decrease.

Patients with artificial sphincters should be followed life-long with increasing intervals between checks. Before discharging a patient a plain X-ray of the prosthesis is performed to serve as a reference for eventual subsequent complications. Fault finding is an important facet of the implant programme. Fig. 3 shows the logical steps to take when the patient complains of incontinence or voiding problems.

Conclusion

The artifical sphincter at the bladder neck offers the severely incontinent and well evaluated patient a good chance of cure. Minute observation of many practical details are all important to achieve good results. Prosthetic surgery of this kind should not be done in departments as an occasional procedure. Only those who are willing to establish an in depth programme should contemplate this type of treatment.

References

1. Scott F.B., Bradley W.E. and Timm G.W. Treatment of urinary incontinence by an implantable prosthetic sphincter. Urology 1 (1973): 252–259.
2. Klarskov P. and Hald T. Reproduability and reliability of urinary incontinence assessment with a 60 minutes test. Scand. J. Urol. Nephrol. (in press).
3. Holm-Bentzen M., Klarskov P., Opsomer R., Maegaard E.M. and Hald T. Objective assessment of urinary incontinence after successful implantation of the AMS artificial urethral sphincter. Neurourology & Urodynamics (in press).

VII.2. Bulbar artificial sphincter

F. SCHREITER

Introduction

The artificial sphincter was introduced in 1973 by Scott, Bradley and Timm [1], and has undergone rapid development since. The result of ten years clinical experience is the latest model of the AMS-artificial sphincter, the AS 800 [4], which is described herein.

Prosthesis design (Fig. 1)

The device consists of an occlusive *urethral cuff* which maintains continence by compressing the urethra. It can be placed at the bulbous urethra or bladder neck. A transfer of fluid within the device is controlled by a *pressure regulating balloon* and a *control pump*. By squeezing the pump, the fluid within the closed system is transferred from the cuff to the balloon, and the urethra is opened for free voiding. After voiding, the fluid runs back from the pressure regulating balloon to the cuff, closing the urethra automatically when the cuff is filled. Thus, the patient has full control of voiding (Fig. 2).

The new AS 800 sphincter device has the option of primary deactivation, whereby a urologist is able to deactivate the device and keep the cuff deflated. By pressing the deactivation button on the control pump, a valve is pushed into place that stops the fluid in the balloon from returning to the cuff. Activation of the device is easily accomplished by giving the pump a strong, sustained squeeze. The advantages of primary deactivation are:
1. The device can be implanted in one procedure, thus minimizing the risk of cuff erosion and infection, even when the cuff is implanted on the bulbous urethra.
2. Healing takes place without pressurizing the urethra, and, when the healing tissue has developed a good blood supply and there is a stabilizing fibrous sheet surrounding the device, activation can be initiated.
3. Cystoscopy, transurethral resection and catheterization are easier to perform, should they become necessary.

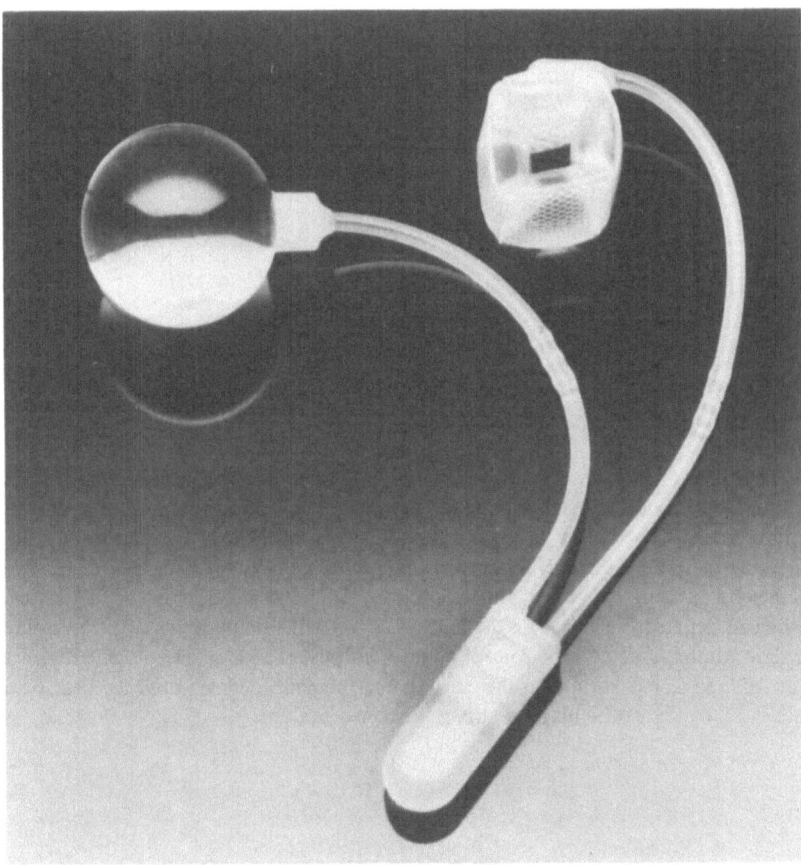

Fig. 1. The AS 800 artificial urinary sphincter. The device consists of an occlusive cuff for compression of the urethra, a control pump which is implanted in the scrotum, and a pressure regulating balloon, which is placed in the prevesical space or intraperitoneally.

The bladder neck is the optimal location for the urethral cuff of the artificial sphincter because of its good blood supply and the thickness of the muscular prostatic tissue. However, after open prostatectomy or radical prostatectomy the bladder neck tissue is often rigid and scarred, and has become fixed to the surrounding layers [3]. Scarring in this area usually involves poor vascularization and the resulting high risk of cuff erosion. Dissection of the bladder neck in these cases is difficult and sometimes impossible, so that it becomes necessary to place the cuff around the bulbous urethra (Fig. 3). Placement at the *distal* part of the bulbous urethra, however, involves not only a higher risk of cuff erosion, but there is also the possibility of the cuff deflating when the patient sits down, resulting in leakage once he stands (Fig. 4a). To correct these problems, we modified the operative technique,

288

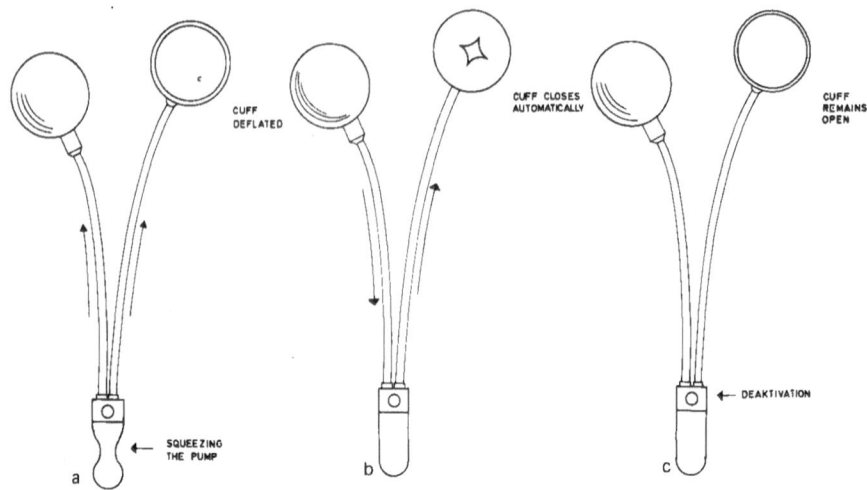

Fig. 2. The hydraulic system. a) To urinate, the patient deflates the cuff by squeezing the pump several times, forcing the fluid in the cuff to transfer to the balloon. b) As soon as the patient stops squeezing the pump, the cuff refills with fluid automatically. This usually takes several minutes, thereby allowing the patient time to void. c) The urologist deactivates the device by keeping the cuff deflated. First, deflate the cuff. Then, after the pump refills with fluid, simply press the deactivation button on the control pump. This pushes a valve into place that prevents fluid in the balloon from returning to the cuff. The cuff remains deflated until the deactivation valve is released by giving the pump a strong, sustained squeeze.

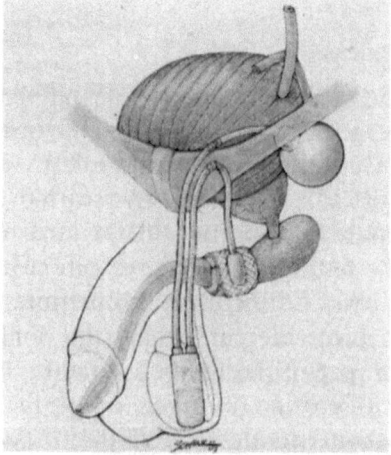

Fig. 3. Artificial sphincter in the bulbous urethra position.

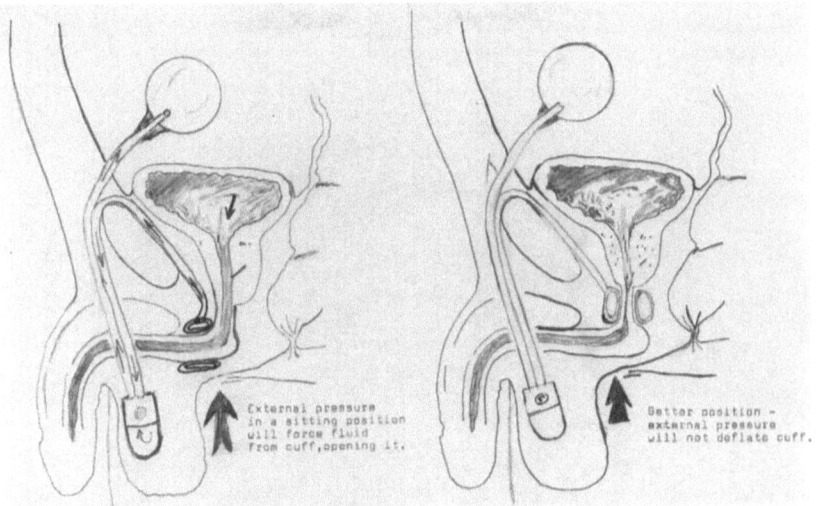

Fig. 4. a) Placement of the artificial sphincter at the distal part of the bulbous urethra. b) Placement of the artificial sphincter at the proximal bulbous urethra.

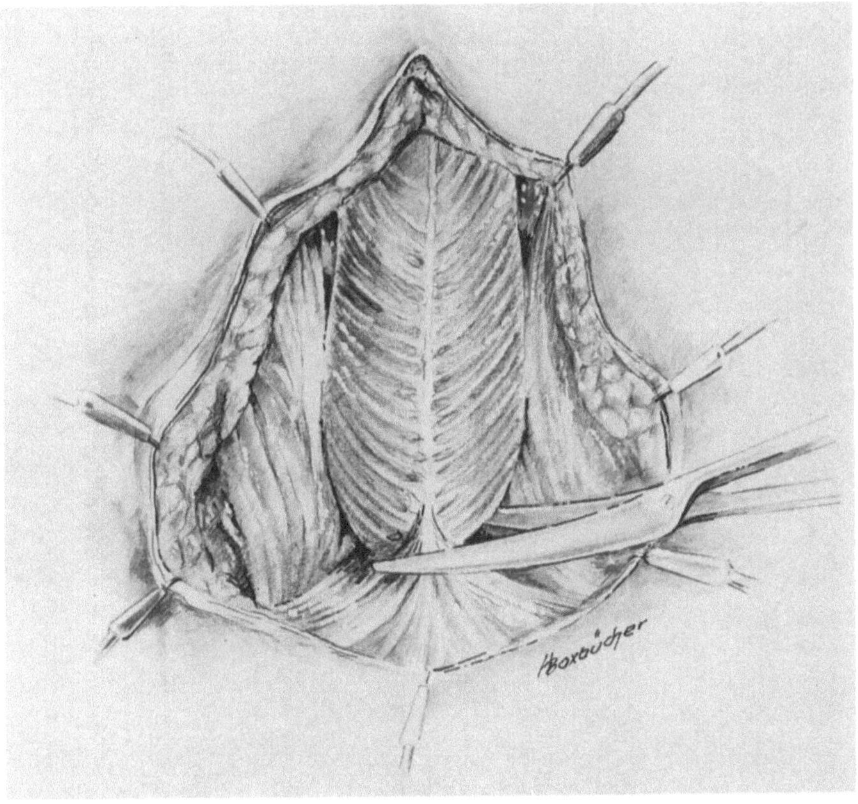

Fig. 5. Operative technique: midline incision, dissection of the bulbocavernosus muscle and central tendon.

290

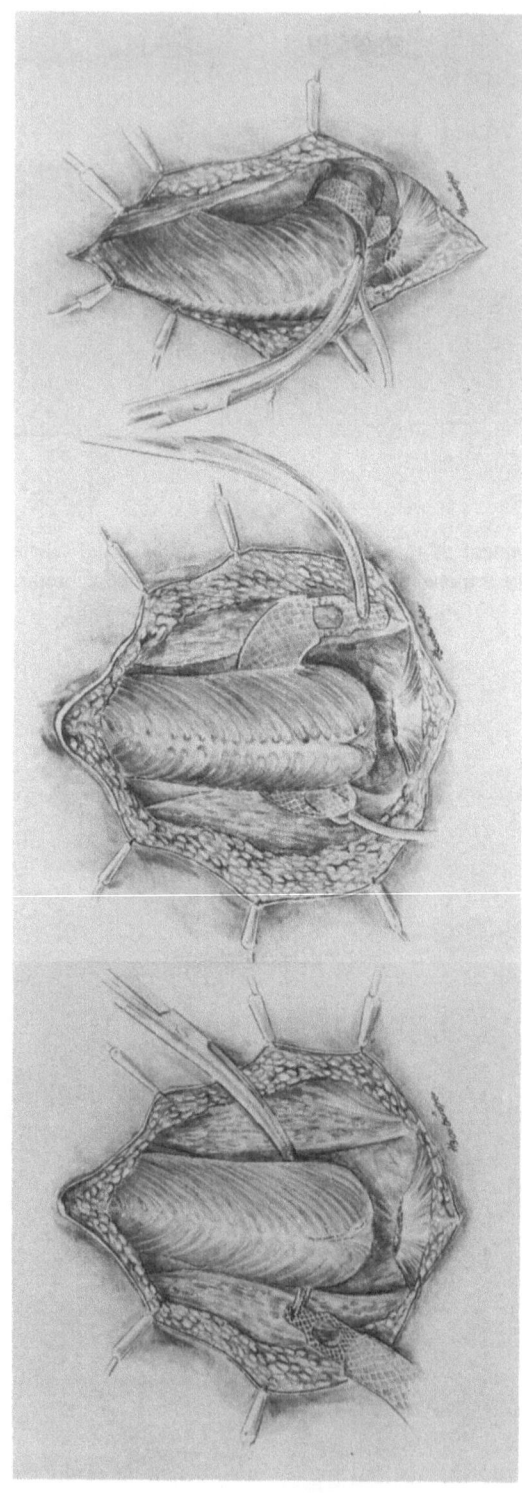

Fig. 6. The cuff is placed around the proximal bulbous urethra, very close to the pelvic floor.

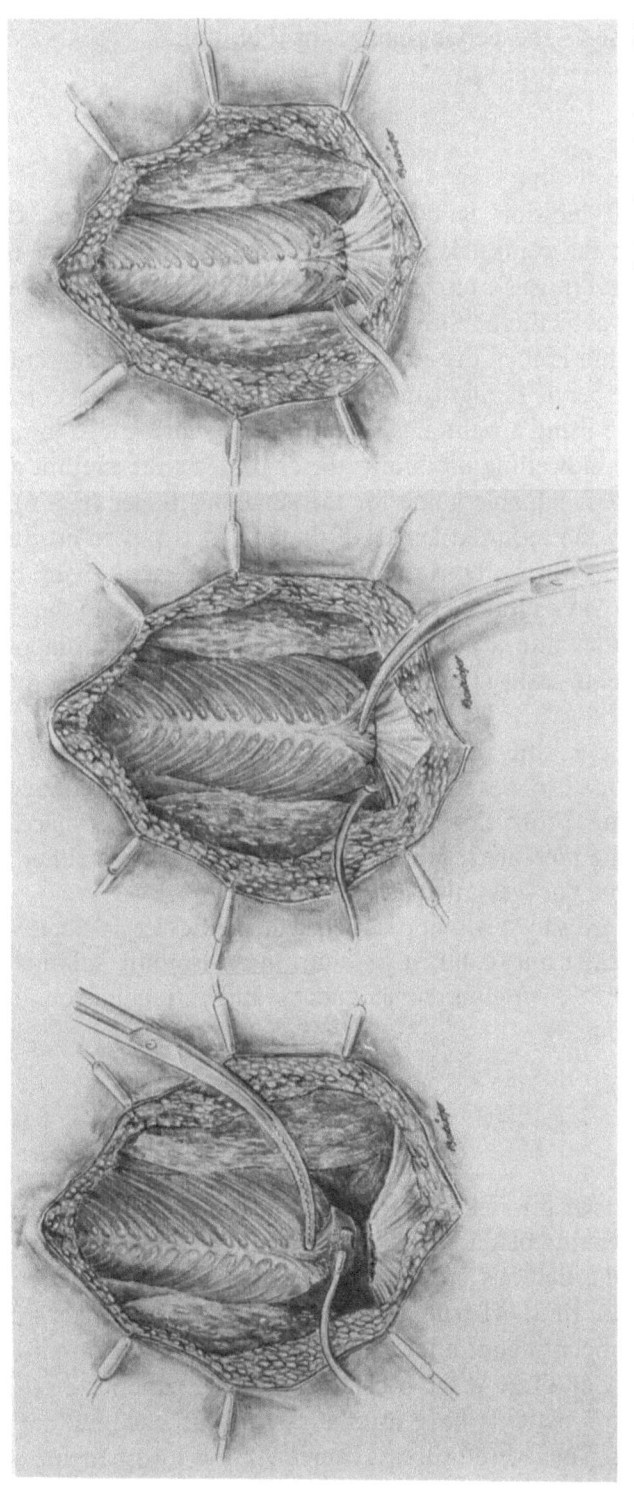

Fig. 7. Suturing of the central tendon brings the cuff in the very deep perineal position, so that emptying of the cuff by sitting down is impossible.

and now implant the cuff at the proximal bulbous urethra, deep in the perineum and very close to the pelvic diaphragm (Fig. 4b).

Operative technique

A midline perineal incision is made and the bulbocavernosus muscle exposed. Thereafter the central tendon of the perineal musculature is dissected. The bulbocavernosus muscle is not divided and later acts as a protective layer to the cuff, thereby preventing cuff erosion (Fig. 5).

The bulbous urethra is then dissected carefully without bleeding until the muscle layers of the pelvic diaphragm are seen. The urethra is dissected free from the pubic bone using a right angle clamp, taking care not to injure the urethral tissue. The indwelling urethral catheter protects the urethra during dissection, acting as a palpable guide for the surgeon's finger (Fig. 6).

After determining the required length of the cuff, it is placed around the most proximal part of the bulbous urethra, covering the underlying bulbocavernosus muscle. After suturing the bulbocavernosus muscle to the central tendon, the cuff settles into a position very close to the pelvic diaphragm. This location prevents leakage caused by the patient's sitting on the cuff (Fig. 7).

The tube leading out from the cuff is then threaded subcutaneously from the perineal incision into a small inguinal incision and placed over the external inguinal ring. From this inguinal incision the pump is placed in a scrotal pouch and the pressure regulating balloon can be placed either intraperitoneally or in the paravesical space (Fig. 8).

Before the tubes are shortened and connected, the device is filled with a mixture of sterile water and contrast medium in an isotonic solution. The wound is closed with a running subcutaneous and intracutaneous suture without drainage (Fig. 9).

Results

A total of 181 sphincter implantations were done at our institution between 1973 and 1984, 140 at the bladder neck and 41 at the bulbous urethra (Table 1). All patients in the bulbous urethra group underwent implantation with primary deactivation. In 31/41 patients the indication for sphincter implantation was urinary incontinence after radical prostatectomy and in 10 cases after adenomectomy or TUR of the prostate. Of the 41 patients, 36 (87.8%) are continent, while 2 patients have mild stress incontinence but are satisfied with the results. The overall success rate is 92.7%. Two patients (4.9%) failed following infection and erosion of the urethra; one patient had cuff

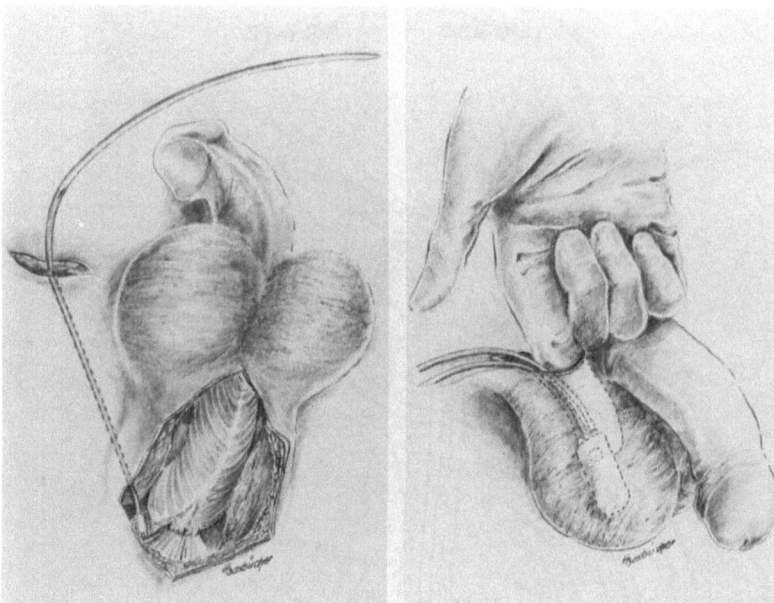

Fig. 8. The cuff tube is passed subcutaneously to the inguinal incision. From the inguinal incision, the control pump is placed in the scrotum and the pressure regulating balloon is placed intraperitoneally or in the prevesical space.

erosion, but was continent after reimplantation; and reoperation is planned in one further patient.

The intra- and postoperative complications are shown in Table 2. In all, there were 29.3% surgical and 12.1% mechanical complications, which resulted in 11 revisions (26.8%) in 8 patients (19.5%) (Table 3). The primary infection rate was 4.9% (2 patients).

Table 1. Results of sphincter implantation at the bulbous urethra (n = 41).

	No of patients	Percentage	
Continent	36	87.8	92.7
Mild stress incontinence	2	4.9	
Failure	2	4.9	7.3
Waiting for revision	1	2.4	

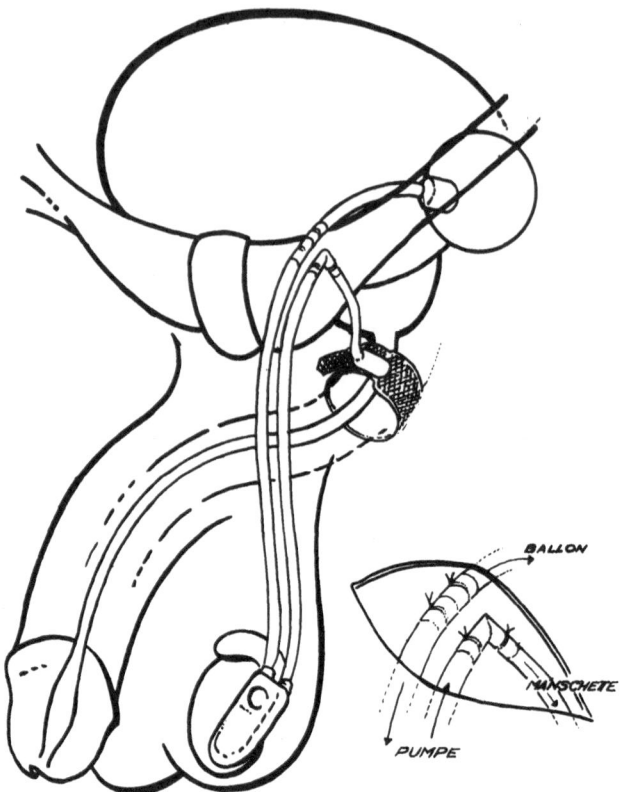

Fig. 9. The tubes are shortened and connected, and the incisions closed by running subcutaneous and intracutaneous 0000 PDS sutures.

Table 2. Complications of sphincter implantation at the bulbous urethra (n = 41).

		No of patients
Surgical		
Urethral injury		2
Hematoma		2
Kinking tubes		4
Cuff erosion/infection		4
	Total	12 (29.3%)
Mechanical		
Balloon leakage		2
Cuff leakage		2
Pump leakage		1
	Total	5 (12.1%)

Table 3. Revision rate (n = 41).

	No of revisions
Urethral erosion/infection	2
Kinking of the tubes	4
Leakage: Balloon	2
Cuff	2
Pump	1
	11 revisions (26.8%)
	in 8 patients (19.5%)

Discussion

A success rate of more than 90% is excellent in patients for whom no other comparable therapy is available for the treatment of their postoperative urinary incontinence. The new AS 800 sphincter with the option of delayed activation minimizes the risk of cuff erosion, as does the modified operative technique of placing the cuff very deep and close to the pelvic floor and leaving the bulbocavernosus muscle in place as a protective muscular layer [4].

While the pressure regulating balloon reservoir is available in a variety of pressure ranges (51–60, 61–70, 71–80, 81–90 and 91–100 cm H_2O), we have consistently used the lowest possible pressure regulating balloon with the range of 51–60 cm H_2O. This has proved sufficient to achieve continence in most patients and further reduces the risk of cuff erosion.

As a consequence of the surgical and mechanical failure rates of 29.5% and 12.1%, respectively, there was a revision rate of 26.8% in 8 patients (19.5). Although this may appear to be high, we have to consider that, with the exception of cuff erosion and infection, the complications encountered were not serious. Furthermore, most of the complications could be corrected by an easy reoperation.

The incidence of cuff erosion and infection is surprisingly low (9.6%) in our experience. In addition, the incidence of mechanical failures has been reduced by the new AS 800 sphincter device as compared to the six-month mechanical failure rate of 50% that Giesy et al. [2] found with the Rosen prosthesis (58% leakage and 42% urethral erosion). In our opinion there is no better alternative operative procedure available today for the treatment of postoperative male urinary incontinence.

In summary, to keep the surgical complication rate low, we recommend consideration of the following principles:

1. In cases of implantation of the cuff at the bulbous urethra, the device must be implanted with delayed activation of 6 weeks.
2. The urine must be sterile and perioperative antibiotic prophylaxis should be done.
3. The lowest possible pressure regulating balloon should be chosen to prevent cuff erosion of the urethra. In most patients, a pressure regulating balloon of 51–60 cm H_2O pressure guarantees postoperative urinary continence.
4. The bulbocavernosus muscle offers a protective layer to the urethra against cuff erosion, if it is not dissected away from the urethra.
5. Dissection of the bulbous urethra should be done very carefully to prevent urethral injury and postoperative hematoma; hemostasis should be done scrupulously.
6. The use of surgical drains should be avoided to make bacterial contamination of the device in the early post-operative period impossible.

Summary

Fourty-one cases of postoperative male urinary incontinence were treated by implantation of the AMS-artificial sphincter Model AS 800 with a success rate of 92.7%, using a modified bulbar implantation technique. The operative technique is described and the complication and revision rates discussed. In our experience the artificial urinary sphincter is a highly effective method of treating severe cases of urinary incontinence, even after radical prostatectomy or TUR.

References

1. Scott F.B., Bradley W.E. and Timm G.W. Treatment of urinary incontinence by an implantable prosthetic sphincter. Urology 1 (1973): 252–259.
2. Giesy J.B., Fuchs E.F., Burry J.M. and Griffith L.D. Initial experience with the Rosen incontinence prosthesis. AUA Meeting, San Francisco, Calif., May 1980.
3. Barrett D.M. and Furlow W.L. Radical prostatectomy incontinence and the AS 791 artificial urinary sphincter. J. Urol. 129 (1983): 528–530.
4. Schreiter F. Ein Jahrzehnt Erfahrung mit der alloplastischen hydraulischen Sphinkter-Prothese AMS. Bericht über das 7. klinische Wochenende, Mainz, BRD, 1.–3. März 1984, S. 325–335.

VII.3. The implantable artificial urinary sphincter in children: a six-year experience

R.L. KROOVAND

Introduction

The implantable artificial urinary sphincter was first used clinically in 1972 by Scott and associates [1] and, after many modifications and improvements, now represents a reliable, universally applicable method to produce urinary continence in children in whom less involved methods have failed [2, 3].

The artificial urinary sphincter* is a hydraulically operated Silastic prosthesis with three components: a cuff, a pressure-regulating balloon and a control assembly (Fig. 1). The cuff surrounds and occludes the urethra. The pressure-regulating balloon transmits sufficient pressure to the cuff to occlude the urethra but insufficient pressure to compromise urethral blood supply. The balloon is positioned in the perivesical space. The control assembly, positioned in the scrotum or a labium majus, permits transfer of fluid from the cuff to the balloon in response to squeezing the pump portion of the control assembly, thus opening the cuff to permit micturition or intermittent catheterization. In addition, the control assembly allows slow return of fluid from the balloon to refill the cuff and control assembly to reestablish urinary continence. Control assembly design permits release of pressure from the cuff in response to nonphysiologic intravesical pressure from bladder contractions or increased intraabdominal pressure.

The current production device, the AS 800*, also includes a deactivation button which permits elective nonsurgical deactivation and activation of the prosthesis.

To operate the artificial sphincter, the child squeezes the pump of the control assembly several times to transfer fluid from the cuff and control device into the pressure-regulating balloon. This opens the cuff and, therefore, the urethra, permitting micturition or intermittent catheterization. The pressure-regulating balloon slowly forces fluid through the control assembly,

---

* American Medical Systems, 11001 Bren Road East, Minnetonka, MN 55343.

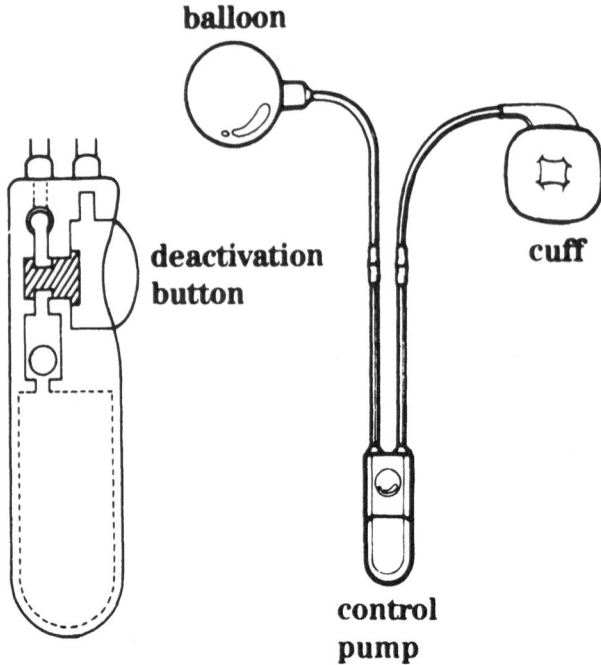

Fig. 1. Schematic diagram of the AS 800.

refilling the cuff and control-assembly pump and reestablishing urinary continence.

Material and method

During the past six years, we have implanted the Scott artificial urinary sphincter* in 44 children and young adults (36 boys and 8 girls) between four and 24 years of age (mean, 10 years; average, 11 years). Follow-up is from three months to six years. The etiologies of the bladder dysfunction producing the urinary incontinence are shown in Table 1.

Criteria for implantation included a high degree of motivation and cooperation in attempts to achieve urinary continence, adequate intelligence,

Table 1. Causes of incontinence.

Sacrolumbar myelomeningocele	38
Sacral agenesis	4
Spinal cord tumor	1
Trauma	1

* American Medical Systems, 11001 Bren Road East, Minnetonka, MN 55343.

good manual dexterity, minimal or correctable vesicoureteral reflux, treatable urinary infection, a bladder capacity sufficient to allow three to four hours of urinary continence, pharmacologically controllable uninhibited bladder contractions, and an understanding of the procedure and potential complications for sphincter implantation. Complete bladder emptying is not considered a requirement for implantation as we use clean intermittent catheterization when necessary to ensure bladder emptying.

Preoperative evaluation included a careful history and physical examination, a urinalysis and culture and sensitivity, an IVP, a VCUG, a cystometrogram, and measurement of residual urine postvoiding. Urethral pressure profile measurements have not been a reproducible and useful study in our pediatric population and, therefore, were not done.

In our series five children required urinary undiversion and four bladder augmentation prior to sphincter implantation. After sphincter implantation two children required bladder augmentation to create sufficient bladder capacity to permit three to four hourly voiding.

After initial evaluation, all children were placed on a program of clean intermittent catheterization, with or without adjunctive neuropharmacology. Those who were not successful in maintaining urinary continence on this nonoperative program were considered potential candidates for sphincter implantation.

All sphincters were implanted around the bladder neck as described by Scott and associates [1], initially employing the AS 742 and later upon distribution the AS 792, and more recently the AS 800. At initial implantation, 24 children had primary activation of the artificial sphincter and 20 primary deactivation (sphincter implanted but not functioning) with sphincter acti-

Table 2. Artificial urinary sphincter — initial implant.

Device activation — initial implant			
Primary activation 24		*Primary deactivation* 20	
AS 742	12	AS 792	7
AS 792	12	AS 800	13
AS 800	0		

Table 3. Artificial urinary sphincter.

Device malfunction 20	
AS 742	6
AS 792	14
AS 800	0

vation four to six weeks after implantation when tissue healing had completed and local site tenderness at the control assembly had resolved (Table 2). Twenty malfunctioning devices were successfully replaced (Table 3).

Primary deactivation was done because of planned (2) or inadvertent entry into the urinary tract (3), or because the sphincter was placed at the time of urinary undiversion (2) and primary activation was considered unwise. With the introduction of the AS 800 and its optional nonsurgical deactivation-activation capability, primary deactivation has become the standard after sphincter implantation (13 children) (Table 4).

For each child follow-up includes pelvic plain and oblique X-rays to document device position and tubing configuration (Fig. 2), checks for residual urine in those not on clean intermittent catheterization, urine cultures, and intravenous pyelogram one month postoperative, and renal ultrasonography at six-month intervals. All children take anticholinergic medication to prevent uninhibited bladder contractions, and those performing clean intermittent catheterization also take prophylactic antibacterial medication. Follow-up after implantation is done at monthly intervals for the first six months postoperatively and six-monthly thereafter unless the clinical course dictates the need for more frequent follow-up.

Results

An excellent result is defined as complete continence for at least three hours and overnight, a stable urinary tract at last examination, and the absence of untreatable urinary infection. As noted, the absence of residual urine is not a criterion for success as we employ clean intermittent catheterization when necessary to ensure complete bladder emptying.

A good result is defined as subjective improvement in urinary continence with episodic leakage generally manageable with one to two pads per day. A failure is defined as no apparent improvement over the preoperative status (i.e., still totally incontinent) or deterioration of the upper urinary system requiring sphincter deactivation or device removal.

Table 4. Artificial urinary sphincter.

Primary deactivation	20 children	
AS 742/792	Urinary tract violated	
	− planned	2
	− unplanned	3
	− undiversion	2
AS 800	Primary deactivation standard	13

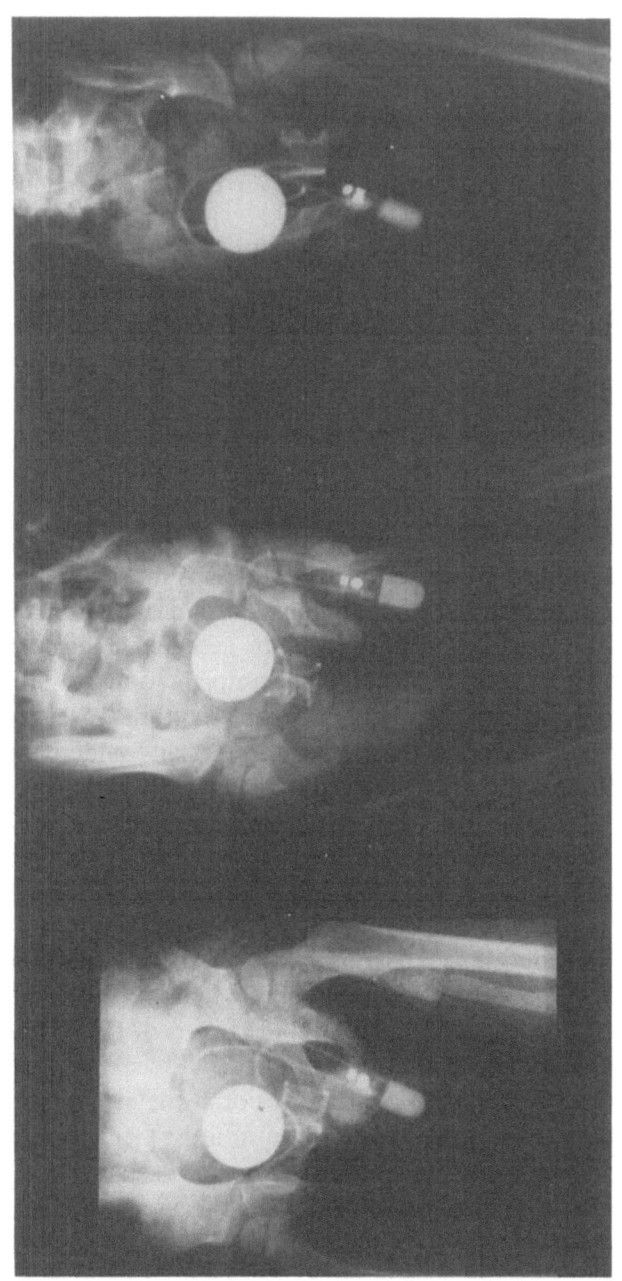

Fig. 2. Plain and oblique pelvic X-rays demonstrating artificial sphincter position (AS 800) and tubing configuration.

Thirty-eight children are continent of urine for at least three hours during the day and are dry at night. Four children have mild stress urinary incontinence requiring a pad or other absorptive device to prevent social embarrassment, and three children have had the device removed because of erosion of the device into the urinary tract. After healing, two devices were replaced, one successfully; however, the other device eroded into the urethra six weeks postoperatively and was removed. This child is incontinent and awaiting further surgery. The third child with device erosion has had a cutaneous urinary diversion. Thus, two children are considered surgical failures.

Of the 44 children, 8 void to completion, 5 void but require supplemental intermittent catheterization to drain postvoid residual urine and 29 depend on clean intermittent catheterization for bladder emptying. One child is incontinent after device removal because of erosion, and one child has a cutaneous urinary diversion.

There have been five intraoperative complications in four children, including inadvertent entry into the urinary tract in three cases (one child in two separate operations) and a vaginal laceration in one girl. All injuries were primarily repaired and sphincters successfully implanted. The bladder injuries necessitated primary deactivation of the device in each instance.

With introduction of the AS 800 and the nonsurgical deactivation-activation option, opening the urinary tract is now an accepted maneuver. An open bladder permits simultaneous ureteral reimplantation or provides direct visualization of the bladder neck and upper urethra to facilitate a difficult dissection between the bladder neck or urethra and underlying rectum or vagina, lessening the risk of postoperative cuff erosion into the urinary tract. Using this option we have done two simultaneous sphincter implantations and ureteroneocystostomies and three urinary undiversions and/or bladder augmentations using bowel combined with sphincter implantation.

Twenty-nine children developed postimplantation complications, eighteen of whom required operative correction. These complications included device malfunction, fluid leaks, tubing kinks, and erosion of the device into the urinary tract (Table 5). Device malfunction and fluid leakage were successfully managed by device replacement and erosion by device removal. Of two attempts at device replacement after erosion into the urinary tract, one was successful and the other complicated by a second erosion.

Eleven children developed postimplantation complications which did not require surgical management. Seven children, all on clean intermittent catheterization, developed acute pyelonephritis requiring hospitalization for parenteral antibiotic therapy. Four of these children had minimal vesicoureteral reflux preoperatively, and three had undergone urinary undiversion (2) or bladder augmentation (1) prior to sphincter implantation. As is customary in children performing clean intermittent catheterization, up to 50 per cent will have bacteriuria; bacteriuria was documented in over half of our sphincter population performing intermittent catheterization and may have contributed to the pyelonephritic episodes cited above.

Four children developed prolonged and unrecognized urinary retention resulting in postoperative hydronephrosis and, in one boy, symptomatic azotemia. All recovered promptly after institution of clean intermittent catheterization. None of the 44 children in our series has developed permanent pyelographic deterioration postoperatively.

We have performed 99 operative procedures to produce urinary continence in 42 of the 44 children in our series (Table 6). Admittedly, this is a tremendous number of operative procedures to have done on such a small group of children; however, this appears insignificant in view of the gratifying results achieved.

Table 5. Postimplantation complications.

1. AS 742   Apparent fluid leak managed by fluid replacement; AS 792 implanted after second malfunction. Actual problem: patient noncompliance.
2. AS 742   Pump valve failure misdiagnosed as a tubing kink; AS 792 implanted after second malfunction.
3. AS 742   Component leaks in 24 children involving 7.
   AS 792   AS 742 and 17 AS 792 devices. All sphincters successfully replaced.
4. AS 792   Postimplantation seroma requiring operative drainage followed by postoperative tubing kink requiring tubing repositioning.
5. AS 792   Cuff erosion through the neobladder neck in a child with caudal regression; device removed; cutaneous urinary diversion.
6. AS 792   Probable infection and erosion of deflation pump through scrotum; device removed. AS 800 successfully implanted.
7. AS 792   Erosion of AS 792 into urethra; device removed.
   AS 800   AS 800 implanted and eroded into urethra 6 weeks postimplantation; device removed.
8. AS 792   Posttraumatic urethral stricture contributing to recurrent epididymitis; TUR of stricture.
9. AS 792   Tubing kinks in two children; operative repositioning.

Table 6. Artificial urinary sphincter.

Operations to produce urinary continence in 44 children	99
Initial sphincter implant	44
Management of complications	38
Delayed activation	7
Bladder augmentation *	6
Urinary undiversion *	4

* Does not include 3 simultaneous procedures.

The implantable artificial urinary sphincter has become a major contribution toward achieving urinary continence which is applicable to most incontinent children who do not respond to less involved nonoperative treatment. Although controversy exists about the advisability of implanting a prosthetic device in children who are not fully grown, none has required device revision because of somatic growth. Our limited experience, while encouraging, strongly suggests a continued requirement for critical implantation selection and careful and prolonged postimplantation follow-up in this patient population.

References

1. Scott F.B., Bradley W.E., Timm G.W. Treatment of urinary incontinence by implantable prosthetic sphincter. Urology. 1 (1973): 252–259.
2. Kroovand R.L. The artificial sphincter for urinary continence. Developmental Medicine and Child Neurology, 25 (1983): 520–523.
3. Light J.K., Hawila M., Scott F.B. Treatment of urinary incontinence in children: the artificial urinary sphincter versus other methods. J. Urol., 130 (1983): 518–521.

VII.4. The penoscrotal sphincter to treat male sphincter insufficiency

U. JONAS

In a period of 8 years a new artificial sphincter was developed, a rather simple device which was implanted at the penoscrotal angle and acted as a sort of 'internal penile clamp'. The silicone device (Fig. 1) is positioned around the urethra at the penoscrotal angle and closed using a stainless steel clamp.

Activation and deactivation happens simply by exceeding pressure from both sides to the sphincter (Fig. 2), therefore no remote control is necessary in order to open and close the sphincter.

The teflon ball (arrow, Fig. 1) was used to deactivate the device in the immediate postoperative phase.

Table 1 shows the first (preliminary) results of 12 implantations since November 1983.

It becomes evident that 7 out of 12 sphincters had to be removed due to erosion (n = 3) as well as impossible activation and deactivation (n = 4).

The reasons for this rather unsatisfactory results were partially operative faults (intraoperative lesion of the corpus spongiosum during implantation, (n = 1), as well as too proximal implantations which made the manipulation impossible (n = 4).

Table 2 shows the results of the other 5 patients, 3 of the 5 were continent.

For further improvement the sphincter S9 was developed (Fig. 3), which was similar to S8, however 2 modifications were adapted:

Table 1. Preliminary results of the clinical application of the penile scrotal sphincter (n = 12).

Postoperative follow-up: 4–13 months

Explantation: 7/12

— intraoperative lesion of the corpus spongiosum → erosion	1
— inability to operate	4
— significant inhibited manipulation → erosion	2

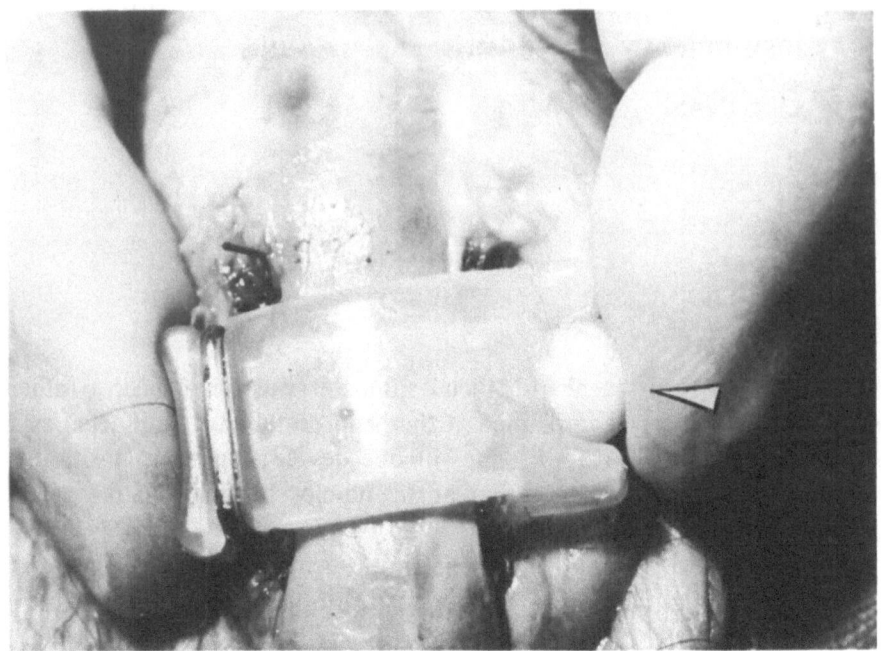

Fig. 1. Implantation of the sphincter at the penoscrotal angle. The arrow marks the teflon ball which can be pushed between both branches in order to deactivate the device.

1. a rather large teflon mesh was left in place in order to have a good fixation of the sphincter at the tunica albuginea and the corpora cavernosa.
2. Instead of 1 teflon ball, in this modification 2 teflon balls were used for activation and deactivation (Fig. 4 as marked by the arrows). In contrary to S8, where only one teflon ball had to be pushed (towards the urethra) in order to deactivate the sphincter, in S9 the manoeuvre had to take place from both sides, thus parallel to the urethra, as also seen in Fig. 5.

Table 2. First preliminary results sphincter in situ: 5/12.

	Postoperative follow-up (months)	Results
S-8-1/2	13/8	Partially continent
S-8-1	13	Partially continent
S-8-2	9	Continent
S-8-3	5	Continent
S-8-3	4	Continent

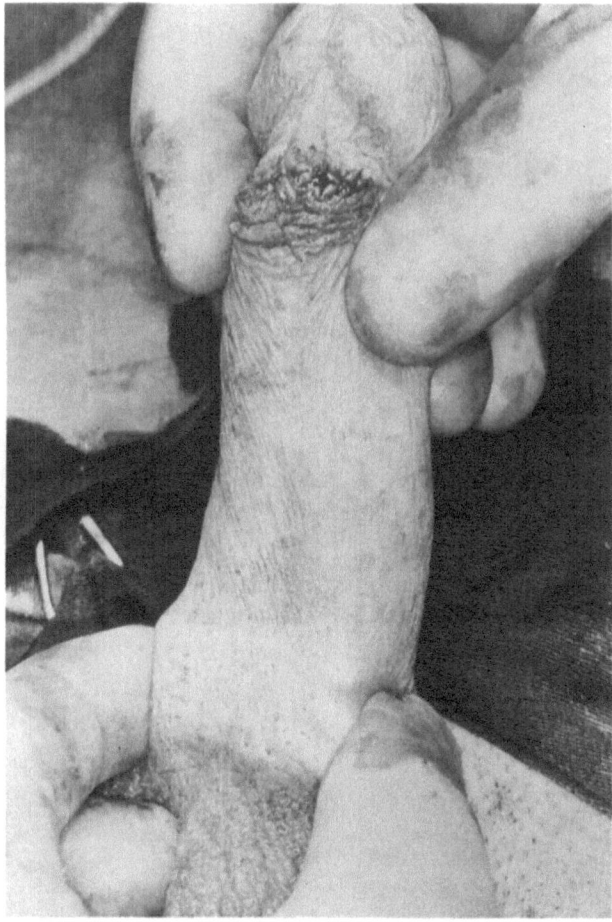

Fig. 2. Handling of the device after implantation by exceeding pressure from both sides.

This led to a better fixation of the sphincter between the two fingers and an easier operation.

Longer postoperative follow-ups however are necessary for definite conclusions on the value of this new artificial sphincter.

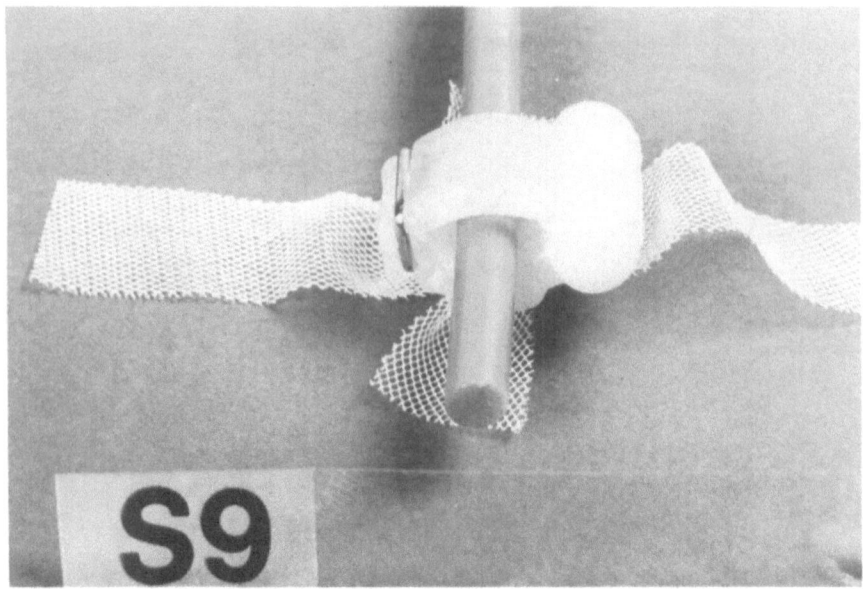

Fig. 3. Penoscrotal sphincter, modification S-9: note that now 2 teflon balls were used in order to (de)-activate the device.

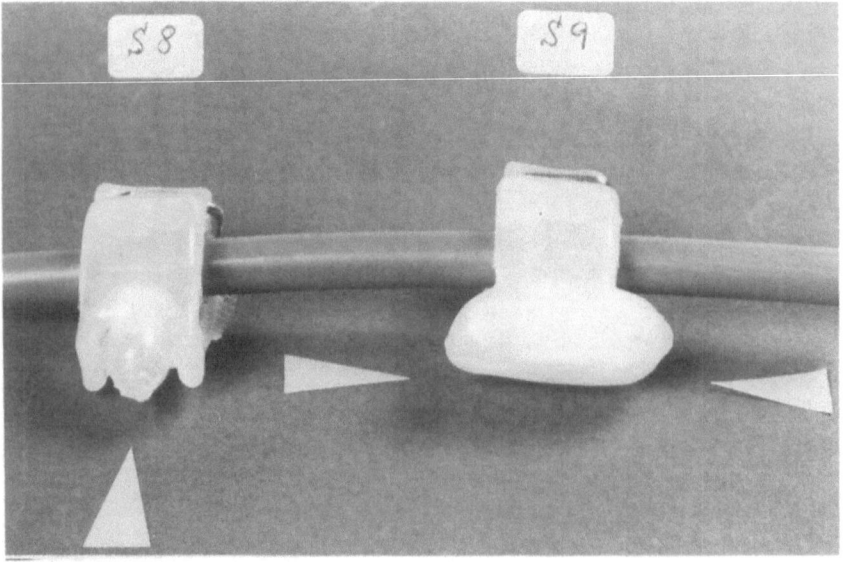

Fig. 4. Comparison between sphincter S8 and S9: while in S8 the (single) teflon ball had to be pushed in direction to the urethra (arrow) in order to deactivate, in S9 two teflon balls were moved by exceeding pressure parallel to the urethra (arrow). Therefore no pressure towards the urethra is further necessary.

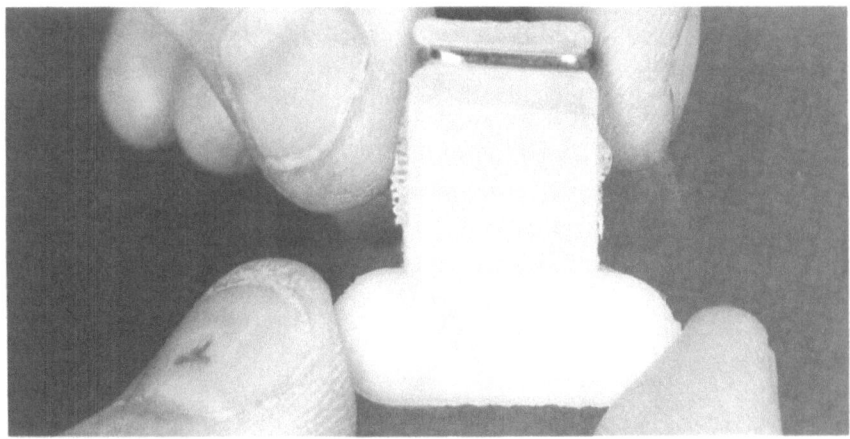

Fig. 5. Activation of the 2 teflon balls by exceeding pressure for both sides. With this arrangement a good fixation of the sphincter between the two fingers during manipulation was achieved.

References

1. Jonas U. Neuer künstlicher Schliessmuskel zur Behandlung der männlichen Inkontinenz – experimentelle Untersuchungen. 7. Symposium für experimentelle Urologie, Tübingen, 6–8 April 1984.
2. Jonas U. Operative Behandlung der männlichen Sphinkterinsuffizienz: Experimente zur Entwicklung eines neuartigen alloplastischen Sphinkters. Akt. Urol. 15 (1984): 280–286.

CHAPTER EIGHT

Past and future of
urinary incontinence

VIII.1. A review of 35 years experience in the management of urinary incontinence

W.A. MOONEN

My review will be historical rather than scientific. Moreover, it concerns the way that I, during almost 40 years, have experienced this history. And, as is usual in a review article, I have gathered some personal and perhaps opinionated concepts. It is, by the way, a dubious privilege to have been able to observe Urology for such a long period of time. I would like to focus on stress incontinence, especially in women.

For a long time it was the most frequently seen type of incontinence, and its treatment has been the most successful, the urogenital fistula excepted. As far as the treatment of urine incontinence in men and the treatment of urge incontinence in women is concerned, I do not want to go into that.

Until the 1940s stress incontinence was almost everywhere the territory of the gynaecologists. Why was there a shifting toward Urology? In my opinion there were 3 reasons for this.

In the first place, the gynaecologist almost never treated stress incontinence according to the principles of suspension described by their masters Goebell (1910) and Stoeckel (1917). These men had advised pulling up the bladder neck by means of the dissected musculi pyramidales. At that time most gynaecologists resorted to various vaginal operations. These 'push up' operations had only a moderate success and then only when performed by skilled hands. In unskilled hands these vaginally performed operations led to catastrophes and calamities. Too often an untreatable urge incontinence developed. Every urologist knows these patients who frequent their clinics for years.

There is a second factor which brought the stress incontinence closer to the urologist. In 1945 Terence Millin proposed his retropubic prostatectomy. It was a rediscovery because in 1908 the Rotterdam surgeon Van Stockum had already performed the operation frequently and had advised it at a meeting of the Dutch Surgical Society. He, however, received such a harsh rejection by the Amsterdam Prof. Lanz that the operation had been discredited. The cavum Retzii was forbidden area. Infections of this cavum and bleedings of the plexus Santorini became nightmares. However, due to work by Terence Millin the taboe associated with the retropubic area disappeared.

Millin himself was looking for more ways of applying the retropubic method and, encouraged by the gynaecologist Charles Read, he applied himself to the retropubic bladder neck suspension. Together they invented the complicated double fascia sling suspension, the so called Millin-Read sling. This was in 1947. At the same time Millin thought of another use for the retropubic surgery. Inspired by the old ideal of Hughes Young, Millin started to work on the radical retropubic prostatectomy.

A third factor in favour of the urologists is that they had applied themselves to urodynamics much sooner than the gynaecologists. They already had experience with the measurement of pressures in neurogenic bladder disturbances, and were soon attempting to improve the diagnostics of stress incontinence with this technique. From the year 1955 on, all bladder function disturbances were investigated urodynamically in my department.

In 1945 I started my surgical and urological training at the University of Leiden. As was done at all university clinics in Holland at that time, the Professor of Surgery also taught Urology. In those days Professors of Surgery were convinced that they had much better control of the operative urology than the urologists themselves. In 1946 in Leiden we switched from the barbaric Fuller-Freyer prostatectomy to Millin's retropubic prostatectomy. However, the stress incontinence and the retropubic suspension remained unknown there. This also turned out to be true of pure urologic wards which I visited in Holland and abroad, including the U.S.A.

There was, however, one exception. During a residency in 1950 at the urological ward of Roger Couvelaire in Paris, I encountered the suspension operation with stress incontinence. The French spoke, and of course they still do, of 'incontinence orthostatique' or of 'incontinence d'effort'. Couvelaire called his suspension 'Cravate aponévrotique' which is a very expressive description because the rectus fascia indeed was trapped like a necktie around the bladder neck. He ascribed the operation to Louis Michon who had published it in 1947 as 'suspension aponévrotique du col de la vessie'.

The introduction of the sling suspension of Michon-Couvelaire in 1950 has for more than 20 years ruled my own way of thinking about stress incontinence and its treatment. All those years I spoke of 'incontinence orthostatique'. Until 1959 the 'suspension aponévrotique', that is the sling suspension, remained for me the only way of suspension. From 1960 to 1970, however, I also performed the MMK operation because it was easier, it had less postoperative complications, that is to say less urine retention, but it nevertheless remained a second choice operation, because I did not like the perforation of the urethra and I feared the osteitis pubis.

Yet the operation of Marshall-Marchetti-Krantz had been described in 1949 and it was becoming a popular operation in the middle of the 1950s in

Holland with urologists as well as gynaecologists. Of course, you ask why this loyalty to the French nomenclature and to the sling suspensions? In fact it was 1970 before I gave in and used the cliché 'stress incontinence'. Then I was convinced that the Colpo-Coopero-pexie of Burch was the most logical, the most simple and the best operation, except in some cases in which the sling was preferable.

Was it nostalgia? Maybe. Was it a jurare in verba magistri? Partially. Was it a francophilia? Un peu. Or was it the aphorism of Horatius 'usus est tyrannus? (which means habit becomes tyranny). I am sure it all played its own role.

What was it that attracted me to the adjective 'orthostatique'? This nomenclature has always appealed to me. The word expresses very explicitly something about the symptomatology. Even more it says something about the pathogenesis and particularly in a phylogenetic way. When the Greek words 'anthropos orthostaticos' are translated into Latin one gets 'homo erectus'. Once man changed from a four footer to homo erectus, as did the Gods, he started to walk on two legs. Undoubtedly, it must have been Prometheus who inspired him to do this in spite of Zeus, the father of Gods. But Zeus punished man for this 'hubris'. He punished him with nephroptosis, with genital prolapse and with ptosis of the pelvic diaphragm.

I purposely do not use the words pelvic floor here because this organ turned out not entirely unsuitable as a floor at all, with orthostasis. And with the ptosis of this pelvic diaphragm the bladder neck sank under the influence of the abdominal cavity and so orthostatic incontinence developed. But why did Zeus only punish the woman and especially her who had been through a difficult delivery? We do not know. But Zeus was, if we concur with the feministic theologists, an androcentric God. He did not pay attention to feminist idealogy and emancipation. With the orthostasis the foundation had been made for the gynaecological urology or female urology, to speak in modern terms.

So I preferred the epithet orthostatic. In the beginning I also had difficulties with the word 'stress'. I associated it with surmenage, overwork, psychosomatic illness. And patients still do use the word in that context. Even when I explain explicitly what the connection is between 'stress' and a sudden rise of pressure in the abdomen, they reject it with a statement that they are not under any stress.

But let us return to the year 1952. I became an independent urologist, treating stress incontinence and performing sling suspensions. This got me into trouble with the gynaecologists. The condition was their territory. Finally a compromise was reached and definite arrangements were made. Stress incontinence combined with a clear prolapse of the foremost vaginal wall belonged to the gynaecologist. He would then perform a colporrhaphy anterior. The urologist was allowed to treat stress incontinence without prolapse. Fortunately, my patients very seldom had prolapses especially not after a suspension.

In the same year (1952) I wrote my first article about stress incontinence in the 'Nederlands Tijdschrift voor Geneeskunde'. At the same time I argued the case for the loop suspension for stress incontinence during a meeting of Dutch urologists (1952).

The reaction of the chairman Dr. Van Capellen was very disappointing. His comment made it clear that it was not done, that the urologists had started to move in on an area traditionally accepted as gynaecological. 'The gynaecologist treats this disease', were his words, 'and he is performing a good job. Let's keep it that way and respect each others territory'. In 1955, I was able, to report the outcome of 50 sling suspensions. In 44 of these cases there was an obvious connection between the incontinence and the partus. And these were the patients with good results. In the remaining 6 cases the indications were disputable and results were disappointing. One case was counted a failure at first, but later seemed to have been a successful operation. This case shows that there is nothing new under the sun. Therefore, allow me one case report.

Mrs. D., a 39 year old, unmarried and childless patient, consulted me in 1954. Due to an accident she had suffered a fracture of the third lumbar vertebrae. She had severe problems with walking and had a large noncontractile bladder which she could partially empty by manual expression, leaving a retention of 200 cc. Lying down she could remain dry for an hour. However, she was continually incontinent when standing. This orthostatic factor prompted me to perform a sling suspension. After this operation she was completely dry, but could not void one drop. A bladder neck incision, luckily without any effect, was performed. Finally, she was catheterised twice daily and when after a while micturition did not start spontaneously the possibility of self catheterisation was considered.

I connected a kind of mirror to a steel feminine catheter and soon our patient could manage the procedure and eventually did not need the mirror at all.

Recently I saw the same patient, now 69 years of age, for a check-up and an I.V.U. was made after 30 years of self catheterisation. Although the kidneys are somewhat small, the I.V.U. was perfect. This report also has another interesting side. From 1954 to 1967 the patient had catheterised herself twice a day with the same metal catheter. This catheter was stored away carefully every time and she carried it with her in a glass test tube with a sublimate solution covered with an ordinary cork. Nevertheless, she seldom had an infection and could have continued in the same manner indefinitely.

However, in 1967 we had reached prosperity with free medical care. Welfare organizations pointed out to her that this kind of catheterisation – with one and the same catheter – is no longer acceptable in these times. So the patient has used disposable catheters ever since, also to full satisfaction, and infections are sporadic; no more and no less than they used to be with the steel catheter.

I kept advocating the suspension operation and remained loyal to the sling. Time was with me. In the first place, the 1950s and 1960s provided many cases of stress incontinence. Those were the years with increased birth rates. Contraception had not yet been accepted, and large families were common. The years with many grand multiparae. Obstetrical care was probably less optimal than today.

In the second place, the diagnosis 'stress incontinence' was made more easily in those years, although the urodynamic investigations were only made in the beginning stages. We know that urge incontinence and especially mixed incontinence can sometimes have an orthostatic factor. But even with the modern, up to date urodynamics, it can still be difficult to make a diagnosis and to advise or advise against a suspension. But these active incontinences were less frequent in the 1950s and 1960s. Why? Because society was more stable. Hard labour was done, by the men outdoors, by the women indoors. Unemployment, divorces, problems with children were less frequent. I am convinced that in those days we saw fewer patients with urge incontinence, less bladder instability, fewer women with inexplicable bladder atonia, which today function in life by means of self catheterisation. Many of these bladder disturbances I see are in fact neurosis of the bladder. Often I spot them at first sight.

And a third point. The gynaecologists in the 1950s and 1960s had had a less thorough surgical training. They operated less frequently. Fewer colporrhaphies were performed. Also fewer hysterectomies. When a hysterectomy was performed, this was more often done transabdominally than vaginally. Nowadays we encounter patients for whom a vaginal hysterectomy has been performed and at the same time a colporrhaphy anterior singely because the patient was already in surgery. In good hands these vaginal operations may have considerable advantages over abdominal operations. But in less skilled hands – and I know them – transvaginal operations provide more cases of active incontinence. And these are the most difficult to deal with.

In the 1950s we were already looking for objective criteria for the diagnosis 'stress incontinence'.

1. In our department from 1955 on all bladder function disturbances were investigated urodynamically. We used the so called Lewis cystometer. All of you who have been raised with the ultramodern urodynamic examination methods will consider the word 'urodynamic' to be an exaggerated euphenism when referring to the Lewis cystometer. But what else did we have? By the way, my statement still stands: 'the man behind the machine

is more important than the machine itself'. And I did have such a man. My co-worker Dr. Ausems could show with this simple apparatus that there were bladders which were heavily burdened by an overdose of parasympathetic stimulii. He then spoke of hyperreflectory or hyperaesthetic bladders, bladders with a poor adaptibility. You would now call this 'low compliance'.

The therapy for these bladders, we now say 'unstable bladders', was with medication such as Atropine. Of course, no suspension operation. He suggested that we should do a superselective parasympathetic resection (1956). But how did it work? We still do not know, although we seem to be close. He also provided evidence in 1955 that some patients with urine retention seem to have an overdose of sympathetic stimulii. Sympatholytic drugs would be better for stimulating micturition than the Doryl or Carbachol which are parasympathicotonic drugs. Of course we did not have Dibenyline in those days.

You will understand how frustated I became once when an American urologist visited my ward and said to me, while looking at the Lewis cystometer: 'That instrument is far too expensive (it cost 2000 guilders) and furthermore it can never function. We made an X-ray of it and there is hardly anything in it'. However, our cystometries did say: 'do not operate here'. But these measurements did not provide a pathognomonic criteria for stress incontinence.

2. Another attempt to view stress incontinence objectively was the cystourethrography. Sideways pictures were taken in order to measure the urethro-vesical angle and to be able to see the ptosis of the bladder under the SCIP line. These pictures did not prove much. Front to back polycystograms were made while resting and while pushing and also while urinating. However, extreme ptosis of the bladder neck could also accompany complete continence. Not until 1959 did I concentrate on the MMK operation which, and this I must admit quickly, caused less postoperative complications. That is, less dysuria.

In 1961 my co-worker Pierre Valcke compared 93 sling suspensions with 20 MMK operations. It was not the type of operation, that is to say sling or pexy, that was of interest, but the indications. If there was a clear relation between partus and stress incontinence, then 75 per cent where cured, while 15 per cent experienced improvement. However, when there was no such connection, for instance with nulliparae, then only 22 per cent were cured and 44 per cent improved.

Conclusions were that the sling suspension:
— had better results with re-interventions,
— was the operation of choice, whenever self catheterisation was the final goal,
— is a better operation in cases in which one must deal with a short medi-

cally-caused mutilated vagina,

— is better protected than the MMK operation against possible future partus.

In 1964 a retrospective investigation was again performed and the conclusions were identical: the indication is far more important than the kind of suspension. On that occasion we compared 120 sling suspensions, 45 M.M.K. operations and 40 simplified suspensions.

The last form of sling suspension must be mentioned because we used it frequently. In 1957 the Frenchman Pierre Delinotte described the socalled 'suspension simplifié' (the simplified suspension).

A small button hole-like incision was made suprapubically up to the fascia. The same kind of incision was made vaginally just under the bladder neck. After that a needle was inserted blindly left and right of the urethra. With the help of this, the sling could be pulled through and tied suprapubically. During this procedure the bladder and urethra were checked for perforations cystoscopically. We experimented with all sorts of materials that were being used for a sling: there were fascia lata, ribbon catgut, calves tendon, chirodka band, skin strip, dacron prothesis, Zoedler band. Only fascia and Zoedler band were satisfactory. Later on we simplified this operation even further by using just a nylon thread, and not pulling it through under the bladder neck, but simply attaching it to the vagina on both sides of the bladder neck. In 1974 we discontinued these operations because retrospective investigation by Frans Debruyne showed that the results were disappointing. The operation itself seemed to be a precursor to the Stamey-Pereyra operation. However, we did not give the latter a fair chance. The indications were poor but we did perform this operation on patients in a poor general condition. If the incontinence after apoplexia, rectum amputation, etc. had only an orthostatic component, then the simplified suspension seemed justified to us. Indeed the operation deserved a better chance.

After 1970 the Burch suspension was introduced in our department. This operation was so logical and simple that it finally became, with stress incontinence, the operation of first choice. For the sling suspension only 3 indications remained:

1. difficult re-operations,
2. the goal of self catheterisation,
3. short, mutilated vaginas (for instance after a prolapse operation).

After 1970 I was marching to the same tune as other urology departments. The urodynamics were modernized and as far as the stress incontinence itself is concerned, I can say that things have stabilized here.

I recently had a discussion with a young colleague. He said to me: 'Recently I came across an article of yours from 1967. You used the word "incontinence orthostatique" and you argued for the sling suspension at a time in which everyone was performing the MMK operation. You intro-

duced then an apparatus to make the sling suspension easier. That means that the operation was not all that simple'. I then asked him which suspension he performed, to which he answered: 'I only know the Burch'. I asked him: 'Is this a reproach because I was so obstinate in refusing to use the word stress incontinence for such a long time or because the sling operation was so important for me until 1970?' He said: 'Not at all. Once in a while I send you a patient for a sling operation because I do only the Burch'. In spite of these words I thought, like every believing person does at the end of his life, I have at the end of my urological life to think about what I did wrong. Maybe I should say, what the French poet Margod de Rennes wrote in his Latin of the middle ages, at the end of his long life (1123): Quae juvenis scripsi, senior, dum plura retractor, poenitet ....
(Now, when I am getting old and think about everything that I have written in my youth, there is a lot that I regret)

And when young urologists are doing a nice colpo-pubo-pexia, they can, like maestro's, make a bow to their patients to receive their ovations. But Destiny has decided: for me the sling suspensions are only for fat females who have already had 5 previous operations in the area of the bladder neck. It is not certain whether she will thank me later, or not. And in a depressive moment doing another sling operation I think of the Bible, which teaches that the sinner will be punished in the way he has sinned.

VIII.2. Future aspects in the management of urinary incontinence

F.M.J. DEBRUYNE & Ph.E.V.A. van KERREBROECK

Introduction

To predict the future management of a disease is an almost impossible task. Particularly in the field of urinary incontinence, it is largely speculative to indicate in which direction the diagnosis and therapy will further develop. On the other hand current treatment remains insufficient. Although we presently know how to deal with genuine stress incontinence in a satisfactory way, we still remain more or less empty-handed in the management of conditions such as bladder instability, urge incontinence, recurrent incontinence and incontinence associated with other diseases, such as Parkinsons disease, multiple sclerosis, diabetes, meningomyelocele, etc.

From our present achievements we can probably predict some directions in which the future might develop. This article will describe the future perspectives of eventual value for the diagnostic and therapeutic management of urinary incontinence.

Future perspectives in diagnosis

Diagnosis is based on the fundamental knowledge of the anatomical, physiological and physiopathological features associated with urinary continence and incontinence. The development anatomy, neuroanatomy and innervation of the lower urinary tract have been studied extensively. The process of storage of the urine and emptying of the bladder, two essential features of normal continence, depends on a complex interaction between the bladder and its sphincters controlled by complicated neurophysiological mechanisms.

Further insight into these mechanisms will certainly contribute to a better understanding and management of the symptoms encountered in the difficult forms of urinary incontinence. With regard to the (neuro)physiopathological bases of bladder instability further fundamental research in the central neurological mechanisms is necessary.

Many patients with a diagnosis of bladder instability (motoric urge incontinence) have a history of enuresis which is assumed to be based on immaturity of the central neurological control of the detrusor activity. The underlying mechanisms are similar and still remain unknown. This is the reason why drug therapy fails in the majority of cases.

Urethral pressure profile (UPP) and electromyography (EMG)

The urodynamic work-up of patients with urinary incontinence is now well standarized. It includes urethral pressure profiles (UPP), cystometry and sphincter electromyography (EMG). The value of cystometry is at present well defined. The value of UPP and EMG remains a point of discussion. The therapeutic consequences of both examinations are still unclear in the majority of cases.

Can we improve these investigations? With regard to UPP, no further developments can be expected as long as we measure indirectly the pressure and pressure-transmission in the lumen of the urethra. More information is needed on what actually happens in the muscles, smooth or striated, responsible for the sphincter closing pressure. It is still difficult to obtain this information. Intracellular and intramuscular smooth muscle potential measurement is still speculative and difficult to perform in a reliable way. Continuous static pressure measurements can eventually add some additional information with regard to urethral functioning, but again remains an indirect method of pressure registration.

External EMG of the striated muscles is more reliable but only gives information on one part of the total continence mechanism, an anatomically indistinguishable entity of smooth and striated muscles. The help of neuroanatomists and neurophysiologists is indispensable to obtain further progress in this field.

Indication for urodynamic investigation

For the future we have to define more precisely which patients should undergo urodynamic investigations and how thoroughly our urodynamic work-up should be. Urodynamic investigation is time-consuming and very costly. The same holds true for roentgenological examination of the incontinent patient. On the other hand it is stated that no patient with micturition problems should be withheld from complete urodynamic analysis.

The necessity for urodynamic investigations depends in the first place on the validity and reliability of anamnestic and clinical findings. In a prospective study we were able to establish an exact diagnosis by the patient's history alone in 85 % of the patients with primary stress incontinence [1]. Conversely, we feel that missing the diagnosis by omitting urodynamic investigation holds more risks for the patients.

In every patient, even with a clear history of stress incontinence, it has to be proven urodynamically that the bladder is stable. This is the first step in improving the results of surgery for stress incontinence and holds true for every day urological and gynaecological practice.

We do not feel however, as stated by Coolsaet [2], that a urodynamic examination is mandatory in every patient with signs and symptoms of urinary obstruction due to prostatic enlargements. Here, in our view, the risks are greater than the benefits. A urodynamic examination can not differentiate between instability secondary to infravesical obstruction or inherent to the detrusor muscle itself and the patient with severe symptoms has to be operated upon anyway.

Many micturition disturbances, especially bladder instability in women, seem to be related to prior pelvic surgery. Turner-Warwick noted in 1979 [3] that as these patients did not undergo preoperative objective evaluation, it is most probable that the effect of the surgery, especially hysterectomy, was to unmask a *latent* abnormality rather than to create a new one. Therefore a statistically supported study to prove this assumption is necessary and will define more exactly the necessity for urodynamic investigation of all females undergoing pelvic surgery.

Vaginal surgery is thought to be the cause of onset of sensory urgency in a substantial number of patients [4]. The underlying mechanisms are unknown. Probably neurophysiological disturbances account for the complaints which eventually lead to insupportable situations. Research to elucidate this phenomenon is hardly possible since no reliable methods are available.

The same problems remain with the management of idiopathic urge incontinence. The clarification of these problems is no longer in the hands of clinicians but should be afforded by more fundamental research in the field of pathophysiology of sensoric and motoric urgency. Recent experiences with forced diuresis urodynamics indicate a relation between diuresis and bladder instability [5]. This leads to the need to study the role of the uretero-vesical junction in the induction of detrusor activity. Furthermore, improving experiments with evoked potentials can differentiate and clarify the nervous pathways in the aetiology of sensoric and motoric urgency.

Evoked potentials already play a role in the study of micturition disorders associated with neurological diseases and diabetes. Further studies in this field, to be conducted in close collaboration with neurophysiologists, will probably hand the clinicians new tools in the management not only of these conditions but also in the approach to patients with so-called non-neurogenic neurogenic bladder and those with so-called idiopathic bladder instability.

Telemetry is another method to improve the differentiation between bladder instability and sensory urgency. With the advent of more refined and handy equipment, telemetry will play an increasing role in the diagnostic work-up of more complicated cases of urinary incontinence. In a growing number of cases we could demonstrate by 24 hours ambulant monitoring bladder instability not detected by ordinary urodynamic examination [6].

Further experiments with telemetry will improve the methodology and also define more precisely its value not only in the diagnosis but hopefully also in the management of bladder instability.

Urethral instability

Urethral instability is described as an inappropriate relaxation of the bladder outlet during filling, similar to that which occurs during normal voiding but without an active bladder contraction [7].

The role of this phenomenon in the origin of urinary incontinence remains obscure. Does it really exist and if so, what are the consequences? How do we measure it and interpret it? Continuous urethral pressure measurement will probably be able to bring further classification in this phenomenon. Many questions, subjects for further research, remain open. Here again only the development of direct measurements of urethral potentials (and pressure) will contribute to the answers. These developments will hopefully be achieved in the near future.

Future perspectives in therapy of urinary incontinence

Stress incontinence

Stress urinary incontinence is now well defined. It is primarily a failure of transmission of intra-abdominal pressure (and consequently intravesical pressure) to the urethra.

Genuine stress incontinence. The most common cause of primary stress incontinence is a change in the anatomical position (descensus) of the vesico-urethral junction and the proximal urethra. Consequently it is obvious that the most appropriate treatment is the restoration of the correct anatomical relationship. A wide variety of surgical procedures to achieve this goal have been proposed.

We still favour the Burch retropubic approach as the method of choice [8]. This technique seems logical, safe and effective. It affords a good overview of the operative field and an 'à vue' reconstruction of the anatomical situation without damage to the bladder neck or urethra.

Several other methods have proved to be as effective and probably more simple (at least for the patient). In particular the modifications of the suprapubic-vaginal suspension first described by Pereyra [9], as proposed by Stamey [10] and later by Raz [11], will increasingly be popularized among urologists in the coming years. By these alterations endoscopic control of the suspension has been introduced. This demands cystoscopic experience of the surgeon and will certainly hamper the popularisation among gynaecologists.

The obturator shelf procedure as promoted in this book by Turner-Warwick, seems a logical procedure when a concomitant descencus of the uterus is present or when one has decided to combine a bladder neck suspension with a hysterectomy, a procedure sometimes favoured by gynaecologists. This technique is surgically more difficult and more prone to per- and postoperative complications.

The success rate of surgical treatment of genuine stress incontinence depends more on a proper selection of patients than on technical errors, especially since a substantial number of patients have a combination of stress and urge incontinence. Even with careful preoperative evaluation and attention to surgical detail, approximately 10 % of the operations still fail. Numerous modifications of the bladder neck suspension technique have been – and probably will be – developed in an attempt to cure these failures.

The use of intra- and peri-urethral teflon injections as promoted by Politano [12] is on its way back and will probably be reserved for minimal stress incontinence in young women. The question here remains if non-surgical measurements are not preferable in these cases. New non-surgical therapies for primary stress incontinence will not arise in the near future. With the advent of new and more simple surgical techniques the importance of these methods, such as alpha-adrenergic drugs, physiotherapy, mechanical compression and estrogen therapy, will probably decrease.

Recurrent urinary stress incontinence. The therapeutic approach to recurrent stress incontinence will remain difficult and perhaps controversial. If the failure is due to improper diagnosis, the patient usually deteriorates after an operation. Urgency, in particular, will become yet more difficult to treat. If failure is due to a technical error, a more proper re-suspension can be envisaged. If recurrent stress incontinence proves to be caused by recurrent anatomical descensus, a re-operation will effect a cure.

We prefer the combined suprapubic-vaginal approach (Raz procedure) as the method of choice in cases where no previous vaginal operations have been performed. Sling techniques are also promoted for secondary operations. Here again meticulous preoperative diagnosis is as essential as the surgical technique.

Bladder instability

The future perspectives of the management of bladder instability (motoric urge incontinence) seem to be disappointing. All drugs and methods used so far have a limited (maximum 30–40%) and temporary success. No new achievements are possible unless a break-through is obtained in the aetiology of this condition.

In the field of pharmacological therapy anticholinergic agents will remain the first choice. Pharmacological research must offer more specific drugs with fewer side effects.

More aggressive therapy for bladder instability resistent to drugs (approximately 60–70%!), such as bladder overdistention and bladder denervation have insufficient results. The future of these procedures is very limited. Two methods however should be further explored: first the bladder drill and biofeedback training alone or in combination with psychotherapy and secondly the functional electrical stimulation. The latter method is still experimental but it is assumed that electrical stimulation of the striated muscles of the pelvic floor results in a contraction of the sphincter with bladder inhibition. When properly applied this method could be used in the management of bladder instability. Many problems, theoretical and technical, still have to be solved but the first steps in this field have been taken and will probably open a way for telemetrically guided stimulation of the pelvic floor. For this goal an intravesical device registering the bladder pressure and telemetrically transmitting pressure change to an external pelvic floor stimulator is in development research.

Artificial sphincters and urinary diversion

Severe cases of incontinence of difficult and complex origin are no longer curable by pharmacological manipulation or 'simple' surgical procedures. But during the last decade, improved devices for sphincteric replacement have been developed.

The indications for the implantation of the Scott sphincter prosthesis [13] have become more and more clear. The implantation technique is rather complicated. With growing experience and improving devices the number of reinterventions will further decrease. Moreover, the limitation of the implantation to experienced centers will reduce the complication rate. Future developments in the field of prosthetic surgery are forthcoming. The simple Jonas incontinence prosthesis is one example. More complicated is the idea of a valvular intra-urethral prosthesis which is being developed.

In patients with locally intractable urinary incontinence and symptoms, eventually a urinary diversion can be taken into consideration. Many methods have been described. 'Internal urinary diversion' such as ureterosigmoidostomy generally affords urinary continence, but has major disadvantages in the long run such as chronic pyelonephritis, renal failure and malignant degeneration of the colon.

'External' urinary diversion replaces the problem of bladder incontinence to 'stomal' incontinence. Improvements in the stomal appliances facilitate stoma care, reducing significantly urinary leakage and skin problems.

The late risks for chronic pyelonephritis and renal failure remain with all classical types of urinary diversion such as uretero-sigmoido-cutaneostomy or uretero-ileo-cutaneostomy and their different variations.

Recently the continent stoma according to Kock et al. [14] the continent ileostoma – or to Mänsson and Sundin [15] the continent coecal reservoir – have been promoted and will certainly be popularized in the near future. Thüroff et al. [16] combined an ileocoecal reservoir with a modified Scott sphincter prosthesis to obtain a continent stoma (the Mainz pouch). It remains speculative if in the long-term the complication rate, especially for the kidneys, will be better compared with the incontinent stoma. The first long-term results recently presented [17] are promising. The disadvantage of this technique is the high number of reinterventions even in experienced hands necessary to obtain and maintain continence. Therefore its use will remain restricted to a limited number of patients to be operated upon in only a limited number of experienced centers.

Intractable urinary incontinence

Unfortunately the treatment of many patients, especially females, with urinary incontinence of complex origin is unsuccessful and a majority of them end up with intractable incontinence. This condition is socially unacceptable and leads to tremendous psycho-social implications for the patient and relatives.

In the near future much attention must be given to these psychological and social consequences of intractable urinary incontinence. In some European countries (Sweden, United Kingdom, The Netherlands) foundations have been started to take care of these aspects. Incontinent patients are supported by these institutions to organize for themselves better social conditions which allow them to break through their isolation and to participate again in the social activities of their environment.

One way to prevent isolation is to restrict the disturbing consequences of urinary leakage. Better absorbant materials haven been manufactured and will continue to be developed. Health care services and insurance companies are starting to refund the expense of these materials, taking over the financial burden from the incontinent patient. The progress obtained in this field so far has to continue and extend in the future and physicians must play an important role in further achievements.

Conclusions

As stated at the beginning of this article, the description of future perspectives in the management of urinary incontinence is hazardous and speculative at the same time. However, some future directions which we think are important have been indicated. The list of possible future achievements is certainly not complete. We feel that the ideas put forward seem to be realistic although it is impossible to predict which aims will be realised and what goal will be obtained first. Hopefully the coming decade will bring such progress that we are able to reduce safely and significantly the number of patients quoted in the last category 'intractable incontinent'.

References

1. Delaere K.P.J., Moonen W.A., Debruyne F.M.J. and Renders G.A.M. De waarde van de anamnese bij urine incontinentie. Tijdschr. voor Geneesk. 35 (1979): 175.
2. Coolsaet B.L.R.A. Ouder worden met de prostaatklier. Ned. Tijdschr. Geneesk. 127, 46 (1983): 2094.
3. Turner-Warwick R. and Brown A.D.G. Urinary incontinence in the female. Urol. Clin. N. Am. 6 (1979): 203.
4. Delaere K.P.J., Moonen W.A., Debruyne F.M.J., Michiels H.G.E. and Renders G.A.M. Anterior vaginal repair, cause of troublesome voiding disorders? Eur. Urol. 5 (1979): 190–194.
5. Blok C., van Venrooij G.E.P.M. and Coolsaet B.L.R.A. Detrusor instability in relation to diuresis and physical bladder properties. Proc. Intern. Cont. Soc. '14th Annual Meeting', Innsbruck, Sept. 13–15, 1984.
6. Valcke A.A.P., van Waalwijk van Doorn E.S.C., Kimmich H.P. and Debruyne F.M.J. L'examen urodynamique télémétrique de la vessie. Acta Urol. Belg. 52 (1984): 220.
7. McGuire E.J. Reflex urethral instability. Brit. J. Urol. 50 (1978): 200.
8. Burch J.C. Urethrovaginal fixation to Cooper's ligament for correction of stress incontinence, cystocele and prolapse. Am. J. Obstet. Gynaecol. 81 (1961): 281.
9. Pereyra A.J. A simplified surgical procedure for the correction of stress incontinence in women. West. J. Surg. 67 (1959): 223.
10. Stamey T.A. Cystoscopic suspension of the vesical neck for urinary incontinence. Surg. Gynaecol. Obstet. 136 (1973): 547.
11. Raz S. Modified bladder neck suspension for female stress incontinence. Urology, 18 (1981): 82.

12. Carrion H.M. and Politano V.A. Periurethral polytef (teflon*) injection for urinary incontinence. In: Raz S. (ed) Female Urology. W.B. Saunders company, Philadelphia, (1983) 213.

13. Scott F.B., Bradley W.E. and Timm G.W. Treatment of urinary incontinence by implantable prosthetic sphincter. Urology 1 (1973): 252.

14. Kock N.G., Nilson A.E., Norlèn L., Sundin T. and Trasti H. Urinary diversion via a continent ileum reservoir. Clinical experience. Scand. J. Urol. Nephrol. Suppl. 49 (1978): 23.

15. Mänsson W. and Sundin T. Experience with a continent coecal reservoir in urinary diversion. Scand. J. Urol. Nephrol. suppl. 48 (1978): 4.

16. Thüroff J.W., Alken P., Engelmann U., Riedmiller H., Jacobi G.H. and Hohenfellner R. Der Mainz-Pouch zur Blasenerweiterungsplastik und kontinenten Harnableitung. Akt. Urol. 16 (1985): 1.

17. Kock N.G., Nilson A.E., Nilsson L.O., Norlèn L.J. and Philipson B.M. Urinary diversion via a continent ileal reservoir: clinical results in 12 patients. J. Urol. 128 (1982): 469.

INDEX